Principles of
Neuropsychological
Assessment with Hispanics

Issues of Diversity in Clinical Neuropsychology
Series Editor: Elaine Fletcher-Janzen, Ed.D., San Angelo, Texas

Principles of Neuropsychological Assessment with Hispanics:
Theoretical Foundations and Clinical Practice
Edited by Antolin M. Llorente

Forthcoming:

Neuropsychological Assessment with Asian Americans
Edited by Tony Wong

Mild Traumatic Brain Injury: Onset, Consequences, and Outcomes
Edited by Barbara P. Uzzell, Nils R. Varney, and Gregory J. O' Shanick

The Neuropsychology of Women
Edited by Elaine Fletcher-Janzen

Neuropsychology of Poverty
by Elsa Shapiro

Principles of Neuropsychological Assessment with Hispanics

Theoretical Foundations and Clinical Practice

Edited by
Antolin M. Llorente

Department of Pediatrics
University of Maryland School of Medicine

and

Mount Washington Pediatric Hospital
Baltimore, Maryland

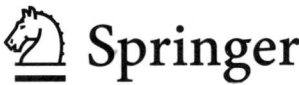 Springer

Editor

Antolin M. Llorente, Ph.D.
Department of Pediatrics
University of Maryland School of Medicine
Baltimore, MD 21201
USA
allorente@mwph.org

Series Editor

Elaine Fletcher-Janzen, Ed.D.
San Angelo, TX
USA

ISBN: 978-0-387-71757-9   e-ISBN: 978-0-387-71758-6

Library of Congress Control Number: 2007926245

Printed on acid-free paper.

9 8 7 6 5 4 3 2 1

springer.com

"La educación empieza en la cuna."

Don José de la Luz y Caballero

[We] "live from birth to death in a world of persons and things which is in large measure what it is because of what has been done and transmitted from previous human activities. When this fact is ignored, experience is treated as if it were something which goes on exclusively inside an individual, body and mind. It ought not to be necessary to say that experience does not occur in a vacuum. There are sources outside an individual which give rise to experience."

John Dewey

"As long as our brain is a mystery, the universe, the reflection of the structure of the brain will also be a mystery."

Santiago Ramón y Cajal

"I have sworn upon the altar of God, eternal hostility against every form of tyranny over the mind of man."

Thomas Jefferson

"Bestir thyself therefore on this occasion; for though we will always lend thee proper assistance in difficult places, as we do not, like some others, expect thee to use the arts of divination to discover our meaning, yet we shall not indulge thy laziness where nothing but thy own attention is required; for thou art highly mistaken if thou dost imagine that we intended when we begun this great work to leave thy sagacity nothing to do, or that without sometimes exercising this talent thou wilt be able to travel through our pages with any pleasure or profit to thyself."

Henry Fielding

Dedicado con amor agape, eterno aprecio y sincero respeto
a la
Sra. Armanda R. Fernández

Preface

The scientific purview of neuropsychology is to understand healthy and dysfunctional brain-behavior relationships. As our knowledge of such relationships increases incrementally, our understanding of their broad scope and complexities exponentially increases. Whereas it was once thought that specific disorders, such as dyslexia, only implicated one of the cerebral hemispheres (Orton, 1937), research has suggested a more complex interaction between stimuli processing and reading ability, expanding our conceptions of hemispheric specialization affecting healthy and impaired brains (cf. Delis, Kiefner, and Fridlund, 1988; Efron, 1990). Over time, it became clear that intricate brain functions and underlying behaviors, including reading, required linguistic and visual perceptual functions, and necessitated the support of both hemispheres, and therefore, disordered brain functions, including dyslexia, were usually the result of problems affecting both cerebral hemispheric regions. Programmatic research further indicated that the right hemisphere is responsible for processing select aspects of a stimulus (e.g., nonlinear, novel aspects, overall gestalt such as faces), in conjunction with components of the stimulus processed by the left hemisphere (e.g., linear, familiarity of stimulus, details), and the synthesis of these two components subsequently yielded an overall representation (cf. Efron, 1990; Robertson, Lamb, and Knight, 1988). In fact, studies have suggested that information processing in healthy and dysfunctional brains is most likely the result of "contributions from both hemispheres entering into every activity and emotional state" (cf. Lezak, 1995). Therefore, as advances emerged in our understanding of hemispheric specialization, creating paradigmatic shifts and transformations in our conceptualizations, an evolution occurred, altering our previous, incomplete, and "infantile" perceptions about brain functions and their relationships to comportment.

Brain-behavior relationships are not necessarily unidirectional or linear in nature. Neuroscientific and psychoneuroimmunologic studies have demonstrated the intricate nature of these bi-directional and nonlinear relationships. For example, musicians (string players) exhibit thickening and increased cortical representation in their motor strip region underlying string maneuvering secondary to endless hours of practice leading to asymptotically exponential performance and expertise (Elbert et al., 1995). Such cortical structural changes additionally have been noted with learning in general (cf. Kleim et al., 1997). Support for such a bidirectional and nonlinear view of brain-behavior relationships also has been supported by studies in language development (Bates, Thal, and Janowski, 1992). A specific behavior is capable of altering brain structure, and such transformation is associated with enhanced performance, including new acquisition, competence, and expertise. These examples suggest that the relationship between central nervous system structural alterations and behavioral competence or expertise appears to be exponential and nonlinear in select circumstances. Similarly, psychoneuroimmunology most recently has demonstrated the intimate nature of brain-behavior relationships and their bidirectional interaction. This branch of neuroscience has shown unequivocally that the level of functioning of individuals suffering from AIDS-related dementia was enhanced as a result of interpersonal contextual variables (Kemeny and Gruenewald, 2000). Enhancements in patients' adaptation and functional level was shown to be associated with increments in immune system response, and an increase in T-cell response led to a reduction in viral load and associated changes in brain functions leading to neurobehavioral benefits (e.g., affect, cognition). In this case, the effect of an infectious disease with neurological involvement capable of infringing upon behavior was diminished by an intervention (e.g., touch) with significant impact on immune system response and indirectly on neural substrates and underlying functions.

The relationship between culture and brain also is bidirectional, and in some instances, nonlinear. With regard to our current understanding of neuropsychiatric disorders, lest we are willing to admit intellectual bankruptcy, it is a well-known fact that cultural context is inextricably intertwined with the expression of such phenomena (cf. Mezzich and Lewis-Fernández, 1997). In this regard, and despite its simplistic approach, the *Diagnostic and Statistical Manual of Mental Disorders-Fourth Edition (DSM IV, Appendix)* acknowledges the impact of culture and its modulation on the manifestations of abnormal brain-driven affect, behavior, and cognition (American Psychiatric Association, 1994, 2000). For example, the expression of neuropsychopathology in two different Hispanic patients, or in the same patient at distinct points in time, may vary depending on whether the patient(s) attribute their problems to "*nervios*" a common cultural description of psychological problems or to a known medical condition found in his or her family (Guarnaccia, Lewis-Fernandez, and Marano, 2003). Regardless of the fact that neuropsychopathology in both patients (or in a patient), may have the same neurobiological etiology (e.g., endogenous clinical depression consequent to diminished 5-HT availability in brain), their individual expressions and personal interpretations may be different as a result of their distinct attributions as a consequence of cultural contextualization. In other words, cultural context provides patients, metaphorically speaking, a license that permits them to navigate through the maze of attributions to reach the one that is perceived as most self-preserving, indirectly impacting neural substrates with less negative effects on functional level. Such a context also is critical in the rehabilitation of the Hispanic patient and plays a major role in treatment outcome.

Culture pervades all aspects of an individual's functioning (cf. Luria, 1976, 1979). Culture defines an individual and the individual, beginning early in childhood, constructs his self within such a backdrop, much like an artist who paints with oils a luscious landscape on a canvas. An individual also reactively impacts all societal "institutions" that bear and form his or her definition(s) of the self (cf. Wartofsky, 1983). Most recently, it appears that our brains and culture are interwoven by biological mechanisms, and humans may actually posses "culture" genes that mediate a complex interaction between biology and the environment, providing an interactive mechanism capable of allowing human brains to assimilate cultural characteristics (cf. Kohler et al., 2002; Lai et al. 2001). Therefore, culture is not something to be sprinkled upon our diagnostic considerations, theoretical formulations, clinical impressions, or neuropsychological inferences as if it were of secondary importance or an afterthought, as realism might have been to the impressionist movement. Instead, culture should be an intricate part of all those components in neuropsychological thought and practice, not because it is, as some may argue in our intellectually broken zeitgeist, "politically correct," but because culture is in "our brains" (Ardila, 2003), and culture is to brain what color is to light on the canvas of the impressionists.

Consequently, neuropsychology, a fledging yet maturing discipline, must struggle with culture and ethnicity if it is to remain a viable and comprehensive science of brain-behavior relationships. *Principles of Neuropsychological Assessment with Hispanics: Theoretical Foundations and Clinical Practice in the Neuropsychology and Culture Series* (Spring Science + Business Media) provides a forum in which to examine and explore the influences of cultural factors on brain-behavior relationships from theoretical and applied viewpoints with Hispanics. From a theoretical standpoint, this book will attempt to provide research-based evidence for the impact of culture on brain-behavior relationships while exploring key factors and issues (e.g., assimilation, cultural identity, demographics) partially responsible for such influences. From an applied perspective, clinical issues such as competence and minimal standards associated with appropriate assessments of these populations will be discussed, including ethical approaches to the assessment of Hispanic patients and the development of neuropsychological procedures capable of reducing bias, indirectly leading to accurate and valid evaluations, inferences, and interventions.

Acknowledgments

This book partly emerged out of necessity as a way of educating attorneys, graduate students, interns, fellows, and some colleagues who over the course of the years developed a genuine interest in cognitive processes and culture, particularly in neuropsychology; in some instances, instruction in such issues was required by their professions, educational curriculum, or other personal circumstances. However, during the course of such interactions, unbeknownst to most of them, they indirectly contributed to my own education and professional growth as it related to this topic, and they thus surreptitiously contributed to this volume. Others contributed much more directly, and even a book as small as this, and of so modest a contribution to the rapidly evolving scholarly area of cross-cultural neuropsychology applied to Hispanics, could not have been produced without the unselfish assistance and encouragement of several individuals. Dedicated students and colleagues unselfishly provided assistance, time, and guidance. I greatly appreciated the support and contributions of Professor Elaine Fletcher-Janzen, who convinced me that writing this book, or as she called it, this "labor of love," was meritorious from several standpoints, including scholarly and humanitarian reasons, and who encouraged me in the first place. Also, I want to acknowledge the contributions of my early mentor, Professor Vicki Green, for originally introducing me to the field of cross-cultural psychology as she supervised my first case as a clinician-in-training while assessing an unaccompanied child from Central America who, fearing for her life, had immigrated to the U.S., seeking asylum in an American court. I additionally would like to express my sincere appreciation to Professors Paul Satz, Louis D'Elia, and Wilfred van Gorp for supporting my career goals as a neuropsychology fellow while at UCLA, Professors Christianne Cox, Keith Slifer, and Gina Richman for providing excellent role models of scholar-practitioners when I was an intern at Kennedy Krieger Institute/Johns Hopkins University School of Medicine, and Professors Robert S. Schlottman and David Thomas for introducing me to neuroscience and neuropsychology as a graduate student at Oklahoma State University. I also would like acknowledge Professor Tony Wong for constructive criticisms that have been included in this book from our "cross cultural conversations." I am additionally and particularly indebted to Professor Jossette Harris for allowing me to use portions of "our" chapter which appear in different areas throughout this book, because I could not have expounded specific points without her assistance. I also like to thank my coauthors, all committed young students of brain-behavior relationships. I express my humble gratitude to Ms. Sara A. Lawless (Chapter 1), Mr. Christian von Thomsen and Ms. Lori Gallup (Chapter 4), Dr. Deborah Weber (Chapter 7), Dr. Brian Potter (Chapter 8), and Dr. Erik Lane (Chapter 6). I also want to acknowledge the contributions of postdoctoral fellows whom I have trained and who contributed to this volume, including Dr. Christine French (Chapter 5) and Dr. Peter Smith (Chapter 6), individuals who carry upon their shoulders the burden of assisting and educating future neuropsychologists about Boas, Dewey, Luria, and Vygotsky and the impact of culture on the human brain and indirectly on neurocognitive mechanisms.

I am also grateful to my colleagues for their assistance and for taking on responsibilities beyond those specified in their job descriptions, which allowed me to have "free" time to complete this volume particularly Dr. Julie Ries (Chapters 1 and 8). My special thanks also are extended to Springer and Kluwer Publishing for their patience during the period of time it took to produce this work. In particular, my sincere appreciation is extended to Ms. Janice Stern for her executive editorial assistance and for her willingness to keep foreboding forces at bay while I completed "the volume." Finally, I want to express my gratitude to Ms. S. Geethalakshmi, production editor, for her assistance in the timely delivery of this manuscript.

Although significant limitations were placed on manuscript length, precluding a comprehensive review of the subject matter, I alone take full responsibility for the content of this book, and my colleagues must be exonerated from literary weaknesses or shortcomings in style or substance encountered in the same. Mea culpa.

Finally, I extend my special gratitude to my lovely confidante and North Star, Tina M. Llorente, a bright Abigail Adams of our times, for her continued support and patience when I was absent while writing this book, in spite of my physical presence.

Antolin M. Llorente
Seven Valleys, Pennsylvania
December 2006

Contents

Contributors List

Christine L. Castillo (French)
University of Texas Southwestern Medical Center
and
Children's Medical Center of Dallas
Neuropsychology, B3244
Dallas, TX 75235

Lori Gallup
Argosy University
Washington, DC
Baltimore, MD 21237

Eric LaneJ
Loyola College, Maryland
Sparks, MD 21152

Sara A. Lawless
Loyola College, Maryland
West Springfield, MA 01089

Antolin M. Llorente
University of Maryland School of Medicine
and
Mount Washington Pediatric Hospital
Baltimore, MD 21209

Brian Potter
Texas Children's Hospital
Houston, TX 77030

Julie K. Ries
Mount Washington Pediatric Hospital
Baltimore, MD 21209

Peter Smith
Mount Washington Pediatric Hospital
Baltimore, MD 21209

Christian von Thomsen
Loyola College, Maryland
Baltimore, MD 21211

Deborah Weber
Children's National Medical Center
Department of Neuropsychology
Washington, DC 20010

List of Tables

List of Figures

Chapter 1
Introduction and Theoretical Foundations

Sara A. Lawless, Julie K. Ries, and Antolin M. Llorente

Neuropsychology faces an intimidating and unparalleled challenge in the 21st century. This specific challenge arises out of the need to develop theoretical frameworks and applied methods and instrumentation that are capable of explaining and assessing complex brain-behavior relationships, including cross-cultural constituents and components of such relationships. Considering that many neuropsychological theories and methods emerged out of scientific and applied endeavors conducted with the majority populations in the United States (U.S.) and abroad, particularly Western Europe, neuropsychologists should not presume that such theories, methodologies, or instrumentation are appropriate or valid for populations that differ in key demographic features. Such theories and applied methods may not necessarily apply to all individuals, including Hispanics,[1] as if such a science and applied methods were universal despite diverging cultural or ethnic background (cf. Nell, 2000; Wong, Strickland, Fletcher-Janzen, Ardila, and Reynolds, 2000) and in spite of significant evidence to the contrary (Anger et al., 1993; Ardila et al., 1989, 1994; Irvine and Berry, 1988; LaRue et al., 1999; León-Carrión, 1989; Luria, 1976; Nell, 2000; Olazaran, Jacobs and Stern, 1996; Verney et al., 2005; Wong et al., 2000; Yeats et al., 2002; Zindi, 1994). In fact, variables such as socioeconomic status and extremely complex cultural, ethnic, and linguistic factors most likely moderate and modulate neuropsychological functions.

The challenge associated with the inclusion of cross-cultural factors in neuropsychology, at least in the U.S., also arises out of formidable and large-scale transformations that have taken place in the nation's population, leading to the creation of one of the largest Hispanic societies on the face of the earth. According to the U.S. Census Bureau (2001, 2004), almost 50% of the population will be comprised of ethnic minorities by 2050, of which approximately 24% will be Hispanic. It is clear that the need to provide neuropsychological assessment services to such

---

[1] See below for a comprehensive explanation of the use of the term *Hispanic* throughout this volume.

diverse and large populations has been growing at an exponential rate as the result of the aforementioned changes in the composition of American society. The need to provide services to such populations encompasses all aspects of society but most critically educational settings, public policy environments, health care, and the civil and criminal justice systems. Moreover, the nonrandom, ever-shifting immigration trends of the U.S., and their impact on neuropsychology, further complicate attempts to respond to a challenge of such scope and magnitude (cf. Llorente, 1997; Llorente et al., 1999, 2000). Countries of migrational origin, and the reasons for immigrations, particularly large-scale migrations, have changed globally and within the U.S. as a result of alterations in sociopolitical and economic climates, and this shift has significant implications for neuropsychology (Llorente, 1997; Llorente et al., 1999, 2000). With those changes, varying occupational status, educational attainment, and patterns of geographical settlement of immigrants in the U.S., as well as other parts of the globe (e.g., Australia, China, France, Turkey), have been observed, which likely affect *observed* brain-behavior relationships (Llorente et al., 2000).

Efforts have been made to increase cultural competency among educators, researchers and practitioners, including awareness, language skills, and standardized training and assessment procedures, methods, and instrumentation to address the emerging scientific and applied need. For example, the *Standards for Educational and Psychological Testing* (1999) established by the American Psychological Association (APA), the American Educational Research Association (AERA), and the National Council on Measurement in Education (NCME) has put greater emphasis on ensuring the fairness in assessments of individuals with diverse ethnic and racial backgrounds. The American Psychological Association (APA, 1991, 2001, 2003) has established the *Guidelines for Providers of Psychological Services to Ethnic, Linguistic, and Culturally Diverse Populations*, urging consultations, supervision, and continuing education to increase cultural competency in clinical practice. The Houston Conference on Specialty Education and Training in Clinical Neuropsychology (Hannay et al., 1998) included "cultural and individual differences and diversity" as a recommended area of study under the Generic Psychology Core, and listed "recognition of multicultural issues" under the Assessments and Treatment and Interventions core skills sections (Hannay et al., 1998; Wong et al., 2000). Wong et al. (2000) and others (Pontón and León-Carrión, 2001; van Gorp, Myers and Drake, 2000) have recommended ways in which educators and practitioners could be more sensitive in identifying and understanding cultural, linguistic, and ethnic differences through careful interviews, education, and the clinician's own awareness of his/her biases.

Despite these efforts, a number of salient issues need to be addressed in neuropsychological practice, research, and theory, and universals need to be partially discarded. However, before embarking on a course to address such topics, important fundamental, theoretical, nomenclatural, definitional, and ethical issues require attention.

Analysis of the History of Science and Paradigmatic Shifts in Neuropsychology

At first glance, the response to the challenges posed to neuropsychology to explain brain-behavior relationships from a more comprehensive context, to include previously ignored cultural factors, could be perceived by individuals outside and within the discipline as a simple addition of knowledge. However, such a response by the discipline may not represent a simple accumulation of facts. To the contrary, such alterations occur within a broader context of change, as is the case for other scientific fields, and can be understood in terms of an overarching model of evolution in the discipline of neuropsychology, or a paradigmatic shift. Although an argument is not being made here that a paradigm shift has occurred of the magnitude and generalization created by the Copernican Revolution, a significant shift, nonetheless, has occurred in the discipline. To better examine such a paradigmatic shift in the field of neuropsychology, a framework that permits an examination of the current and ongoing transformation that has taken place addressing cultural factors is required.

The Structure of Scientific Revolutions (Kuhn, 1962, 1970, 1996) provides an integrative and comprehensive meta-analysis of the history of science. Although Kuhn's (1970) work was originally applied to the natural sciences, his analysis of the progression of natural science also has been elaborated in the past to explain changes in the field of psychology in general by a selected number of authors (cf. Masterman, 1974), and Kuhn's exposition can be easily applied to neuropsychology in its extant and continuing adoption of cultural factors as it evolves as a discipline dedicated to understanding complex brain-behavior relationships. Using this model (cf. Kuhn, 1962, 1970, 1996), for example, the changes that occurred in the neurosciences with the emergence of the explication of brain functions as the byproduct of individual neuronal cells working in consonance by the Spanish histologist Ramón y Cajal (1889) was not a simple accretion of knowledge but a novel approach of understanding the brain and its functions as a collection of cells working in harmony to drive human behavior. The changes in how brain functioning was subsequently viewed by the neuroscientific community superseded the existing explanation espoused by reticular theory, preponderant in the late 19th century, or in Kuhn's words, a paradigmatic shift.

Although space is not available to examine in a detailed fashion the paradigmatic shift that has occurred as a result of the adoption of culture within the discipline of neuropsychology, an examination is made here of selected aspects of Kuhn's (1962, 1970, 1996) model and its application to neuropsychology. In Kuhn's (1970) work, science, including neuropsychology, undergoes periods in which scientists, realizing that a "crisis" is present in the discipline (e.g., existing models and methods are unable to account for phenomena), begin to explore new ideas and alternatives (e.g., inclusion of culture in models) to traditional and strongly held beliefs (e.g., universals), which he termed "revolutionary science," in opposition to "normal science," or a period of time in a discipline in which solutions to problems occur using well-established methods and ideas (paradigms). A paradigmatic shift occurs, over a period of time, when new ideas or paradigms become established and accepted, replacing old ones (Kuhn, 1962, 1970).

According to Masterman (1974), Kuhn (1970) identifies three chief categories of paradigms that are critical and, in this review, readily applicable to neuropsychology. As noted by Masterman (1974), paradigms can be metaphysical, artifactual, or sociological. Masterman characterized metaphysical paradigms as new perspectives, or "organizing principles of reality" of a discipline. This is clearly a more abstract definition of a paradigm than an artifact paradigm, which is more palpable – such as the methods, instrumentation, and textbooks of a discipline. Finally, a sociological paradigm included the recognized achievements within a discipline, or social changes or legal aspects that help define a discipline. Similar to Masterman's sociological paradigm but more restrictive, Kuhn's theory (1996) includes the 'disciplinary matrix,' a broadened definition of theory or set of theories concerning the collective decisions within a specific scientific profession or community (Eckberg and Hill, 1979). These collective decisions include but are not limited to symbolic generalizations, beliefs, and values within the specialized scientific area (Kuhn, 1996). Within the disciplinary matrix, a more restrictive use of the word paradigm exists, namely the term *exemplar*. According to Kuhn, the term means, "initially, the concrete problem-solutions that students encounter from the start of their scientific education, whether in laboratories, or examinations, or at the end of chapters in scientific texts" and "at least some of the technical problem solving found in periodical literature that scientists encounter during their post-educational careers and that show them by example how their job is to be done" (Kuhn, 1996). The importance of the exemplar lies within its function, which is to think about the discipline in a concrete manner in order for problem solving to occur (Eckberg and Hill, 1979). Thus, the exemplar paradigm is an important piece within the disciplinary matrix and is crucial to a specialization's problem-solving ability. All these definitions of a paradigm are applicable to neuropsychology, as an explanation of its adoption of cultural factors into its very essence and fabric.

Although it could be argued that its philosophical and theoretical origin had its early beginning in radical environmentalism and, in particular, in the work of Vygotsky and Luria (cf. 1930/1993) and Luria (1976), from a theoretical perspective, a "crisis" leading to a paradigmatic shift, particularly in the metaphysical paradigmatic realm, occurred within neuropsychology with the emergence of findings suggesting the importance of cultural factors on cognition (Luria, 1976) and its impact on neuropsychological processes (cf. Vygotsky and Luria, 1930/1993; Luria, 1976). These new conceptualizations and notions demonstrated, for example, that culture is able to modify cognition and neuropsychological performance and, as such, led to the onset of a new paradigm shift incorporating cultural factors into psychology. In the 20th century, one of the chief proporients, the Russian psychologist Vygotsky, advocated a perspective that provided an appreciation for culture in human development and cognitive processes. According to Vygotsky, culture separates humans from animals, as well as plays an important role in our history (cf. LeFrançois, 1995) stating:

because humans can use tools and symbols; as a result, they create cultures, and cultures have a vitality, a life of their own. They grow and change and exert a very powerful influence on their members. They determine the end result of competent development – the sorts of things that its members must learn, the ways they should think, the things they are most likely to believe. (p. 84)

Vygotsky, however, was clearly not the first person to appreciate the importance of culture in the understanding of illness, injury, and intervention, but provided a greater understanding of the impact of one's environment, and indirectly culture, on development. According to Christensen and Castano (1996), Luria also made significant contributions to these new conceptual models, which like Vygotsky's, were in essence cultural-historical models (Luria, 1979; cf. Wartofsky, 1983).

Although not related directly to neuropsychology, and unfortunately forgotten, yet significantly influential from a theoretical standpoint, the German (and later American) cultural anthropologist Franz Boas was an early and strong proponent of theories underlying the forces of culture on behavior and indirectly on the brain. According to Boas (Kuper, 1999), considered the father of modern American anthropology, based on his studies of the Inuit in the latter part of the 19th century, it was culture that shapes humans, not their physiology or psychology. In addition, culture was not a linear or "upward" mechanism, but an emergent characteristic acquired from art, rituals, songs, traditions, and customs.

In the U.S., from a philosophical perspective, another view leading to a metaphysical paradigmatic shift in psychology, and indirectly on neuropsychology, was provided by the neopragmatist philosopher, psychologist, and educator John Dewey, the founder of the Chicago School of Pragmatism. According to Dewey, whose moral epistemology is contextualist (see Boydston, 1981; Dewey, 1938), contextualism discarded the idea that values and norms were void of external influences and practices. He rejected any notion of intrinsic value as a property that has value in itself, regardless of context. As noted in page v of this book, he stated that:

individuals "live from birth to death in a world of persons and things … transmitted from previous human activities. When this fact is ignored, experience is treated as if it were something which goes on exclusively inside an individual's body and mind. It ought not to be necessary to say that experience does not occur in a vacuum."[2]

A Kuhnian "crisis" was further exacerbated by investigators who began to conduct empirical studies, revealing that normative data for the general population were not appropriate for certain groups of individuals, particularly for ethnic minority individuals (e.g., Padilla et al., 1982). They also discovered that other factors could account for neuropsychological performance, aside from cognition (cf. Wechsler, 1950),

---

[2] It is poignant to note that the philosophical foundations of radical environmentalism, and to some extent, contextualism, were affected, or at least perceived in the U.S., to be impacted by the ideas and writings of Marx and Engels, and coupled with the Cold War such theoretical foundations, were not part of the core educational expositions in American neuropsychological educational circles. As noted by Lezak (1995), "neuropsychology is a child of its time and place."

indirectly leading to an artifactual paradigmatic shift. Using the definition of artifact paradigm, this is most likely one of the chief areas that led to a paradigmatic shift in neuropsychology and to the study and greater understanding of the impact of cultural and ethnic factors in the field. These changes included the emergence of significant and unparalleled developments of new instrumentation, such as new tests and procedures to be used with ethnic minority populations, Hispanics in particular (e.g., Batería, WISC-RM). They also included the development of new normative sets for such populations, as well as the emergence of new texts and writings addressing cross-cultural neuropsychology, particularly in neuropsychological assessment. Finally, changes in ethical guidelines occurred leading to the paradigmatic shift (sociological paradigms) in the field of neuropsychology, requiring the adoption of culturally relevant models in education, research, training, and so on. In this regard, for example, the *Ethical Principles of Psychologists* (APA, 1992, 2002) and the *Standards of Educational and Psychological Testing* (1985, 1999) clearly noted the importance of considering cultural factors and ethnicity when interpreting test results of individuals from diverse cultural and ethnic backgrounds. Position papers and guidelines from major organizations and conferences within the discipline also emerged that addressed the importance of such factors. For example, educational and training guidelines require that neuropsychology "attempt to actively involve (enroll, recruit) individuals from diverse backgrounds at all levels of education and training" (Hannay et al., 1998). Finally, internationally recognized nosological manuals such as the *Diagnostic and Statistical Manual of Mental Disorders-Fourth Edition* (DSM-IV) (APA, 1994) included cross-cultural factors in the interpretation of psychiatric conditions. Organizations dedicated to supporting the efforts of Hispanic neuropsychologists in the U.S. and abroad also emerged (e.g., Hispanic Neuropsychological Society), further buttressing the view that a sociological paradigmatic shift had occurred within the discipline.

As a result of the sociological paradigm shift in neuropsychology, attempts to advance the study and understanding of culture's impact on the brain have not ceased. The aforementioned accomplishments have made it clear that neuropsychology has evolved its disciplinary matrix to include cultural and ethnic factors. Now these factors must be developed and researched to better comprehend the mechanisms involved. With regard to a paradigmatic shift, neuropsychology has created a new exemplar paradigm, the affirmation and incorporation of cultural differences, which require further problem solving to take place. With the strides of new instrumentation, normative sets for minority populations and ethical considerations demonstrating the need for culturally relevant models, scientists within the field are embracing the exemplar paradigm in an attempt to understand possible neural organization-associated culture. Although it is obvious that no single individual could ever adequately represent an entire culture, efforts have been made to comprehend cultural influences on brain organization. Kennepohl (1999) has proposed a "cultural neuropsychological model." This model attempts to explain a "culturally sensitive brain" that simultaneously interacts and reveals its involvement in a multitude of environments while constricted by developmental and evolutionary restrictions through the acquisition of a perceptual filter and schemas during and throughout neural development (Kennepohl, 1999). Although there has been limited empirical support, Kennepohl's model provides new avenues for continuing research concentrating on cultural and ethnic factors in neuropsychology. Kennepohl's model is another example that demonstrates neuropsychology's ability to endure a paradigmatic shift and pursue problem-solving solutions relevant to such a shift.

Why are these fundamental, theoretical, philosophical, and historical antecedents important? It is critical to recognize that neuropsychology as a discipline has an underlying epistemological and natural history and that its evolution, in many respects, is similar to that of all other scientific disciplines. It is also critical to understand that as a discipline, neuropsychology is not free of underlying roots and zeitgeist (cf. Lezak, 1995), which in essence has an architecture and structure of attitudes, beliefs, methods, practices, skill sets, and values that define it and that shape its present and future. As a discipline, neuropsychology is not impervious to a process of alteration, evolution, and metamorphosis, as is evident for all other sciences, natural or social. Finally, such alterations are the results of shifts in those characteristics that define neuropsychology, leading to evolutionary phases in the discipline and the adoption of new ideas and explanatory frameworks and changes in theory and clinical practice, including the inclusion of cultural factors and ethnicity, in essence a paradigmatic shift.

Culture and Brain: Bridging the Gap Through Genetics

Although space constraints limit its exposition, this chapter must address the relationship between the brain and culture through genetics, as such a relationship supports a hypothesis suggesting that genes (and indirectly brains) and culture are closely intertwined. This is particularly true from our vantage point at the onset of the 21st century, when great advances have emerged in genetics, particularly during the last part of the 20th century as a result of the Human Genome Project and other investigations.

However, before we address the topic in humans, let us examine for a moment a very important yet often forgotten experiment, conducted with animals in the 1960s in Russia by the geneticist Belyaev. Belyaev was interested in taming wild, and aggressive, foxes which were being used for their coats in his fur business. To do so, Belyaev began by selecting tamer wild foxes from his breeding stock, those that were most approachable, less shy, and less likely to flee when in his presence. As he proceeded with his breeding program, he discovered that he indeed was producing tamer animals, and in some instances he produced foxes that would actually approach him and his staff. However, these alterations in behavioral characteristics (tamability) were accompanied by an unforeseen result, namely that the tamed foxes' fur also had been altered. More important, as far as neuropsychology is concerned, the tamed foxes had the behavioral and physical characteristics of domesticated dogs, such as tamed comportment, floppy ears, rolled tails and shorter snouts, and <u>brains</u> that were smaller than those of wild foxes. In other words, by selecting a specific, desirable behavior (approachability, tamability), and genetically selecting for it over many generations (over 20 to be precise), Belyaev not only impacted the physical and behavioral characteristics of the animals, but also their brain! [Belyaev, 1979]

Unfortunately, an animal study does not support a hypothesis suggesting that genes, the environment, and culture are inextricably related in brain development in humans. Therefore, let us examine human studies. One study involves the work of the neuroscientist Rizzolatti and his colleagues (c.f., Kohler et al., 2002), who researched brain functions using functional MRI scans of the brain. These researchers have demonstrated that "mirror neurons," which have been speculated to be responding to an "action," also respond to the "vision of an action," most likely a mechanism of brain function involved in imitation, a critical aspect of the transmission of cultural variables. In fact, in another study they have shown that these types of neurons may not respond to the observation and enactment of a behavior or action, but respond in a similar fashion to a noise associated with the action (Kohler et al., 2002). Another recent finding involves language, a domain closely involved with culture and brain functions. In this study, reported by Lai et al. (2001), investigators discovered a mutation responsible for a severe type of speech and language disorder. This gene, known as forkhead box P_2, is a gene responsible for modulating other genes, and when abnormal, leads to language and speech disorders, because the gene is necessary for the normal development of speech and grammar, language closely associated with the transmission of culture through narrative, songs, and other factors closely associated with language.

In sum, it is clear from these examples that brains, through genetic mechanisms and culture, and through a myriad of mechanisms, including imitation and language, are closely intertwined. As we stated in the Preface, there appears to be a bidirectional relationship between brain and behavior, and because behavior is partially shaped by the environment, particularly in humans, and because humans are impacted by their culture, culture affects brain.

Definitions, Terminology, and Ancillary Issues

Although several of these concepts and terminology will be covered in greater detail in subsequent chapters, an introduction to some definitions and terms is provided here to familiarize the reader with various topics.

There has been significant confusion in the psychological literature related to *culture, ethnicity,* and *race*. In fact, psychology and neuropsychology have lagged in the accurate and timely incorporation of such constructs. The field of anthropology provides better and more comprehensive expositions of such terminology. It is also interesting, yet unfortunate, to note that the confusion has become part of everyday linguistic expression and even some dictionaries indicate that race "often has been replaced in the scientific literature" with ethnicity or ethnic group (not to mention governmental agencies; see Chapter 2). Therefore, the confusion in neuropsychology, though understandable, is neither proper nor acceptable, with significant, and in some instances, detrimental repercussions (see Chapters 2, 3, and 6). Unlike race, ethnicity is a complex construct. Within the realm of anthropology, particularly cultural anthropology, ethnicity and race are very distinct terms, ethnicity referring to a characteristic that defines an individual based on his or her ancestry, language, geography, history, religion, rituals, and values (cf. Applebaum, 1987). To a certain extent, ethnicity is an individual characteristic that develops over time, and may evolve over time in an individual as a result of many factors, including assimilation of a new, distinct ethnicity and simultaneous discarding or diminishing adoption of existing ethnic characteristics. Unlike ethnicity, many writers view race as an attribute in an individual that is assumed to have a biological origin. Most original description(s) in readily available dictionaries (e.g., Webster's) defined race as "one of the different varieties of mankind." In other words, ethnicity can be perceived as a demographic based to a certain extent on cultural traditions, while race, whether or not wholly appropriate, is seen as chiefly a demographic based on biological traits. While ethnicity develops around similar features as cultures, race is not derived from beliefs, history, and so on. Whereas a specific ethnicity involves the constant adoption of an ethnic identity and may require differentiation from other ethnicities, racial differentiation is determined not by the individual but by his or her genetic attributes. Finally, Jalali (1988) defined ethnicity as "the culture of [a] people [that] is thus critical for values, attitudes, perceptions, needs, and modes of expression, behavior, and identity" (p. 10). Although race may be easier to discern in an individual, his or her ethnicity is not, and in some instances, it is even difficult for some persons to readily identify themselves with a specific ethnicity.

Culture, on the other hand, can be thought of as a set of unifying beliefs, behaviors, ideas, and values that connect symbols to form a cultural integration in a group of individuals. A culture is composed of smaller subcomponents that transmit symbols such as family, groups, and institutions. Cultural characteristics and patterns of behavior, including beliefs, language, institutions, technology, and values, are transmitted across generations as culturally learned traits leading to the very cultural definitions of its components (childhood, e.g., cf. Wartofsky, 1983). It is interesting to note that unlike other animals humans have, to a certain extent, replaced biological instincts with individually, culturally defined characteristics. Although biologically based responses and behavior are common in all humans, such as the ability to learn a language, cultural factors modulate such mechanisms and functions, leading to significant and individual differentiation and to cultural factors leading to learned specific functions such as distinct languages, including Urdu, Spanish, and others. However, the question remains, how are culture and ethnicity different? Although culture and ethnicity can be considered to be similar because they are learned and flexible (Smedley, 1993), culture, as noted above, can be perceived as a complex manifestation or expression or as symbolic elements that define a group of individuals or society from which individuals may adopt specific characteristics which over time lead to their own ethnic identity (cf. Smedley, 1993; Nagel, 1994, Shorris, 1992). Whereas ethnicity is in the individual, there can be many ethnicities represented within a culture.

It is also critical to note that ethnicity, culture, and race are not related to nationality. Individuals with the same nationality or region of origin may have different races, ethnicity, and cultural characteristics, and this is particularly true for Hispanics (cf. Shorris, 1992). It is also critical to understand that Hispanics, as will be noted later, may have multiple racial and ethnic backgrounds.

Within the context of culture, ethnicity, and race, the concept of *Hispanic* is better defined. The term *Hispanic* is used throughout this text to refer to all individuals perceiving themselves to be Latino, Spanish, and Spanish-speaking individuals. Puente and Ardila (2000) note that some dictionaries, such as the *Merriam-Webster's Dictionary*, include individuals from Portugal as Hispanics. In that sense, individuals who speak Portuguese or dialects thereof may be considered Hispanic, and thus the term would include individuals from Brazil and other regions of the world. They also note that *El Diccionario de la Lengua Real Española* (*Real Academia Española*, 1984) is more restrictive, limiting the term Hispanics to individuals from Spain or Spanish-speaking Latin America. As noted by Puente and Ardila (2000), such a restrictive definition may be incorrect. Therefore, the term Hispanic in this text is intended to represent individuals from Latin or Central America and the Caribbean (i.e., Latino), as well as from Mexico and from other Spanish-speaking (e.g., Spain) origins and the U.S., and individuals who identify themselves as such because they perceive themselves as "Hispanic." As might be expected, and as noted by Harris and Llorente (2005), "Hispanic individuals living in the U.S." and other parts of the world "share many of their institutional and societal structures, including values, political, economic, and general educational systems." However, groups of Hispanic individuals vary greatly with regard to "country of origin, educational attainment, religion, use of language(s), and other important variables, and the pan-ethnic label "Hispanic" fails to include these unique individual attributes."

Although an argument could be made that any ethnic group living within the U.S. may represent a heterogeneous cohort, this is especially the case for "Hispanics" living in this country. Aside from issues related to language differences to be covered in detail in Chapter 5, significant heterogeneity emerges even if language is excluded. In order to understand the genesis of such heterogeneity, it is critical to learn that the pan-ethnic label "Hispanic" fails to include unique attributes, and race unfortunately often, but inappropriately, has been used as an ethnic category, even by governmental entities, which creates significant confusion and problems, particularly for neuropsychology (see Chapters 2, 3, and 6; cf. Llorente et al., 1999). Although as noted by Harris and Llorente (2005), "the identification as a separate race stems from the blending of races within the history of some Hispanic peoples," including "the result of intermarriage of the European Spaniards with the indigenous Indians, producing the "mestizo," many a Mexican-American peoples favor the distinction of the term *Chicanos*. This preference represents certain political and ethnic perspectives and emerges because they often consider themselves to be descendents of this "new" race that migrated northward to the U.S. from Mexico. However, others prefer the term *Mexican-American*. As noted by Harris and Llorente (2005), "even within a specific nationality/ethnic grouping, such as the largest category in the U.S. ("Mexican"), there are additional factors to take into consideration, including the fact that the term Mexican encompasses both U.S.-born and Mexican immigrants.

Evidently, the term Hispanic is in fact a pan-ethnic term used to identify a number of cultural or ethnic groupings, and Hispanic individuals can claim one or more of many racial origin(s) as well as any Spanish-speaking country of origin, nationality, or ethnicity. Even within an intra-ethnic definition, individuals emigrating from Mexico may identify themselves with any of many ethnic groups that reside in that country (Vázquez, 1994). In addition to traditional Spanish, many of these individuals may use languages which exceed over 200 different indigenous living languages, including Mayan, Náhuatl, and Tamaulipeco (Harris and Llorente, 2005). Similar considerations, for example, are applicable to "Hispanics" from Guatemala and other nations. Therefore, Hispanic "individuals within the U.S. may consequently be of any race, any ethnicity or combination of ethnicities (e.g., parents with Puerto Rican and Colombian nationalities), and may be monolingual Spanish speakers, monolingual English speakers, bilingual (e.g., Spanish-Mayan), or multilingual (e.g., Náhuatl-Spanish-English), even if English is not yet a proficient language" (Harris and Llorente, 2005). At one end of this continuum Hispanics may represent recent immigrants, "monolingual Spanish-speaking individuals," and "at the other end of the" spectrum "they may represent children whose ancestors have been living in the U.S. for multiple generations and whose parents may not share the same ethnicity (Hispanic or other), and may not even speak the Spanish language" (Harris and Llorente, 2005).

Pontón (2001b) provides an intriguing, although simple, model of the diversity of the Hispanic population, one that is useful when interpreting assessment results during the course of neuropsychological evaluation. He proposes to view the population as a cube with variation along three dimensions, namely (a) years of exposure to education, (b) country of origin, and (c) language proficiency (English, Spanish, or bilingual). Although such a model is a good starting point, clearly it could easily be made more complex and comprehensive by adding more factor values, such as proficiency in indigenous languages, acculturation (Pontón, 2001b; Roysircar, 2004), region of origin or residence (urban/rural), or migration history (Llorente et al., 1999).

In the final analysis, it is sincerely hoped that the reader realizes that the terms culture, ethnicity, and race encompass different constructs that are not interchangeable. It is also hoped that the reader surmises that the term Hispanic is being used in this text as a literary term to refer to individuals of a Spanish or Latino background who identify themselves as Hispanic, yet in no way are these individuals being characterized as a homogenous group, since heterogeneity is the rule within this population (cf. Harris and Llorente, 2005; Puente and Ardila, 2000; Shorris, 1992). Hispanics can be of many races and ethnocultural backgrounds, and even within the same ethnic group, there are interethnic differences. The term Hispanic, or that of other groups of individuals for that matter, such as "Cuban" or "Mexican," is being used for ease of expression, not any other reason, and the authors hope that individuals understand the diversity encompassed by such pan-ethnic terms.

Acculturation occurs when foreign cultural traits and values are adopted by a society on a large scale or when a minority group or an individual adopts, assimilates, or conforms to and integrates the characteristics, norms, and values of another culture (cf. Berry, 1997; Portes and Rumbaut, 1990). In the process, the culture of the receiving society is altered as a result of such acculturation, as in changes in American society associated with large-scale migrations of Hispanics and other ethnic minority groups (e.g., Italians), yet the emerging culture is not completely new, but rather an interrelationship of amalgamations leading to the union of the existing traditional and foreign traits. Within this context, acculturation and assimilation are being used to described the adoption of values and foreign cultural traits by an individual, in this case, Hispanic, as result of immigration or residence within a foreign culture (U.S.). In this context, for example, a Hispanic individual from the Dominican Republic adopts new values and traits over the years after his arrival in the U.S., and in this sense a certain degree of assimilation occurs in this individual. As is the case for many of these variables, acculturation can exist and occur in varying degrees along a spectrum. For example, some Hispanic individuals, upon arrival in the U.S., as result of desire or necessity, exhibit little if any acculturation to American society, whereas others extensively acculturate to American society en masse. It is critical to note that many variables influence degree of acculturation, including age of the individual or residential area of preference (Portes and Rumbaut, 1990). In this regard, it is easy to realize how there is no need for a Hispanic individual who immigrates to Miami, Florida, to assimilate American culture unless it is desired or perceived to be beneficial, whereas the opposite may be required if a Hispanic individual, upon arrival to the U.S., were to reside in Bismarck, North Dakota. In some instances, some of these individuals partially or completely may discard their Hispanic identity, or may never become acculturated as measured by bilingual status along with other acculturation traits.

From an applied standpoint, the issue of acculturation is important for cross-cultural neuropsychology. As noted by Pontón (2001a), level of acculturation is critical because it assists the clinician to make important pragmatic determinations related to the assessment process. When necessary, acculturation should be assessed formally during the course of a neuropsychological examination, if at all possible. Acculturation scales have been shown to predict generational cohort, degree of acculturation, and other factors (Marin et al., 1984). These scales depend on test items that tap into preferred language use, language spoken in the home, language use during leisure time, or friendships. Aside from the fact that there are scales that permit the objective assessment of acculturation for Hispanics (Marin et al., 1984), assessment is helpful because it helps guide the process in terms of its components, including language use during the assessment, the selection of assessment procedures, and test performance interpretation to name a few factors (cf. Pontón, 2001a). If formal assessment is not possible, acculturation also can be gauged through the use of similar information, including language spoken in the home, the nature of friendships, and leisure activities. Aside from measuring language dominance and literacy, readily published formal reading, reading comprehension, and phonemic processing tests can also be used to address the degree of acculturation of a client.

A number of neuropsychologists (cf. Ardila and Moreno, 2001; Nell, 2000) appropriately and coherently have argued that *literacy* plays a major role in the differences sometimes observed between Hispanics and members of other ethnic minority and nonminority groups. Although such a viewpoint is not considered objectionable in this volume, it is only part of the puzzle, particularly if illiteracy is not defined in the traditional sense in which it has been described and used in the clinical neuropsychological literature, such as the inability to read and/or write.

Literacy is in itself an extremely complex area of inquiry. The term *literacy* has evolved over time, and currently there are significant controversies as to what defines literary fluency and competency, namely cognitive processes, inability to read text, social literacy, technological literacy, and other factors (Kress, 2003; Tannen, 1980). The term literacy also has to be examined with care because it describes varying degrees of this construct along a continuum (Tannen, 1980). Whereas some individuals may be able to simply sign their names and have a rudimentary mastery of reading, their reading fluency and other aspects of this skill (e.g., reading speed), and any other skills used to define literacy, may be more or completely limited. To complicate matters further, many individuals who report certain degrees of literary mastery may not be sufficiently literate to undergo evaluation in a specific language (e.g., Spanish; see example in Chapter 6). What is unequivocally documented in the literature is the fact that illiteracy has significant consequences for neuropsychology and neuropsychological practice. For example, related to Hispanics, Ardila and colleagues (1989b, 1994) have spent a great deal of effort attempting to examine the effects of illiteracy on neuropsychological performance. In their work with illiterate clients, using a brief neuropsychological battery, Ardila et al. (1989b, 1994) examined visuospatial and memory abilities in "extreme educational groups" (illiterate and highly educated individuals). The results revealed statistically significant differences in all visuospatial tasks, and all but one memory task, between the two groups. Aside from noting differences between these groups, these investigators concluded that "cognitive skills are usually examined by neuropsychological tests" that require "highly trained abilities," such as those provided by a formal educational system.

As noted above, the concept of literacy is actually an evolving construct, and in its current usage, it is becoming more complex because of advances in information processing and the emergence of new technologies. Therefore, Kress (2003) and others (cf. Lankshear and Knobel, 2003) argue that new forms of literacy are emerging and are constantly required in our society. *Technological literacy* would be considered one of those emerging in our society. Although such an issue may be thought of as irrelevant to neuropsychology, it is critical because many tests and procedures administered to Hispanic patients, whether adult or pediatric populations, are technology-dependent (e.g., computerized neuropsychological tests), yet many Hispanic patients come from backgrounds where technological illiteracy is commonplace.

Lack of formal education and the interaction between education, literacy, and culture also are important to consider. Although it is tempting to equate lack of education with illiteracy, these two variables represent different constructs and most likely play distinct roles in neuropsychology. For example, not every literate Hispanic individual has received formal education in excess of a few years of schooling or any at all. Therefore, although literacy can have significant impact on neuropsychological assessment, or cognitive development and mechanisms for that matter, lack of education can have independent effects that are not associated with illiteracy and that are capable of accounting for "problems" sometimes observed in neuropsychological performance. Although Heaton et al. (1986) have made a strong argument as to the importance of education in neuropsychological test performance, research addressing culture and education merits attention, particularly for Hispanics. In this regard, Ostrosky-Solis et al. (2004) examined the influence of education and culture on neuropsychological performance in indigenous and non-indigenous populations in Mexico. Although sample sizes were small, their results suggested that culture and education exert independent effects on neuropsychological performance. Culture reportedly "dictates what it is important for survival" and "education could be considered as a type of subculture that facilitates the development of certain skills."

From an applied standpoint, the issue of education will be explored in more detail in later chapters. However, it is sufficient here to note that many tests and procedures, including those considered by many practitioners as gold standards in instrumentation, have significant deficiencies in this regard, and many do not have normative data for specific groups of individuals, particularly Hispanics, with limited or very advanced educational backgrounds (Ardila, 1998; Llorente, 1997; Llorente et al., 1999, 2000; Puente and Ardila, 2000). Even more perplexing is the fact that such data may not even be available for individuals from the mainstream culture, yet clinicians continue to use such norms without questioning the validity or reliability of the inferences derived from them. For example, the reader is asked to determine how many 75- to 79-year-old Hispanics who came from educational backgrounds with 9 to 11 years of education are found in the WAIS-III standardization sample, or more relevantly, how many 10-year-old "white" children who came from backgrounds whose average parental educational is ≤8 years are found in the WISC-IV's standardization sample?[3]

With regard to test construction, as noted by Harris and Llorente (2005), there are significant implications for level of education associated with the standardization of cognitive and neuropsychological procedures when applied to Hispanics. They note that "normative studies comprised of examinees with lower mean education, or in the case of children, lower parental education," are important to scrutinize because "Test publishers typically stratify socioeconomic status within ethnic

---

[3] Because education plays such a pre-eminent role in neuropsychology and its clinical practice, and because low levels of educational attainment have been implicated in poor neuropsychological performance in some instances, it is given special attention in several chapters throughout this text. However, the reader should not assume that all Hispanics come from impoverished backgrounds with low levels of educational attainment, as such an assumption is far from actuality in the U.S., the fifth largest Hispanic population on the face of the globe.

groupings to reflect the characteristics of the country's population. This is often accomplished by utilizing parental education as a proxy for socioeconomic status because of the strong relationship between these two variables" (Prifitera, Weiss, and Saklofske, 1998, 2005). In the case of intellectual tests, "When IQ scores are compared across ethnic groups, the overall reference group, which is overwhelmingly represented by the non-minority cases, will tend to have higher mean SES and parental education than the subgroups that are the focus of the comparison (Prifitera, Weiss and Saklofske, 1998). The lower performances of individuals from ethnic minority groups reflect both the correlation between SES and IQ (Prifitera et al., 2005), as well as the composition of the normative sample.

Another important variable is worth mentioning, namely, quality of education (Byrd, Sanchez, and Manly, 2005). Although this variable is not given enough attention in the literature or in daily clinical practice, it is critical because not all educational systems are able to provide the same quality of education. Even in the U.S., where specific guidelines and standards for teacher education and qualifications as well as curriculum guidelines abound, stark discrepancies in quality of education are sometimes evident, in some instances, within the same school district and, as noted by a colleague who is a former teacher, sometimes within the same school. Differences also are sometimes observed between private and public educational settings, and between suburban educational settings relative to poor inner city schools in the U. S., the latter with high enrollment of Hispanic youths. Another frequently encountered problem that impacts quality of education is the fact that many youth are promoted on the basis of their chronological age rather than as a result of academic mastery, leading to poor levels of academic achievement and competency. This factor impacts Hispanics and should be given due weight. In the U.S. and abroad, quality of education affects large numbers of Hispanics, be they children or young adults. Chapter 2 will show how, for children, immigration factors impact residence in the U.S., and how such preferences sometimes lead to large numbers of children being enrolled in metropolitan inner city schools, where the problems described above are frequently encountered or exacerbated. In adults, educational level and quality of education issues are often encountered as a result of higher school dropout rates for adolescent Hispanics than for other ethnic minority or majority populations (see Harris and Llorente, 2005). Although not applicable to all individuals, educational level and quality of education relates to Hispanics from abroad, particularly those individuals who have immigrated as adults to the U.S. from rural and/or impoverished backgrounds from underdeveloped countries, who have received academic training in a poor educational system. For example, their educational levels sometimes may lead to the same number of years of education as individuals in the U.S. Yet, despite having attended the same number of years as have individuals living in the U.S., they may have experienced a significantly lower quality of education. Although at first glance issues related to quality of education may not be seen as important to neuropsychologists, they are critical because most neuropsychological tests and procedures, used in daily practice with Hispanics, employ normative data that have been stratified according to years of education, without attention to "quality of education."

Pragmatic test development and application issues also deserve attention. Chapter 6 provides a more thorough review of procedures and methods that can mitigate the effects of test bias during the course of test development for Hispanic populations, particularly monolingual Spanish-speaking individuals. Therefore, such factors will not be presented here in detail. However, it is appropriate and important to briefly delineate issues that have been raised in the literature related to test construction and application for Hispanics and that have led to negative consequences. The topic merits attention because it addresses important issues and weaknesses in the neuropsychological literature, including the lack of appropriate tests for Hispanics and Spanish-speaking populations.

One topic deserving exposition is test development and the use of simple test translations. As noted above, paradigmatic shifts occur in scientific disciplines that lead to changes in their theory and practice, particularly artifactual paradigms closely associated with palpable aspects of a discipline (Kuhn, 1970). Although it was common and probably appropriate during the early stages of paradigmatic shift to observe the development of tests in Spanish as simple translations of tests from other languages, such a practice has become obsolete over time. Modern test development efforts for Hispanic populations have increased in complexity, and the use of forward and back translations were used to develop procedures in Spanish from other languages. However, a translation of a test is not an adaptation of a test, which is a more comprehensive methodology of test development, and later tests developed for use with Hispanics not only included translations or back translations but a comprehensive adaptation into Spanish. The complexity and arduous task of appropriately adapting a test included an examination of word usage and frequency of word appearance (using existing manuals [cf. Carroll, Davies, and Richman, 1971]) in the culture for which the test was being "adapted," use of similar populations for standardizations, and other adaptations.

However, more recent test development strategies and efforts for procedures in Spanish have seen a diversification and increase in sophistication, rather than a simple adaptation of a test from English or any other language. For example, as will be noted in more detail in Chapter 7, modern tests with Spanish versions (e.g., BASC- II, SENAS; WISC-IV in Spanish, WJ-III) have adopted more advanced methodological postures, including the use of advanced statistical procedures to reduce bias (e.g., item analysis), sampling methods (e.g., over sampling), and test development procedures that have surpassed older methods of test development and validation, leading to new exemplars in the creation of modern tests in Spanish (or any other language for that matter).

Another issue that warrants attention is the development of test norms for Hispanics. Although recent criticism has emerged related to the creation of separate norms for minority populations (Brandt, 2005), including Hispanics, such norms are temporarily necessary, particularly during the early stages of paradigmatic shift. Such norms are required because they enhance the inferential process by attempting to reduce the effects of potential confounds, and such a practice is necessary until unbiased tests are developed that do not discriminate against ethnic minority groups, including Hispanics. It is also critical to realize that according to Kuhn's

(1970) model, this approach is how practice evolves in a discipline, and how paradigmatic shifts eventually become extant models of thought and practice. Criticizing such a posture fails to take into account the natural progression of a discipline, particularly during the infancy of a paradigmatic shift.

Another important factor to consider is the generalization of test data, normative data in particular, that have been collected in other countries, that were developed for groups of individuals different from the individual undergoing assessment (see Llorente et al., 1999), and that are used with such an individual simply because he or she speaks the common language (i.e., Spanish) or other convenient reasons (cf. Mitrushina et al., 1999). Many problems are inextricably related to this assessment posture, including lack of language dominance and ethnic differences (cf. Puente and Ardila, 2000). It also includes cultural factors. For example, norms developed with Spanish-speaking individuals in Spain may not be applicable to individuals who speak Spanish in the U.S., despite the fact that both may be fluent in Spanish. This issue is encountered with greater frequency as a result of increased globalization. As tests are produced in specific countries (e.g., Australia, United Kingdom, and Spain) and applied in other areas of the world, where populations may be inherently different from an ethnic and cultural standpoint yet not linguistically, and it is likely that such instances may become more prevalent, yet not always appropriate. As a case in point, it is not unusual to see a client, pediatric or adult, seem confused with a test stimulus (e.g., Union Jack) from a test developed in another country, leading to failure by the patient on that particular test item in the U.S.

An egregious posture that occurs every so often also includes the use of other professionals acting as health professionals or in a similar capacity without having training in the health sciences, but acting as an evaluator for purposes of assessment because he or she "may be bilingual." Such unethical and illegal conduct does not require or deserve further elucidation. Another problem sometimes encountered in the practice of neuropsychology is the use of a unique and "live" translation of a test published in English into Spanish, a test without a published Spanish version by a bilingual clinician. In this case, a clinician essentially creates a unique, live, on-site, unpublished Spanish translation of a test that does not have an authorized or published version, adding to the problem by referring to existing norms for the English version test. It is clear that such postures should be avoided, and an explanation for such a rationale is not necessary (cf. Artiola i Fortuni et al., 2005).

Another inappropriate approach frequently encountered in practice is the administration of only one scale of a comprehensive test (e.g., WAIS III, Performance Scale). This practice involves administering only one scale of a test with many or multiple scales and subsequently using such narrow information to generalize and inferentially approximate an individual's overall or omnibus score, such as his or her overall intellect. This practice is unfounded and marked by several problems, and it relies on inappropriate assumptions about cognitive processes and psychometric properties of tests. One important misconceived assumption is that cognitive processes may be discrete phenomena. In other words, when administering a visual reasoning scale of a test without administering its accompanying verbal reasoning scale, it is incorrect to assume that visual processes occur independently of verbal processes or that language and verbal reasoning processes do not enter the evaluative process during the completion of a task that predominantly may require visual processing skills (Lezak et al., 2004). Another erroneous assumption is the belief that administering such a scale provides a more accurate interpretation and gauge of the individual's overall skill. Although an accurate measurement may emerge for the scale administered, such a restrictive assessment process fails to assess other major functional areas, areas that actually may be impaired. Although such a practice was used inappropriately for years with individuals with severe sensory (auditory or visual) handicapping conditions, such as deaf and hard-of-hearing persons or the legally blind, such an approach should not be used with a Hispanic individual. Finally, the reader should surmise from the above that we are not arguing against the use of a single test scale (WAIS-III, Performance IQ score) to examine a specific domain, such as visual (nonverbal) reasoning, but rather we are arguing against the misuse of such a scale to infer an individual's *overall* index (WAIS-III, Full Scale IQ score) from his score on the single scale.

From a psychometric standpoint, an assessment posture whereby only one scale is administered is not appropriate for multiple reasons. However, due to lack of space, only major reasons will be addressed here. First, perusal of the correlations between subscales and overall index for most tests reveals that such subscales are incapable of accounting for the overall test variance. For some tests (e.g., WAIS-III), such test scales (e.g., Performance IQ score) account for approximately 79% to 90% of the total variance in overall intellect (FSIQ), depending on specific demographics. Second, it should not be assumed that such a variance is the same for all ages; differences exist in the amount of variance that is accounted for by specific subscales from the total variance as a function of chronological age. Third, as noted by Kaufman and Flanagan (2004), as the difference between an individual's subscale scores increases, the validity of the omnibus index may not be interpretable or its interpretation may become difficult because the subscales may not be measuring the construct they were meant to assess, leading to a spurious omnibus index. Finally, the base rates of such differences are important (cf. McCaffrey et al., 2003), yet sometimes not available, or worse yet, not considered, thus biasing and hindering interpretation. In summary, such an approach should be avoided, and an appropriate, comprehensive measure should be administered.

Although a more comprehensive discourse related to this topic is found in Chapter 5, a narrow summary of specific issues associated with bilingualism applicable to neuropsychological assessment will be provided here. As noted by Harris and Llorente (2005), the "relationship of language proficiency and bilingualism to cognitive performance has long been a sensitive topic but one that has direct bearing on the performance discrepancies observed for some ethnic minority (e.g., Hispanic) versus non-minority groups." Despite their absurd conclusions, early studies suggested that bilingualism might represent a cognitive liability, yet later investigations revealed that such differences were the result of artifact associated with flawed research methodologies, including failure to control for socioeconomic and other variables, heterogeneity in the samples defining "bilingual, and other factors" (cf. Paradis, 1978).

In addition, past research suggests that second language acquisition, particularly English proficiency, takes long periods to reach what might be considered a deep structural level, and that such mastery should not be confused with the simple ability to use English in conversational (social) situations (Cummins, 1979). Cummins (1979) differentiated between "surface fluency" (basic interpersonal communication skills) and more cognitively and profound levels of processing and language proficiency. Cummins (1979, 1984) further argued that in face-to-face verbal interaction, the meaning of the communication is supported by contextual cues (e.g., facial expression), whereas test situations are context reduced, cognitively demanding circumstances, situations which require significant language proficiency in excess of that utilized in basic communication. In studies Cummins conducted in the U.S. and Canada, he found that individuals arriving from another country after the age of six years required an average of five to seven years to approach grade norm levels of English proficiency (Cummins 1981). As noted by Harris and Llorente (2005), it "seems logical, then, to conclude that" Hispanics "acquiring skills in English may not possess sufficient fluency" or deep structural mastery to "effectively perform on more demanding, contextually reduced neuropsychological examinations."

From an applied standpoint, language competency in bilinguals (e.g., English and Spanish) should not be left to arm chair speculation, but rather, a data-based approach should be taken at the onset of evaluation to assess the degree of language proficiency of a client (see Chapters 5, 6). Although it will not be reproduced here, Pontón (2001b) provides a good starting point, and he developed an assessment decision tree that may serve as a charter guide in reaching a conclusion as to whether to test a Hispanic client in English or Spanish. It is also critical not to depend on the client's verbal report related to their degree of fluency in any language, as bilingualism is not a discrete, digital, dichotomous characteristic but rather an analog variable with varying degrees of fluency in English and/or Spanish (or any other language), and a client's report may be inaccurate. Yet, as noted by Mungas (1996), good communication with a client is critical to enhance the validity and reliability of assessments conducted with Hispanic clients.

Although many factors already have been mentioned that should convince the reader that linguistic factors should be strongly considered prior to assessment, another important issue requires consideration because it is inextricably related to neuropsychological diagnostic categorization. In this regard, it is paramount to recognize that the phenomenology of a construct, such as schizophrenia, may be altered in its assessment or interpretation by the examiner due to a lack of language proficiency (Perez-Foster, 2001). As noted before, ethical considerations should prevail in the decision to assess or not to assess a Hispanic client or to seek consultation or supervision (APA, 2002). It is left to the clinician to determine whether their degree of professional competency is appropriate to evaluate a specific Hispanic individual in a specific language (cf. Artiola i Fortuni and Mullaney, 1998).

Another vital topic that requires attention in this chapter is the use of interpreters. Aside from ethical considerations (cf. APA, 2002), there are several factors worth addressing related to the use of interpreters during the course of neuropsychological evaluations or related components such as interviewing or feedback of assessment results. Although at first glance the need for such interpreters is required because large portions of individuals from Hispanic populations are monolingual Spanish speakers or "bilingual" with poor English fluency and mastery, there has been an increase in the number of individuals who are able to conduct neuropsychological assessments in Spanish during the last decade, and the use of interpreters should be avoided. In addition, although the use of an interpreter may be appropriate to schedule an appointment or other clerical components, and in some instances such a posture may be sound in conducting other health-related consultations, it is neither appropriate or sensible to use interpreters to assess complex cognitive skills, some of which might require intricate language abilities or, in some instances, sophisticated processes involving verbal reasoning such as verbal abstraction. Although it is our opinion that interpreters should not be used during the course of clinical interviewing and neuropsychological assessment with Hispanic populations, and taking such a course of action opens clinicians to all types of potential problems, including liability, there may be cases in which the use of an interpreter is unavoidable, such as the unavailability of bilingual neuropsychologists in selected areas within a nation. Therefore, several factors should be considered if interpreters are necessary. First, the quality of the interpretative services should be closely scrutinized and strongly considered. There may be qualified individuals in a community who may be professional interpreters. If at all possible, unqualified interpreters should be avoided, and if possible, interpreters familiar with the content of the work performed by neuropsychologists should be preferred. There are interpreters who have received specialized training in mental health, and preference should be given to these individuals.

The use of family members as interpreters is one of the most pernicious errors during the course of neuropsychological assessments with Hispanics, and this issue has received some attention in the literature. Aside from the fact that these individuals are usually not aware of ethical guidelines related to the process of interpretation or translation (American Translators Association, 1997), as noted by Dodd (1983), the use of family members is inappropriate because employing such individuals for such a purpose may lead to bias during the course of interviewing or other assessment components. Although at first glance the novice clinician may note that there are inherent and perceived advantages associated with the use of interpreters who may be very familiar with the client, individuals who may have a genuine interest in the patient, who are easily accessible, and who serve the client as a buffer related to anxiety-provoking and other assessment-related effects, such perceived advantages easily disappear and become potential liabilities when examined more closely. The reasons that such advantages are misperceived easily become evident when the clinician considers the risks and potential problems that may arise when family members act as interpreters. Although there are probabilistically a myriad of ways that the interpreting family member can hinder the interviewing or assessment process (cf. Blau, 1998; Kayser, 1993), one of the chief factors involved with such a practice is the risk of harm to the patient as a result of intended or unintended misinterpretation by a family member. In some instances such a misinterpretation may be for obvious or not-so-obvious reasons. For example, imagine the assessment of a Hispanic child who has been the victim of abuse, leading to a traumatic head injury, who is brought for neuropsychological assessment or rehabilitation by his father, in this case, responsible for the abuse, or a woman, serving as an interpreter, brings her elderly husband or father or other loved one for a feedback session and has to provide negative information that she perceives may be painful to her kin, such as the disclosure of the presence of a dementia. Will these interpreters serve as unbiased reporters? Clearly, these individuals may not serve as accurate reporters when discussing the cause behind the head injury or when providing negative yet in some instances necessary, prudent, and realistic feedback.

Advents in technology also have decreased the need to use family members as interpreters, and if the use of such resources becomes absolutely necessary, modern interpretative services are readily available through telecommunication systems from local or international telephone companies. Combined with the use of speaker phones and similar technologies, such a posture reduces the need for family participation unless necessary for clinical purposes but not as interpretative resources. Therefore, the use of family members as interpreters should be avoided (Dodd, 1983).

For obvious reasons, the use of interpreters truly becomes a critical factor during the course of civil or criminal legal proceedings. In short, the practice of using interpreters during forensic neuropsychological evaluations also should be avoided at all costs (cf. De Jongh, 1991; LaCalle, 1987). In these cases, important legal dispositions may have significant impact on the client, his family, his community, and in some instances, the establishments of critical legal precedents, and therefore the use of interpreters in such settings is especially inappropriate. From a legal standpoint, the forensic psychology and cross-cultural literatures indicate that evaluations conducted through an interpreter may be invalid and must be avoided, not to mention unethical and easily challenged in a court of law (LaCalle, 1987). The literature suggests that even an accurate translation of test protocols and other components of an evaluation may result in the loss of subtleties and connotational nuances of speech (Cervantes and Acosta, 1992), leading to diminished validity and reliability (see Psychometric Issues below). In fact, some researchers and clinicians argue that simply changing the manner in which a test is administered without restandardizing the tool to meet the ethnic and cultural and linguistic requirements of the individual undergoing assessment leads to challenges of the validity, and reliability, of test results, particularly in the case of forensic evaluations (Melendez, 2001). It is important to realize that such a posture should be taken for ethical reasons, the ultimate reason to take a specific course of action during the course of assessments with Hispanics, but also for pragmatic and legal reasons. In this regard, it is critical to note that there are ethical aspirations and principles (APA, 2002) associated with the appropriate conduct of neuropsychologists when acting in the forensic arena, as well as legal issues to consider concerning admissibility of test results on the basis of their validity and reliability in such proceedings (cf. Daubert v. Merrell Dow Pharmaceuticals [92–102], 509 US 579 [1993]).

A Brief Examination of Statistical and Psychometric Issues

The majority of factors discussed above are common knowledge and have been well articulated in the cross-cultural neuropsychological literature by several authors. One area, however, that is capable of hampering neuropsychological assessments with Hispanic populations that has not been given proper attention is psychometric issues associated with reliability and validity.

Reliability (R_x) is a measure of consistency or the degree of stability or accuracy of test results associated with inferences in neuropsychological assessments. Using traditional psychometric theory, an individual's score on a test ($X_{test\ score}$) is comprised of a true score (X_{true}), representing the actual characteristic or trait under investigation, and error (X_{error}), assumed to be random in nature. Because random error enters the measurement process, a person's true score is not observable on any test (Kirk, 1990). In other words:

$$X_{test\ score} = X_{true} + X_{error}$$

Reliability then represents the ratio of true score variance over the observed score variance. Although a more detailed coverage of this area is beyond the scope of this discussion, and Chapter 6 provides a comprehensive discussion of ways to reduce such error variance, it is important to realize that the reliability of the inferences derived from a battery of neuropsychological test is impacted by each one of its components, and that the use of interpreters, or any other factors, such as an inappropriate measurement as a result of language differences, lack of acculturation, and so on, may lead to increased bias or diminished reliability, thus hindering the evaluative process, particularly nonrandom error.

It is critical to note that, unfortunately, the overall reliability (R_x) of an assessment battery is the multiplicative product of the reliability of each of its components ($1, 2, \ldots n$). In essence:

$$R_x = reliability_1 \times reliability_2 \ldots \times reliability_n$$

where $1, 2, \ldots$ and n represent each test or procedure used in a battery and overall assessment during the course of neuropsychological evaluation. In other words, the reliability of a neuropsychological battery (or evaluation) is, at best, as high as the lowest reliability coefficient of any of the tests or procedures used in such a battery (or evaluation) (cf. Anastasi and Urbina, 1997). Therefore, pretend that a clinician uses an interpreter as part of an assessment but only for one measure of verbal reasoning. Let's pretend that the inference derived from the administration of this test possesses the lowest reliability in the battery during the assessment. The reliability of the entire assessment is at best as high as the lowest reliability of any test or procedure administered to the Hispanic patient regardless of greater reliability of any other tests. If the clinician further uses information from the verbal reasoning test in the inferential process, and such a test was conducted with the aid of an interpreter, possessing a lower reliability coefficient than that of any other test procedure used by the examiner during the course of assessment, then that test will impact the overall test battery reliability during the assessment and will limit the overall accuracy and consistency not to surpass its reliability. It is evident from this exposition that bias, particularly nonrandom effects, should be reduced during the course of neuropsychological assessment. Introducing biased sources of error may exert damaging influences during the course of assessment, and it is imperative to reduce such influences during the course of neuropsychological evaluations with Hispanic populations.

Now that the concept of reliability has been introduced, it is also critical to note a concept that has received limited attention in the cross-cultural literature but deserves scrutiny here. *Validity* refers to a test's ability to measure a construct that it was designed to assess or that it purports to measure (Anastasi and Urbina, 1997). In terms of cross-cultural neuropsychology, one aspect of this issue has been referred to as *cognitive equivalency* (see Puente and Ardila, 2000). For example, as will be noted in Chapter 4, cross-cultural research has demonstrated that specific ethnic minorities may perform better than others in specific cognitive measures such as digit span, a test of auditory simple attention (cf. Kwak, 2003). Although it is possible that specific cognitive strengths and weaknesses in different ethnic minority groups may account for such findings as a result of cultural factors, it is critical to first rule out other factors capable of accounting for such differences, including lack of cognitive equivalency of test measures. For example, using digit span, it is evident that numbers in various languages do not have the same number of syllables, capable of differentially impacting memorization and later recall (Kwak, 2003). Therefore, this factor alone may be capable of accounting for performance differences between ethnic groups, unrelated to actual differences in cognitive abilities. Although this construct has been termed or relabeled cognitive equivalence, it is not new, and it is directly tied to the construct validity of a test, and sound construct validity has to be at the psychometric heart of newly developed measures for Hispanics.

Within this area of inquiry, ethnicity and test *variance* represent another critical topic worth mentioning in neuropsychological assessment. By variance, reference is being made to the statistical concept associated with the amount of variance accounted for by any variable (e.g., age, education, ethnicity/culture, injury type, severity of insult) or combinations of variables on overall test performance during the course of neuropsychological evaluation. This is an intriguing yet critical issue meriting attention because bright attorneys, colleagues, lay individuals, and students, whether in a facetious or heart-felt fashion, often inquire about it. The answer to this question is complex, yet it has received little detailed scientific scrutiny. Figure 1.1 shows graphs that attempt to capture the essence of a rational response to such a complex question. On one hand, the type of trauma or injury and its severity is critical to the formulation of any coherent response. The type of trauma is important because there are insults that require significant repeated exposure before they have significant impact on brain functions with ecological and clinical consequences. Although modern views of the effects of brain injury have advanced (DeBlesser, 1988), early annals of neuroscience noted that severity of an insult is important because the extent of damage

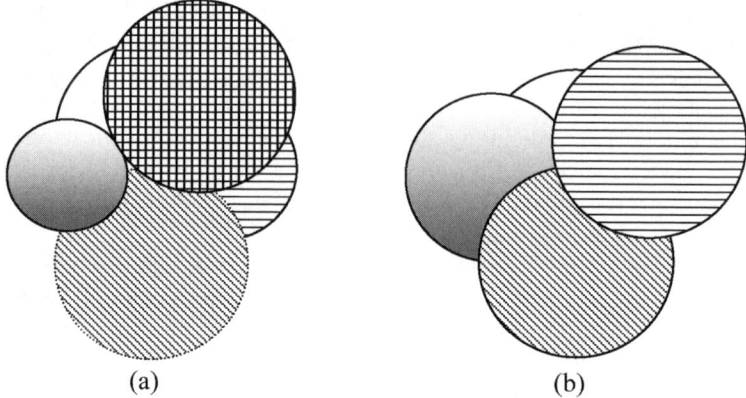

(a)   (b)

Figure 1.1 Venn diagram-culture/ethnicity and total test variance-diagrams displaying diffferent factors posited to account for total test performance variance. Figure 1.1 (**a**) shows total test performance variance (white) accounted for age (slanted lines), culture/ethnicity (grey), education (horizontal lines), and injury (cross-hatched lines) in the case of an individual who sustained severe TBI. Figure 1.1 (**b**) shows the amount of total test performance variance (white) accounted for by age (slanted lines), culture/ethnicity (grey), and education (horizontal lines) in the case of noninjured individual. Note differences in the amount of total test performance variance accounted for by culture/ethinicity in each case, but particularly in the case of the TBI individual

may account for much of the variance in neuropsychological test performance, leaving any other variable(s) little to account for (Lashley, 1938). For example, if a Hispanic patient sustains a severe brain injury with significant loss of consciousness and trauma, extensive posttraumatic amnesia, and objective evidence of injury (e.g., diffused axonal injury, injured galea, remarkable MRI results), it is most likely that the severity of such trauma accounts for a large proportion of the overall test performance variance, and cultural factors, or any other variable(s) for that matter, will account for a small amount of the total performance variance[4] (Figure 1.1a). In contrast, if healthy, uninjured Hispanic individuals are chosen for participation in a normative study, even when controlling for age and education, ethnicity, cultural, and linguistic factors may account for a large proportion of the variance, particularly if there are specific variables confounded with the concept of ethnicity in those individuals, such as literary ability or other variables that partially define ethnic and cultural differences in those individuals (Figure 1.1b). This issue is well exemplified by research addressed in greater detail later (cf. Rey et al., 1999). However, it is interesting to note that despite the fact that ethnicity and cultural factors may account for a small portion of the total test performance variance in the case of the severely brain-injured individual above, his or her rehabilitation, recovery, and attributional factors related to the injury, and its long-term outcome, nonetheless, may be modulated extensively by cultural factors (see Chapter 8).

Finally, while discussing psychometric issues, it is important to address one final issue that is actually applicable to all populations, not just Hispanics. This critical

---

[4] Other variables being held equal such as brain reserve capacity etc.

factor emerges as a result of a lack of understanding of psychometric characteristics of measurement instruments in general, regardless of discipline, and in particular neuropsychological and psychological tests. It is related to the reliability coefficients published in test manuals and their meaning. Here is an example: Consider for a moment that a somewhat astute neuropsychologist performing his duties in a rehabilitation center decides to examine a test manual to determine the test-retest reliability of a neuropsychological instrument prior to administering it to a Hispanic patient who sustained a closed head injury. He wisely decides to look at the psychometric characteristic of the instrument because he realizes that he will have to administer the same test to the same patient on two or more occasions. After a review of the manual, he happily realizes that the test-retest reliability noted indicates that such a coefficient was obtained from a study in which the test-retest interval was approximately (average) four weeks, similar to the schedule of administration that he will require to use with his patient. Although he is not pleased with the fact that such a coefficient was obtained in a healthy population, not a group of traumatic brain-injured individuals, and he realizes this to be a problem, he is exalted by the high test-retest coefficient (.80) noted in the manual. Assuming for a moment that the test-retest reliability study reported included Hispanics, similar to his client, and that the lack of data for injured individuals is momentarily ignored, as well as other important factors, an eminent and salient issue remains that is often, yet sadly, ignored. The problem is related to the fact that the coefficient reported is for a group of individuals, comprising the test-retest study, informing the astute clinician nothing about individual test scores and their variability. Yet, the clinician's role is not to make a decision about a group of patients, but to make critical and important decisions about one individual, his Hispanic client. Unfortunately, test manuals, including those developed by the senior author and his colleagues (Llorente et al., 2003), usually do not address the issue of individual scores, and only group data are usually reported, or the reproducibility of test scores have to be obtained from investigations, sometimes in obscure sources. This is unfortunate, because a measurement device, be it neuropsychological or any other type, may exhibit a high reliability at the group level but not at the individual level. In other words, although the reliability coefficient reported by the test manual may show a "high" reliability for a group of participants in a study, it tells us nothing about the reproducibility of individual scores (see Llorente et al., 2001a). Yet, clinicians, unless conducting research with groups, are not making everyday decisions at the group level but at the individual level. It is also important to be cognizant of the fact that the reproducibility of individual scores varies as a function of other individual characteristics, including overall intellect, and the presence of a specific neuropathological condition. Furthermore, it is not as if such information is difficult to obtain, and there are methodologies capable of examining such an issue (cf. Bland and Altman, 1986). Finally, it is also critical to realize that vital assumptions were made above, including the fact that Hispanics were included in the study and that injured groups were studied. Unfortunately, the problem noted above is accentuated by the absence of Hispanics in such studies, yet those data are used everyday to make, in some instances, very important decisions in their lives, life-and-death decisions in the case of Hispanics undergoing legal proceedings associated with capital punishment.

Ethical Issues, Hispanics, and Neuropsychology

Important ethical issues addressing cultural factors also must be considered in the application and practice of cross-cultural neuropsychology when intervening with or assessing Hispanics. In this regard, the *Ethical Principles of Psychologists* (APA, 2002) and the *Standards for Educational and Psychological Testing* (1999) clearly note the importance of considering cultural factors and ethnicity from several aspects. Although it is beyond the scope of this chapter to address all these issues in detail, a few salient aspects of the *Ethical Principles of Psychologists* as they relate to cultural issues, and Hispanics in particular, will be mentioned. From the standpoint of the *Ethical Principles of Psychologists* (APA, 2002), its Preamble notes:

> Psychologists are committed to increasing scientific and professional knowledge of behavior and people's understanding of themselves and others and to the use of such knowledge to improve the condition of individuals, organizations, and society. Psychologists respect and protect civil and human rights and the central importance of freedom of inquiry and expression in research, teaching, and publication. They strive to help the public in developing informed judgments and choices concerning human behavior. In doing so, they perform many roles, such as researcher, educator, diagnostician, therapist, supervisor, consultant, administrator, social interventionist, and expert witness. This Ethics Code provides a common set of principles and standards upon which psychologists build their professional and scientific work.

Clearly, the Preamble, although general and aspirational, addresses the inclusion of cross-cultural factors in neuropsychology, as it requires a commitment on the part of clinicians, educators, practitioners, and researchers to "improve the condition" of individuals and society. In addition, the Preamble requires the protection of basic "civil and human rights."

Aside from its Preamble, ethical principles and regulations provide more specific guidance related to these issues that are applicable to ethnic minorities including Hispanics. For example, the ethical principle addressing "Respect for People's Rights and Dignity" (Principle E) notes:

> Psychologists are aware of and respect cultural, individual, and role differences, including those based on age, gender, gender identity, *race, ethnicity, culture, national origin*, religion, sexual orientation, disability, *language*, and socioeconomic status and consider these factors when working with members of such groups. Psychologists try to eliminate the effect on their work of biases based on those factors, and they do not knowingly participate in or condone activities of others based upon such prejudices [italics added].

With regard to specific components of neuropsychological assessment and its application with Hispanics, the *Ethical Principles of Psychologists*, specifically referring to the interpretation of test results indicate:

> When interpreting assessment results, including automated interpretations, psychologists take into account the purpose of the assessment as well as the various test factors, test-taking abilities, and other characteristics of the person being assessed, such as situational, personal, *linguistic*, and *cultural differences*, that might affect psychologists' judgments or reduce the accuracy of their interpretations. (9.06 Interpreting Assessment Results) [italics added].

In brief, although specific portions of the *Ethical Principles of Psychologists* (2002) are "aspirational" in nature, it is evident that other portions set by standards for practice have greater specificity, and because of their emphasis and consideration of cultural, ethnic, and race factors are quite applicable to the work that psychologists perform ("teaching, research, clinical," and so on) with clients from diverging backgrounds in general, and more specifically, Hispanics. Although similar to the *Ethical Principles*, the *Standards of Educational and Psychological Testing* (1999) provide specific and detailed guidelines that are applicable to those who work with Hispanic populations. Although a detailed examination of all these issues will not be covered, it is critical to note specific issues addressing the assessment of multicultural groups including Hispanic populations. For example, with regard to test application and construction, according to the *Standards for Educational and Psychological Testing* (1999), such tests should be suitable for the "background" (e.g., cultural) of the test taker. The construction of tests should also include information on validity and reliability of the inferences derived for such populations. In reference to test interpretation, the *Standards* indicate that contextual information should be provided in the interpretation of test scores, and when unavailable, cautions should be raised against the misinterpretation of test scores.

With regard to ethical issues and their interaction with other factors already discussed in this chapter (e.g., language), in addition to professional organizations, several clinicians and researchers have addressed important factors associated with such considerations. Although their point may be too strong, as they essentially propose that the assessment of monolingual Hispanics should be conducted by someone with an advanced degree in Spanish, a practice that does not occur in the U.S. or abroad during the course of most neuropsychological evaluations with individuals from their respective mainstream culture, the point made by Artiola i Fortuni and Mullaney (1998) is important, and if toned down to an ethical and logical level in its application and interpretation, critical and timely. They essentially note that an evaluation of a Hispanic individual should not be undertaken by a clinician who does not have a certain degree of mastery of the language of the individual undergoing assessment, and doing so is unethical. As noted by Artiola and Mullaney (1997), although this point should be a logical step in the assessment process and decision-making process of competency, it is something that sometimes fails to occur, at a rate much greater than one might suspect, including judicial proceedings. Because an ethical course of action has not been followed by large number of practitioners, particularly in the U.S., Pedersen and Marsella (1982) have equated the current status of the field regarding the lack of an ethical posture during the course of cross-cultural psychological assessment and treatment as a crisis. This crisis pervades a large number of settings including educational and legal arenas.

In sum, neuropsychological assessments of monolingual, and in some instances of "bilingual" (see Chapter 5), Hispanics should be conducted in Spanish by a Spanish-speaking expert cognizant of the client's ethnic and cultural background with language fluency adequate to conduct a competent examination. The complexity of such evaluations requires that they be conducted in the language in which the client can dispatch his or her responsibilities most fluently. This is particularly true for educational, legal, or other types of evaluations with significant economic, personal, and social consequences for the client and his society.

Summary and Conclusion

Neuropsychology faces significant challenges if it is to remain a viable science capable of explaining complex brain-behavior relationships that take into account powerful cultural components. From an applied standpoint, such challenges also face the practicing clinician having to deal with an ever-increasing population of individuals from ethnic minority backgrounds living in the U.S., including Hispanics The integration of culture into theoretical models within neuropsychology should be perceived not as a corruption of existing models, or an accumulation of knowledge, but as a drastic paradigmatic shift in the field of neuropsychological inquiry as a result of its progression from normal science as a developing and evolving field of inquiry. Although many contributed to the inclusion of culture into neuropsychology, several individuals within the field, and indirectly outside the field, made significant contributions including Boas, Dewey, Luria, and Vygotsky.

Several definitions and terminology were introduced to allow for an equal footing when addressing topics throughout this text in the subsequent chapters. One of the most important is the fact that culture, ethnicity, and race are three distinct terms that should not be confused with one another, and a similar approach should be taken with the term Hispanic, a pan-ethnic term incapable of accounting for significant heterogeneity in individuals from such a background, despite its use in literary parlance or confusion by governmental bodies, lay people, or the media. Language in Hispanic populations also was presented as a unique and salient characteristic capable of impacting all aspects of neuropsychology. Other topics such as literacy, education, and quality of education capable of modulating individual definitions of "Hispanic" also were addressed. Several pragmatic factors, including administrative and statistical issues important during the course of neuropsychological assessment and rehabilitation, were also discussed because they are capable of impacting inferences from results obtained with individuals from ethnic minorities, with significant negative repercussions in some instances, and because they are not consistent with standards of practice or do not meet ethical standards.

At first glance, it would appear difficult to incorporate cultural components into brain-behavior relationships. However, culture and brain are closely intertwined and are part of a bidirectional relationship, as noted through studies involving genes and neurons. In other words, brain and culture are not opposites or mutually exclusive but different components of our very definitions of human and at the core of our existence. Aside from the factors noted above, it is important for the practicing neuropsychologist to be cognizant of ethical principles and aspirational goals set forth by Ethical Principles of Psychologists that require the practicing clinician to take into consideration in the assessment and intervention of ethnic minority individuals, including Hispanics.

Chapter 2
American Population Estimates, Trends in American Immigration, and Neuropsychology: Influences on Assessment and Inferential Processes with Hispanic Populations[1]

Antolin M. Llorente

A review of the most recent decennial U.S. Census (U.S. Census, 2001) indicates that Hispanics account for approximately 11% of the total American population. The conservative 11% estimate represents a total of approximately 32 million legal individuals of Hispanic origin living in the U.S. Table 2.1 presents a brief description of the most recent census estimates for the U.S. Hispanic population according to country of origin for selected nations (U.S. Census Bureau, 2001). The data collected by the U.S. Census is to a large extent impacted by patterns of American immigration, and although a comprehensive review of such patterns is beyond the scope of this book, a brief examination of American immigration trends for Hispanics will be reviewed.

It is first proper to examine the biased nature of American migrations as they relate to Hispanics, in an attempt to understand with greater insight their subsequent impact on the acquisition and application of neuropsychological norms and standards. Close scrutiny of migrational patterns reveals that American migration, legal immigration to the U.S., is not the product of random mechanisms and processes (Hamilton and Chinchilla, 1991; U.S. Immigration and Naturalization Service, 1991; Portes and Rumbaut, 1990; Portes and Borocsz, 1989). The nonrandom nature of these migratory patterns is the result of selective factors associated with both the host and sending nations (Portes and Rumbaut, 1990). With regard to host country receiving factors, Garcia (1981), and reviews of historical records, convincingly have noted that the U.S. government has had selective immigration aims in the past that are arbitrary by their very nature and that significantly affect current and past immigration patterns. In addition, revisions in American immigration laws and guidelines during the past decades led to significant alterations in migrational patterns. The Immigration and Naturalization Service (U.S. Immigration and Naturalization Service, 1991) notes that the predominant shift occurred due to the elimination of "country specific quotas," replacing them with quotas partially based on "humanitarian concerns" and shifting American migrational patterns from "European to Asian and Latin American immigration." This change in immigration

---

[1] This chapter is largely based on previous work by the author, most notably Llorente et al., 1999, 2000.

Table 2.1 U.S. Census Estimate for the Hispanic Population According to Country of Origin

Hispanic or latino by type	Number	Percent
Mexican	20,640,711	58.5
Puerto Rican	3,406,178	9.6
Central American	1,686,937	4.8
South American	1,353,562	3.8
Cuban	1,241,685	3.5
Dominican	764,945	2.2
Spainiard	100,135	0.3
All Other Hispanic or Latino (e.g., write in Hispanic or Latino)	6,111,665	17.3
Total	35,305,818	100

Adapted from U.S. Census Bureau, 2001.

Note: For the purpose of Census reporting, country of origin is defined by the origin of the head of household, the individual responsible for completing the Census.

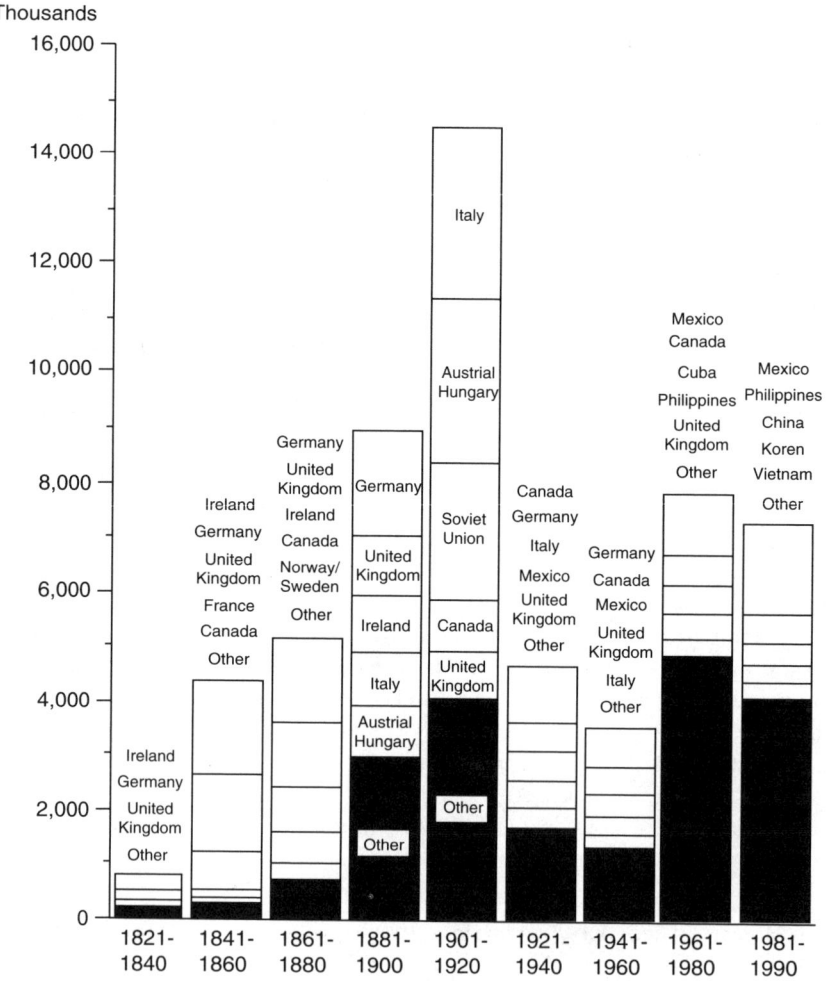

Figure 2.1 Changes in U.S. Immigration (1901–1990)

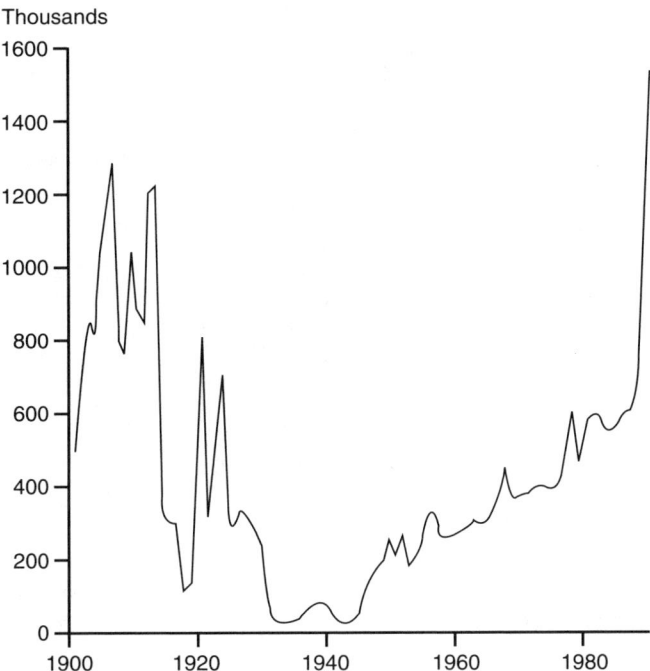

Figure 2.2 Total legal U.S. immigration (1901–1990)

policy altered the profile that typified U.S. migrations for "over 200 years." This shift in migrational trends is best depicted by Figure 2.1.

The substantial variability observed in the number of immigrants allowed to enter the U.S. during the past 90 to100 years is another marker capable of elucidating the nonrandom and rapidly shifting nature of American immigration patterns. Figure 2.2 clearly shows the toll that various socioeconomic and historical events (e.g., the Great Depression, World War II) had on the total number of immigrants allowed to enter the U.S. between the early 1930s and the mid to late 1940s. This figure additionally depicts the increasing number of legal immigrants that have been allowed to enter the U.S. in the last three to five decades and the sudden shifts in total migration that have taken place across time. Although reliable data are not yet available, significant alterations will be evidenced shortly after September 2001, and in particular after the Immigration and Naturalization Service was absorbed by the Department of Homeland Security, which led to new immigration guidelines as a result of governmental restructuring and which, most critically, selectively impacted specific groups of Hispanics.

Although data for level of education are not available, Figure 2.3 shows the reported occupational allegiance of legal immigrants entering the U.S. from 1976 to 1990. These data indicate that the various occupational categories, closely associated with the educational attainment of such legal immigrants, during those two decades were not proportionally represented. Although great variability in immigrants' occupational and educational attainment is observed in the literature, dis-

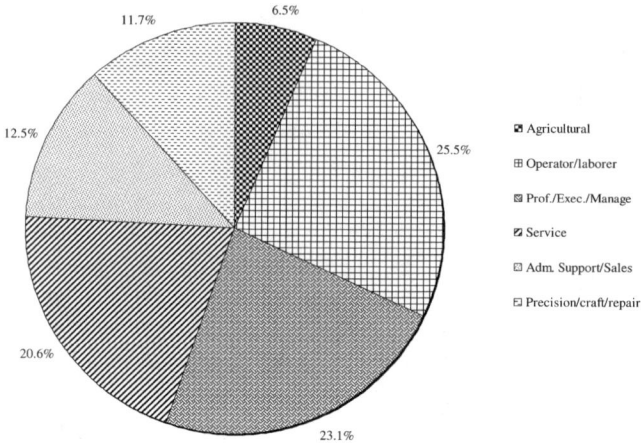

Figure 2.3 Immigration and occupational allegiance (1970)

proportionate occupational representations are more pronounced for certain Hispanic groups relative to others (see Llorente, 1997; Llorente et al., 1999, 2000; U.S. Census Bureau, 2001.)

Absolute and Relative Migrations

Table 2.2 shows the number of legal immigrants entering the United States from Argentina, Cuba, and Mexico, by decades, between 1931 and 1990. Perusal of this table indicates that the total number of immigrants from Mexico surpassed three million during the past 60 years, while the total number of immigrants from Argentina during the same period only reached a total of approximately 131,000 immigrants. During the same time span, the total number of immigrants from Cuba reached an approximate total of 732,000 individuals. A great deal of variability was observed in timing of maximum immigration and the magnitude of maximum immigration. Whereas immigration from Mexico peaked at approximately 1.5 million between 1981 and 1990, migration from Cuba peaked at approximately 264,000 during the 1970s, while migration from Argentina to the U.S. reached approximately 50,000 legal immigrants between 1961 and 1970. With regard to absolute migration, the number of Argentinean immigrants is approximately 24 times less than the number of Mexican immigrants and approximately six times less than the number of Cubans entering the U.S. during the same period. The total number of immigrants from Cuba also is four times less relative to the total number of immigrants from Mexico during the same six decades.

Although analyses could have been conducted to determine whether the expected number of immigrants from each nation under investigation differed statistically for these countries across the six decades, such analyses are beyond

Table 2.2 Total Number of Immigrants (Absolute Migration) Across Six Decades (1931–1990): Argentina, Cuba, and Mexico

Decade	Country and number of legal immigrants		
	Argentina	Cuba	Mexico
1931–1940	1,349	9,575	22,319
1941–1950	3,338	26,313	60,589
1951–1960	19,486	78,948	299,811
1961–1970	49,721	208,536	453,937
1971–1980	29,897	264,863	640,294
1981–1990	27,327	144,578	1,655,843

Adapted from INS, 1991.

the scope of this exposition. However, it should be noted that analyses conducted in the past for Hispanic data easily reached statistical significance (cf. Llorente et al., 1999, 2000 indicating that the expected distribution of absolute numbers of immigrants changed significantly over time and for each country). It is also clear from the data presented above that the interrelationship and intrarelationship for these nations as they relate to absolute immigration is in all likelihood statistically significant. These data also underscore the biased nature of American immigration patterns.

An examination of the absolute number of immigrants was critical in an attempt to understand American migratory patterns. However, the proportion of immigrants for three separate decades (1961 to1970, 1971 to 1980, and 1981 to 1990) relative to the total population of each country at the end of those decades is just as important to our understanding of Hispanic migrations to the U.S. This analysis was thus conducted for each country. In 1970, Argentina had an approximate population of 24,300,000 inhabitants and an approximate migration to the U.S. (1961 to 1970) of 50,000 or 0.2% of its population. In 1970, Cuba and Mexico had respective populations of 8,500,000 and 48,000,000, and approximate American immigrations of 208,000 and 454,000, between 1961 and 1970 or 3% and 1% of their respective populations. In 1980, Argentina had a total estimated population of 27,000,000 and a U.S. immigration of approximately 30,000 or 0.1% of its population, whereas Cuba had a total estimated population of 10,000,000 inhabitants and a U.S. migration of 265,000 individuals, a total of 2.6% of that country's population. Mexico's U.S. immigration was 1% of its total number of inhabitants (total U.S. immigration, 1971 to1980 = 640,294 / total estimated population, 1980 = 72,000,000). In 1990, the relative population percentages for Argentina, Cuba, and Mexico were 0.1%, 1.3%, and 1.8%, respectively.

In summary, in terms of relative immigration, migrations from Argentina have remained relatively constant and small in magnitude over the last three decades. Cuban immigration reached its peak during the 1970s and 1980s, with decreasing American immigration during the 1990s, while Mexico's relative immigration to the U.S. has been steadily increasing during the same period.

Immigration and Occupational Allegiance

Occupational data in Table 2.3 depict the "occupational group allegiance" for legal immigrants during the year 1990 for the indicated nations. It is clear from these data that the occupational and, most likely indirectly, the educational levels of these groups were substantially different. Whereas Mexican immigrants reporting occupation were primarily classified under Precision/Craft, Operator/ Fabricator, Farming/Forestry, and Service categories, with few immigrants from the Professional/Technical, Executive/Managerial, Sales, and Administrative Support sectors, Argentinean and Cuban immigrants reporting occupational status showed greater diversity. Specifically, Argentinean and Cuban immigrants represented the entire occupational spectrum with greater proportionality including those from the Professional/Technical (not as proportional for Cuba), Executive/Managerial, Sales, Administrative Support, Precision Craft and all other occupational ranks. Immigrants from Argentina comprised the most proportional representation across all occupational categories relative to the other countries and to the size of their respective migrations.

Previous studies with Hispanics (cf. Llorente et al., 1999) have revealed statistical significance in reported occupational preferences when a randomly selected year (1990) was chosen for analysis. In that investigation, Argentinean and Cuban immigrants reported occupational allegiance from across the entire occupational spectrum within the range of expectation and with underrepresentation in the Farming/Forestry category; immigrants from Mexico were underrepresented for most occupational categories in the same year, except for the Farming/Forestry category, where they were overrepresented at twice the rate of expectation (cf. Portes and Rumbaut, 1990).

Altogether, these findings suggest that occupational migratory configurations, and probably educational attainment, for these nations are indeed different. These data also suggest that either these nations had been differentially targeted by the U.S. government to satisfy occupational manpower needs in the U.S., the host country, or

Table 2.3 Percentage of Total Legal Immigrants and Reported Occupational Allegiance at Time of U.S. Entry for 1990*

Occupation	Country and percent of total immigration		
	Argentina	Cuba	Mexico
Professional/technical	9.2	4.0	.88
Executive/managerial	7.9	1.7	1.4
Sales	3.6	2.6	1.7
Administrative/support	6.5	4.0	2.7
Precision/craft	8.1	7.7	9.2
Operator/fabricator	6.7	16.2	24.0
Farming/forestry	0.5	0.4	12.0
Service	10.2	10.6	17.4

Adapted from INS, 1991.
*Excludes immigrants not reporting occupation (e.g., Children)

the sending nations had undergone major changes, including socio-political transformations, that required large-scale emigrations. These selective recruitment and emigration impetuses are partly responsible for each country's demographic differences as it relates to occupational status (cf. Portes and Rumbaut [1990] for specific U.S. government recruitment aims of Mexican nationals relating to occupational allegiance). Regardless of the cause or causes for the differences in reported occupational allegiance, it is clear from these data that discrepancies do exist in occupational and possibly educational migratory patterns. It is also interesting to note that such information is typical for many other nations worldwide, including Australia, Canada, France, Saudi Arabia, and Turkey, to name a few, as the result of their own requirements and needs, including occupational requirements.

Immigration and Residential Preference

Table 2.4 shows the number of legal immigrants admitted to this country from Cuba, Mexico, and Haiti (for purposes of comparison) for the year 1990 and their intended area of initial residence for five major metropolitan regions. As noted by Llorente et al. (1999, 2000) these data indicate that immigrants tend to have geographical predilection for certain areas within the United States. Whereas 11% and 34% of Mexican immigrants reported Los Angeles, California, as their preference for initial residence during 1990, only 2.5% of immigrants from Cuba reported this destination as their intended initial residence. In sharp contrast, 72% of Cuban immigrants reported Miami, Florida, as their initial intended destination or residence for the year 1990, whereas only 0.2% of immigrants from Mexico reported this city as their intended initial area of residence (U.S. Immigration and Naturalization Service, 1991). With regard to New York, New York, only 3.4% and 1% of immigrants from Cuba and Mexico, respectively, selected this metropolitan region as their intended residence. Chicago, Illinois, and Houston, Texas, had a relatively low percentage of legal immigrants, although immigrants from Mexico, due to its large absolute migration, had a large number of its immigrants reporting Houston as their intended area of initial residence.

Table 2.4 Percentage and Total Number of Legal Immigrants Reporting Intended Metropolitan Region of Initial Residence for Three Countries for 1990: Five Selected Regions

Metropolitan region	Country, percent, and (total number) of immigrants		
	Cuba	Haiti	Mexico
Chicago, Illinois	0.8 (84)	.98 (199)	6.2 (41,846)
Houston, Texas	0.3 (31)	0.1 (24)	5.2 (34,973)
Los Angeles, California	2.5 (274)	0.27 (55)	34 (231,267)
Miami, Florida	72 (7,7685)	17.9 (3,635)	0.2 (1,273)
New York, New York	3.4 (358)	37.7 (8,066)	0.9 (6,436)

Adapted from INS, 1991.

Distinct patterns of selective immigration were not only observed for the major metropolitan cities listed in Table 2.4, they were also evidenced for other groups of Hispanics from other countries as well. These results suggest that certain Hispanic immigrants have historically selected specific metropolitan areas of residence different from those chosen by other Hispanic immigrants (Portes and Rumbaut, 1990).

The data presented above suggest that the total number of immigrants (absolute migration) to the U.S. varies substantially among countries and fluctuates over time for each nation as a result of variables affecting both the host and sending states. Therefore, migrational patterns must be considered "dynamic nonrandom processes that change over time as a result of selective factors" (Llorente et al., 1999, 2000). As noted by Llorente et al. (1999, 2000), the variability of these patterns of immigration may be the result of various social, political, and economic trends (push–pull factors; see Hamilton & Chinchilla, 1991) affecting all countries sharing migrations (i.e., the host and sending countries). The range of occupational status of foreign immigrants also varies extensively between nations regardless of the total size of their migration. This variation may be the result of selective recruitment policies or similar nonrandom variables adopted by the host country to satisfy certain of its unmet occupational classification requirements as well as other factors (cf. Garcia, 1981 and Portes and Rumbaut, 1990). For this reason, occupational allegiance from immigrants entering the U.S. cannot be assumed to be random, as a certain degree of selectivity for specific vocational groups was observed for some nations. Instead, nonrandom shifts in the occupational choice of immigrants from foreign countries should be expected longitudinally, including the occupational choice of immigrants from the same country, and associated with occupation, differential educational levels. Finally, a great deal of affinity for certain geographical/residential areas was observed for most immigrant groups across the time span under investigation. In sum, and as previously argued (cf. Llorente et al., 1999; 2000; Llorente, 1997), a review of the migrational literature reveals that American immigration is not the result of random mechanisms or processes (Portes and Rumbaut, 1990; U.S. Immigration and Naturalization Service, 1991, 1981, 1975) but rather the result of predominantly shifting and changing biased migrational patterns.

American Migratory Trends and Neuropsychology: Inferences with Hispanics

With regard to the impact of these migrations upon neuropsychology, demographic variables (including age, education, and ethnicity) significantly influence the outcome of neuropsychological assessments, as noted in Chapter 1 of this volume (Adams, Boake, and Crain, 1982; Badcock and Ross, 1982; Botwinick, 1967; Heaton et al., 1986; Rosselli, Ardila, and Rosas, 1990). Therefore, as noted by Llorente et al. (1999, 2000), a phenomenon capable of modulating demographic characteristics of Hispanics comprising normative samples would be of significant interest to cross-cultural neuropsychology. A "logical candidate would be capable of impacting the procurement and application of neuropsychological norms, as well as the overall neuropsychological assessment process. American immigration patterns indirectly influence demographic characteristics, as noted above, and indirectly during the acquisition of normative standards" for Hispanics within the U.S. (Llorente et al., 1999; Llorente, 1997). These influences are the indirect impact of migrational patterns upon demographic characteristics and on the subsequent availability of adequate and suitable reference and comparison groups. Aside from factors associated with the acquisition and application of normative data, U.S. migrations are inextricably associated with levels of acculturation and assimilation (Montgomery and Orozlo, 1984; Portes and Bach, 1985), differences in levels of educational attainment capable of impacting test-taking strategies (Rey et al., 1999; Rosselli et al., 1990), perceptions of the immigrant as an individual and of the immigration process proper (see Chapter 3; Malzberg and Lee, 1956; Ødegaard, 1932; Sanua, 1970), and the clinical inferences made about Hispanics. The normative data acquisition process for Hispanics is not free from potential biases. A host of possible confounds could result in the distortion of these standards invalidating inferences made on their basis.

Potential Confounds Associated with Demographic Characteristics

The effects of demographic variables, including education on test performance, are well established in the neuropsychological literature (Adams, Boake, and Crain, 1982; Ardila, 1993; Ardila, Rosselli, and Rosas, 1989b; Heaton et al., 1986; Laosa, 1984). A comparison in neuropsychological performance between a Hispanic client and a normative cohort differing in educational attainment would be inappropriate under most circumstances. This issue is best exemplified with Hispanics through research recently conducted by Pontón and his associates (1996). In their sample, individuals of similar age attained higher levels of performance on measures assessing neuropsychological functions as a result of greater educational attainment across all groups. Similarly, Rey and his colleagues (1999), while conducting research to develop psychological instruments for Hispanics, have shown that differences in neuropsychological performance existed among Cuban and Mexican normative samples in Dade County, Florida. Although at first glance the differences between these two seemingly similar Hispanic groups could have been attributed to differences in brain functions consequent to ethnic differences (cf. Jensen, 1980), a closer look at the demographic characteristics of the samples revealed *selection biases* associated with lower levels of education in the Mexican cohort available to researchers in Dade County, Florida, relative to the Cuban cohort. The demographic differences of these two groups were most probably the result of distinct immigration patterns, particularly geographical allegiance.

These findings suggest that potential confounds associated with certain demographic characteristics, modulated by migrations in the case of Hispanics, must be carefully monitored to avoid introducing putative sources of systematic error, as noted in Chapter 1, from entering the norm acquisition process. Careful consideration of these factors is also merited to avoid attributing differences in neuropsychological performance in ethnic groups, including Hispanics, to nonexistent abnormal brain-behavior relationships rather than differences in demographic and other characteristics such as a lack of test equivalency. These potential sources of error not only apply to age and education but to other demographic factors as well, as noted in Chapters 1 and 3.

Potential Confounds Associated with Site Selection Bias

Standardization populations differ according to regions (Anastasi and Urbina, 1997; Pontón et al., 1996). Although such is the case for all populations, probably as a result of effects related to demographic variables and other factors, such differences are probably accentuated for Hispanics as a result of the tendency of specific groups of individuals from this background to reside in circumscribed geographical regions within the United States after immigrating to this country. As noted above, such a geographical predilection may affect standardization samples. This issue is best depicted by the intended area of initial residence data presented earlier. These findings are significant for neuropsychology since they suggest that differential geographical migrational patterns and predilection for certain destinations and residential areas may have a substantial impact on the collection and subsequent application of neuropsychological norms for Hispanics (cf. Rey et al., 1999).

Neuropsychological data have traditionally been collected in academic and medical centers in or near metropolitan areas around the U.S. or school districts where the majority of neuropsychologists reside and conduct research with urban ethnic minority populations. Although the observed pattern of geographical settlement of Cuban immigrants has been historically typical of that pattern, the figures in Table 2.4 suggest that neuropsychological data collected in Houston, Texas, will most likely underrepresent individuals from Cuba or of Cuban descent who live in the U.S. because the availability of these immigrants at this geographical site is extremely limited. Consequently, unless procedures are established (see Chapters 3 and 6) during the collection of normative samples in Houston to preclude biases from entering into the acquisition process, such procurement could very well result in invalid inferences were the norms to be applied at a later date with individuals from Cuba or of Cuban origin in Miami, Florida. In Miami, Florida, individuals from Cuba or of Cuban descent comprise one of the largest conglomerations of Cuban immigrants, with their distinct ethnic identities, outside of their native country. Normative data collected in Los Angeles, where the prevalent Hispanic population is of Mexican background, would probably not be representative of Cuban populations, and is hardly available to researchers in Los Angeles.

Site selection bias also has significant implications for making inferences, on the basis of foreign norms, about Hispanic populations living in the U.S. (see Chapter 1; see also Chapter 4 for intellectual tests, particularly the comment on the DAS). As depicted by the migrational data, most populations in the U.S. from foreign countries, or foreign nationals, with their unique ethnic identities, are not represented cross-sectionally in the U.S. Therefore, when foreign norms do not represent minority individuals born in the U.S., or individuals from foreing country living in the U.S., with their specific ethnic backgrounds, the accuracy of the inferences made on the basis of such norms and standardization samples may be compromised due to their lack of inferential validity.

In summary, it should be recognized that ethnic minority groups, including Hispanics, tend to exhibit geographical predilection for certain areas within the U.S. and such geographical affinity or selection bias may impact the acquisition and application of neuropsychological norms. Such a geographical preference may also impact the acquisition process as a result of the effects that specific migratory patterns may have upon the assimilation of American culture by specific ethnic minority groups.

Potential Confounds Associated with Interactions Among Demographic Variables

So far, specific demographic factors such as education and geographical region have been used to show how they are capable of infringing on normative data collection, standardization samples, and inferential processes. However, some demographic variables most probably interact with other demographic characteristics, all modulated by migrations, to create specific patterns of neuropsychological performance capable of encroaching upon subsequent inferences. For example, although "Cuban" populations may be available to researchers in New York City, different levels of acculturation may lead, as a result of poor sampling or other factors, to an inadequate representation of this ethnic group regardless of the number of participants comprising the normative cohort. The same could be said of Cuban populations living in Miami, in spite of the fact that this metropolitan region is host to a large number of individuals from this ethnic group. Other potential confounds, such as level of acculturation as noted in Chapter 1 (Marin and Marin, 1991), interacting with demographic characteristics known to impact neuropsychological performance (cf. Heaton et al., 1986) and modulated by the immigration process, may play a moderating role in the acquisition and inferential process (see Chapter 3).

Immigration, Acculturation, and Assimilation

The process of immigration is inextricably intertwined with acculturation (cf. Portes and Rumbaut, 1990) and with the acquisition and application of neuropsychological procedures with Hispanics. Llorente et al. (1999, 2000) and Harris and Llorente (2005) have argued that depending on the level of acculturation and assimilation, norms acquired in the United States for certain minority groups may not be representative of individuals from their respective country of origin, or specific ethnic group, if the standardization group differs from the recent immigrant in levels of acculturation. "All other variables held constant, norms ascertained from individuals living in the U.S. whose countries of origin are cross-sectionally represented in the U.S. with greater levels of acculturation would probably make for a more valid inferential tool (cf. Harris and Llorente, 2005). In contrast, normative data for minority groups of foreign nationals, or individuals born in the U.S. of foreign ancestry, may be representative of such populations.

Level of acculturation and assimilation is also closely associated with language, particularly for ethnic minority groups, including Hispanics, who reside in the U.S. and whose language of origin is not English. It is clear that immigrants with greater levels of assimilation and acculturation would in all likelihood have adopted greater levels of English proficiency. Although such an assessment posture is not being advocated here, greater levels of language proficiency, in turn, allow for a more valid neuropsychological comparison with existing norms from mainstream populations.

It is also vital to note that bilingualism is capable of impacting neuropsychological test performance (cf. Paradis, 1978), and thus (as noted in Chapter 1 and in subsequent chapters within this volume) the level of acculturation and language proficiency should not be left to armchair speculation. Instead, a data-based assessment approach should be used in establishing level of language proficiency and acculturation for each patient. Several investigators have also developed instruments capable of providing an index of acculturation for specific minority groups (adults and children; cf. Franco, 1983, or Marin, Sabogal, Marin, and Otero-Sabogal, 1984; Suinn, Richard-Figueroa, Lew, and Vigil, 1987). These instruments take into consideration variables known to significantly impact acculturation and assimilation, such as timing of immigration, generational differences in migration, ethnic identification, and length of U.S. residence.

In sum, neuropsychologists serving Hispanic populations should be cognizant of the effects of acculturation on neuropsychological evaluations. They should be aware of the methods available to them to determine the level of acculturation and language proficiency of a specific patient prior to beginning such an examination. It is also critical to recognize that individual variables, such as level of education, are capable of infringing on the assessment process, but that the interaction of multiple variables also should be given due weight.

Special Populations – Unaccompanied, Hispanic Immigrant Children[2]

Despite the fact that adolescents and children account for approximately half of the world's immigrant population (Cole, 1998), there is a dearth of information in the literature addressing the specific mental health needs of immigrant youth (Hicks, Lalonde, and Pepler, 1993), particularly unaccompanied children, including Hispanics. In spite of this limitation, there is convergence in the literature suggesting greater prevalence of neuropsychopathology, particularly posttraumatic stress disorder and depression, in unaccompanied immigrant children. In addition, unaccompanied children may exhibit greater psychological vulnerability and risk factors as a result of trauma than other children or adults, in conjunction with underdeveloped adaptive, cognitive, and neuropsychological resources secondary to their early developmental stage. Risk, resiliency, and personality characteristics also appear to serve as moderating variables. Finally, immigration context, including community assimilation and integration, have been shown to play a major role (Portes and Rumbaut, 1990).

Adding to the complexity of the problem, any dialogue addressing neuropsychological problems faced by unaccompanied immigrant children and adolescents also should take into consideration serious health problems observed with greater prevalence among this population. Malnutrition, developmental disabilities, medical illnesses, injuries, and central nervous system involvement are often encountered with greater prevalence in these children (Westermeyer, 1991). Given the psychological and physical trauma that some unaccompanied Hispanic or other children experience prior to entering the U.S., many of them migrate with a history of traumatic stress (Almqvist and Brandell-Forsberg, 1997; Portes and Rumbaut, 1990). More important, as it has direct bearing on this chapter, it is vital to note that unaccompanied Hispanic immigrant children represent one of the largest groups of youth entering the U.S.

Posttraumatic Stress Disorder

Research focusing on the impact of trauma on neuropsychological functioning in immigrant children and adolescents has predominantly concentrated on the prevalence and expression of posttraumatic stress disorder (PTSD) (DSM-IV-TR, APA, 2000). For example, studies with school-aged children have shown a correlation between quantity of traumatic exposure and PTSD prevalence (Almqvist and Brandell-Forsberg, 1997; Pynoos, Steinberg and Wraith, 1995). The relationship

---

[2] This portion of the chapter substantively appeared in Llorente (2004).

between severity of exposure (amount and proximity) of experienced trauma and the presence of PTSD in children and adolescents may be a cross-cultural phenomenon and has been observed in different ethnic groups, including Cambodian (Mollica et al., 1997), Middle Eastern (Montgomery, 1998), and most directly relevant to this chapter, Hispanic children from Central America (Espino, 1991). In addition, the chronic impact of such experiences on psychological functioning post trauma has been documented in the literature (Kinzie et al., 1989). It is interesting to note that the severity of PTSD and its persistence over time in the aforementioned studies is consistent with studies investigating PTSD in children following exposure to other types of trauma, such as natural disasters (cf. Hodes, 2000). Finally, students of immigration have noted the emergence of PTSD in different centuries in European and Hispanic (Latin American) migrations despite the divergent nature of the cause for such immigrations, historical context, or the period of time during the ensuing immigration (cf. Llorente et al., 2000, 2004). Thus, reports exist of immigrant Irish children having experienced PTSD during their large-scale migrations to the U.S. as a result of famine during the last century, similar to that experienced by large-scale migrations to the U.S. by Mexican and Central American children seeking better economic opportunities or escaping physical or sexual abuse and/or oppression during the last century.

Consistent with the research literature (cf. Thabet and Vostanis, 2000), during the course of clinical neuropsychological and psychological assessment, unaccompanied immigrant children and adolescents, including Hispanics, who present with PTSD sometimes exhibit symptoms of this disorder, including altered mental status, confusion, alterations in verbal and visual memory systems, and dampened intellect. As a result of past traumatic events, these youth may exhibit alterations in their psychological status, personality changes, and in some instances may imitate violence similar to what they experienced in the past (cf. Hicks et al., 1993; Llorente, 2004). Although symptoms vary across age groups, they may be manifested as aggression, conduct problems, delinquency, exaggerated startle responses, flashbacks, heightened anxiety, irritability, nightmares, physical ailments and psychosomatic problems, poor concentration and focus, sleep disturbances, and interpersonal withdrawal (DSM-IV, APA, 2000; Hicks et al., 1993).

Depression

Aside from PTSD, a high prevalence of clinical depression and depressive symptomatology also has emerged in the literature as a frequent and significant neuropsychopathology affecting unaccompanied immigrant children (McCallin, 1992; Mghir et al., 1995), including Hispanics. Although much of the current literature concentrates on the comorbidity of PTSD and depression, and some studies suggest a higher prevalence of PTSD than depression, the proportion of individuals with depressive symptoms has a high probability of meeting the diagnosis for clinical depression (Heptinstall et al., 2004). Common overlapping symptoms of the two disorders in immigrant children additionally include reports of sleep disturbance, somatic complaints, constricted affect, impulse control, and difficulties concentrating (Thabet et al., 2004). However, findings from better-controlled investigations indicate that PTSD symptoms are distinct from symptoms of depression, and the latter appear to be unique manifestations of trauma, contrary to previous beliefs perceiving depression as a corollary of PTSD (cf. Sack et al., 1995). A study supporting such a hypothesis was reported by Laurel and Zimmerman (2001), indicating that while PTSD and depression are frequently comorbid, the two disorders often follow different paths. It is believed that while both disorders are initially linked to traumatic experiences, depression is more related to the current living situation than past experiences (Sack et al., 1996).

Depression has been found to be more prevalent in youth that had experienced parental separation than in youth that remained in contact with their parents or caretakers. In a study conducted in Hong Kong, McCallin (1992) observed depression in a majority of immigrant children in his investigation. However, aside from reporting symptoms of depression, which constitute clinical depression in many instances, unaccompanied children reported greater severity of symptoms than accompanied children.

Other Issues (Risk and Resiliency)

Other variables have been shown to moderate psychological outcomes of unaccompanied Hispanic immigrant children. A number of these variables are associated with the process of immigration prior to and after arrival in the host country. With regard to risk, resiliency, and protective factors prior to or after immigration that are capable of affecting unaccompanied Hispanic children and adolescents, their unaccompanied status alone has been found to be a risk factor. Unaccompanied children and adolescents have been shown to be at greater risk for neuropsychiatric problems than their accompanied peers (Ajdukovic and Ajdukovic, 1993; Hicks et al., 1993; Rumbaut, 1991). In fact, children and adolescents accompanied by their families during the process of immigration were less likely to receive a psychiatric diagnosis at a later date than those who immigrated alone, including Hispanics (Arroyo and Eth, 1996). In the same vein, greater positive psychological outcomes following migration have been reported in children who immigrated with family members than in those children who immigrated unaccompanied (Melville and Lykes, 1992).

Parental and familial psychological stability and health prior to immigration of the unaccompanied child may be an important factor (Sack et al., 1994). Because psychological problems in the family of origin are related to childhood neuropsychopathology, the role of these variables, particularly maternal mental health prior to immigration, may be an important moderating factor of psychological outcome in immigrant children (Ajdukovic and Ajdukovic, 1993). Studies have shown that mothers' emotional health is the best predictor of mental health and emotional stability outcomes of immigrant children. Aside from maternal psychological well-being, Almqvist and Broberg (1999) and Rumbaut (1991) have suggested that family climate and cohesion before and after migration may represent some of the best predictors of mental health outcome and psychological adjustment in immigrant children. Familial psychological dysfunction and quality of family life prior to immigration also have been shown to be critical and influential aspects modulating posttraumatic stress and resiliency in young immigrant children, including Hispanics.

Another important factor that has been identified as a significant risk factor capable of affecting the psychological well-being of unaccompanied Hispanic immigrant children is exposure to trauma in the child or members of his family (Berman, 2001; Hicks et al., 1993). Along with the absence or presence of child and parental psychopathology, trauma itself has received a great deal of attention.

Other major risk and resiliency factors include child personality characteristics. A child's unique adaptation strategies to trauma and stress, as well as psychological makeup and resources (e.g., intellectual level) are important variables capable of moderating overall mental health factors of unaccompanied immigrant children. For example, good temperament has been shown to limit and reduce vulnerability to psychological disturbances (Almqvist and Broberg, 1999).

The immigration context and reception environment also have been shown to impact the psychological adaptation of immigrant children and adolescents, and difficulties in this area have been known to be associated with poor psychological outcomes in different ethnic groups including Hispanics (Portes & Borocsz, 1989, 1990). For example, greater risk of poor psychological adaptation has been noted in the childhood immigration literature in youth that perceive rejection from the assimilating society. Immigrant children who experienced conflict and similar negative events in shelters and communal housing after immigration have exhibited poor mental health outcomes. Negative experiences associated with government interactions during the process of immigration, such as detention, incarceration, and trauma within the receiving country, also have been known to represent further risk to poor psychological outcomes.

As noted above, and as hinted in Chapter 1, assimilation and acculturation are directly associated with the immigration context. In this regard, problems associated with acculturation as immigrant children adapt to stress in their host society place unaccompanied children at greater risk for psychological morbidity. For example, academic difficulties, and from a neuropsychological standpoint, problems in language acquisition have been shown to predict poor adaptation (Rousseau, 1995). Conflict in the development of identity among immigrant adolescents also has been noted to be related to poor psychological adjustment (Rousseau, 1995).

Accessibility and availability of community support systems have been known to facilitate adaptation with less psychological distress even in immigrant children and adolescents who had survived significant trauma prior to their migration (Fox, Cowell, and Montgomery, 1994). The maintenance of close cultural and ethnic community bonds also has been noted to be a psychological protective factor in children and adolescents, along with involvement in cultural and religious traditions (cf. Rousseau, 1995; Sack et al., 1995). Other factors known to have a negative influence on mental health outcomes of unaccompanied youth include poverty and low SES (Howard and Hodes, 2000), school problems, and discrimination (Hyman et al, 2000).

Summary and Concluding Remarks

In conclusion, although the effects of certain demographic variables have been known to significantly affect neuropsychological performance (cf. Adams et al., 1982; Laosa, 1984; Heaton et al., 1986), the etiology behind differences in demographic characteristics have not been well researched, especially among ethnic minority groups including Hispanics. The present chapter examined a plausible candidate capable of modulating demographic variables, namely, American immigration trends.

With regard to migrations, examination of this process revealed nonrandom, shifting, selective, and dynamic mechanisms affecting patterns of U.S. immigration. Regardless of the causes for the nonrandom nature of immigration (e.g., economic, immigration laws of the host country), absolute and relative migration to this country were observed to vary drastically. Fluctuations in such migratory patterns over time within the same country of origin were also evidenced. Similarly, the occupational affiliation of immigrants from foreign nations to the U.S. varied extensively. More important, occupational status, and most probably, educational attainment differed significantly for immigrants from various nations over time independent of absolute migration. Parenthetically, such factors can even vary for immigrants from the same country, and therefore represent an intracountry variation over time. Such migrations can be observed when subgroups of individuals arrive from the same host country at distinct periods of time, and who thus have distinct demographic characteristics. Finally, selective patterns of geographical settlement within the U.S. were observed for most immigrant groups across time.

These results have significant implications for neuropsychology. They suggest that migrational trends are capable of modulating demographic characteristics, partly infringing upon inferential processes for Hispanic groups. This infringement could possibly bias normative data and their application, including assessment or rehabilitation. Such plausible biases could potentially invalidate or place into question studies comparing intellectual functioning or other neuropsychological domains in research participants or patients between sites. Similarly, such selective factors could potentially render invalid norms or research comparing Hispanic groups at the same or different geographical sites.

The present findings also suggest that differences in demographic characteristics, modulated by immigration patterns, are capable of mimicking abnormal brain-behavior relationships (cf. Rey et al., 1999). Therefore, care should be exercised not to attribute neuropsychological differences to nonexistent brain-behavior relationships when those differences can be accounted for by more objective variables, such as demographic characteristics from inappropriate standardization samples modulated by U.S. immigration trends for specific ethnic minority groups, including Hispanics. In addition, it is clear that unaccompanied Hispanic immigrant children represent a high-risk group deserving special attention, but particularly related to specific factors associated with neuropsychological functioning and mental health.

Finally, these problems underscore the limitations of assumptions neuropsychologists may be able to make when using standardization samples for Hispanics. Under most circumstances, it would be inappropriate for neuropsychologists to assume that norms ascertained in one geographical region of the U.S., or in a foreign country, would be applicable to individuals and interchangeable with norms from other geographical areas in the U.S. – solely because the normative cohort was predominantly similar (e.g., Hispanics) to that of the patient undergoing assessment. A decision to use the most appropriate norms and tests remains the responsibility of the practicing clinician (cf. Mitrushina et al., 1999).

Chapter 3
Hispanic Populations: Special Issues in Neuropsychology

Antolin M. Llorente

For many members of ethnic minority and non-minority groups living in the U.S., Hispanics included, the interrelationship between neuropsychological test perform- ance and education, socioeconomic factors, and other specific variables, such as nutrition, access to health care, and stress, is particularly complex, with significant implications for a science of brain-behavior relationships and its practice. While educational attainment to a large degree dictates, and certainly facilitates, income potential, it is also the case that socioeconomic advancement facilitates educational attainment and other specific advantages, and both of these variables have been shown to impact neuropsychological performance. These are important factors meriting attention, and many investigators have noted that it is these factors, rather than cultural or ethnic factors, that require attention.

Socioeconomic Factors

Socioeconomic status (SES), sometimes proxied by neuropsychologists through education, occupation, economic opportunities, daily living conditions, poverty, and so forth (cf. Hollingshead, 1957), plays a paramount role. With regard to pov- erty, Hispanic children represent approximately 18% of all children living in the U.S., yet they constituted 30% of all children living below the poverty level in 2002 according to the U.S. Census Bureau (2003). With regard to adults, Hispanic adults represent approximately 13% of the total U.S. population, yet 24% of Hispanic adults were living below the poverty level in 2002 – almost three times as many as the 7.8% of white, non-Hispanic population living below the poverty level accord- ing to the U.S. Census Bureau (2003). However, this is not an American phenom- enon. It is critical to note, particularly for clinicians whose practice includes the assessment of foreign born patients, that Hispanics living outside the U.S., particu- larly those living in developing countries who may eventually immigrate to the U.S., also may come from impoverished backgrounds, and global estimates note that Hispanics are one of the largest populations living in poverty worldwide (World Health Organization, 1998). These data, aside from providing testimony to the economic disparity and challenges facing Hispanics in the U.S and globally, are critical to note, because they are factors that impact quality of life and brain development that have significant impact on current and later neuropsychological functioning (see below).

Harris and Llorente (2005) note that parental income of Hispanic "children is often constrained by the lack of legal residency," further "limiting employment and educational" opportunities. "Data on the number of "illegal" residents who graduate from high school each year and are unable to enroll in college are not readily available, but it is estimated that there are approximately 1.6 million children living without legal residency status in the U.S. (Passel, Capps & Fix, 2004). Only 7.3% of Hispanics of all ages who entered the U.S. between 1990 and 2002 had become citizens by 2002, compared with 73.3% of those entering before 1970 (U.S. Census Bureau, 2003). Certainly, this circumstance partially contributes to the low percentage of Hispanics graduating from college in the U.S. and indirectly affects their socioeconomic status. Harris and Llorente further note that "These realities conspire to depress the SES" for Hispanic groups as a whole. As a given minority group gains an economic foothold, educational and other opportunities tend to increase" (Harris and Llorente, 2005; cf. Portes and Rumbaut, 1990).

The interaction between SES and other factors also is important to examine because it has significant and critical repercussions for neuropsychology. Variables such as nutrition, access to medical care, educational attainment, and the presence of CNS or other physiological diseases are vital, as they have a pivotal impact on neuropsychological functioning.

Nutrition

Nutrition in Hispanic populations living in the U.S. and abroad, aside from humanitarian concerns, represents an important topic for neuropsychology. In this regard, before addressing data from the scientific literature, we would like to present three scenarios from experiences that the senior author has had that underscore the importance of nutrition and neuropsychological assessment with these populations.

The first is based on an experience encountered both in the U.S. and abroad, as the senior author conducted seminars to train graduate students and professionals. During such seminars, the information presented to participants from all walks of life (medical and neuropsychology students, neurologists, pediatricians, psychiatrists, psychologists, social workers, and others) was welcomed. However, on several occasions, the attendees, although happy to be exposed to recent advances in the neurosciences and neuropsychology, indicated that the greatest problem encountered in their practice was related to a lack of appropriate nutrition in patients undergoing medical, neuropsychological, or psychological assessment. When asked to expound on this point, conference participants unequivocally indicated that they consistently discovered a history of nutritional deprivation or malnutrition, in many instances with childhood onset and covering a large portion of their patients' lives.

The next example is more painful to describe because it affects individuals, particularly children, in large scale. During the senior author's research collaborations with colleagues investigating the effects of specific *nutraceuticals* (i.e., essential fatty acids) on cognition and disease, he came across a seasoned and distinguished colleague with a significant history of consulting experiences for the nutritional industry in the U.S. and abroad. On one of those trips, he consulted for a company that produced and sold nutritional products that was about to introduce a product in a country abroad with an extensive Hispanic population. When the senior author queried his colleague why such consultation was necessary, particularly when the company produced the "same" product in the U.S., his response made it clear to the senior author that the company included different levels of the minerals, vitamins, and other nutritional contents in the product sold abroad than it did for the "same" product sold in the U.S. In fact, the levels of minerals, vitamins, and other nutrients for the product sold in the U.S. were higher than those of the "same" product sold overseas. Remaining incredulous, the senior author compared the actual products only to learn that differences in the composition of the two formulas indeed existed. More important, the contents for the product sold overseas would not meet USDA minimum daily requirements for some of the contents.[1]

The final example also is difficult and disturbing to describe, partly because it is one that is recurrent in the U.S., unquestionably one of the wealthiest nations on the planet. It is also more personal, affecting daily clinical practice. Prior to the start of each assessment, the senior author always queries his clients whether they enjoyed a good night sleep prior to the beginning of a potentially fatiguing and extensive day of assessment. In addition, eating habits are often assessed. During such preassessment periods and interviews, it is not uncommon to find large numbers of Hispanics who have experienced a protracted history of nutritional deprivation, including recent episodes – in some instances, the night before the day of neuropsychological assessment. This finding has prompted "breakfast sessions" (providing breakfast for the client prior to the start of the assessment). Such experiences unfortunately have included children and adults. However, the information presented above is based on personal experiences without scientific scrutiny.

From an evidenced-based approach, it is clear that appropriate nutrition plays a preeminent role in brain development (DeLong, 1993) and, indirectly, on chemical brain functions underlying neuropsychological skills. The importance of nutrition, particularly appropriate intake of essential fatty acids, metals, minerals, and vitamins, is critical for healthy brain development and functioning. In fact, an analysis of the brain's composition and metabolism reveals that a large proportion of the brain is made up of essential fatty acids and other nutrients (Sastry, 1985). One of the reasons why such nutrients are considered essential, aside from the

---

[1] Many factors impact costs and their subsequent affordability. This information is not included as a criticism but as an educational fact which neuropsychologists should recognize, since many factors conspire to create such a set of unique circumstances.

obvious reason, is because they can only be obtained from daily diet, yet poor diets are "the catch of the day" in the U.S. and abroad in many settings (e.g., schools, homes). In addition, lack of appropriate nutrition, including metals and other nutrients, in a diet has been associated with brain dysfunction in humans and animals, a fact with a long historical record of support (cf. Winick and Noble, 1966; Winick and Rosso, 1969). Because Hispanics, as noted above, have a greater probability of coming from impoverished backgrounds where lower SES affects their ability to rise above the poverty level, with potentially significant nutritional implications and indirect implications for brain functions and neuropsychological skills, this is an issue that deserves special attention when working with such populations.

Access to Health Care

Specific and unique cultural expectations and experiences also play a major role that impacts factors such as access to health care and, indirectly, neuropsychology and its application with Hispanic populations. For example, although a two-tier medical system encompassing private and public providers (quality of care aside) may exist in their native countries, the majority of Hispanics come from countries such as Mexico or countries in the Caribbean, Central America, and South America, where a socialized medical system is available to the majority of the population using relatively simple access mechanisms and low out-of-pocket costs. Therefore, many Hispanic individuals have difficulties accessing and traveling through the complex maze associated with the third-party insurance systems encountered in the U.S. This difficulty limits their access to health care, particularly mental health services and advanced specialty services such as neuropsychology. Others, including those who are U.S. citizens or born in the U.S., including children, the elderly, and specific Hispanic populations such as veterans of foreign wars, do not have any health care insurance, which clearly places constraints on accessibility and services. The lack of regular and scheduled medical care has led indirectly to problems and to the overwhelming use of emergency medical services (with devastating consequences for emergency services in selected hospitals) in selected communities throughout the U.S. This occurs partly because limited access to regular and preventive care often have led to the need for emergency medical and mental health care (Baker et al., 1996). This can be surmised from the increasing rates of emergency room admissions and utilization by Hispanics in the U.S. in the last two decades.

Socioeconomic status, sociopolitical climates, and sheer societal economic realities and constraints also have significant impact on access to health care and medical services by all U.S. citizens. Unfortunately, either as a result of the issues mentioned thus far, including poverty, or language barriers, or a combination of both, it is well known that Hispanics, including those born in the U.S. or foreign-born U.S. citizens, have less access or seek less dental, medical, and mental health services (cf. Weinick, Zuvekas and Cohen, 2000). Data from the U.S. Department of Health and Human Services (USDHHS) makes clear that significant health disparities exist in the U.S. between Hispanics and individuals from mainstream culture, and this has significant impact on American neuropsychology. From a data-based standpoint, the USDHHS published a report noting the presence of such disparities (U.S. Department of Health and Human Services, 2004).

Education

As briefly noted in Chapter 1 and above, education is a critical factor. Aside from the fact that education has been shown to impact neuropsychological functioning (cf. Heaton et al., 1986; Ostrosky-Solis et al., 2004), it is crucial to examine this variable as a special factor because large numbers of Hispanics living in the U.S. have achieved low levels of education. For example, Harris and Llorente (2005) note that in the "Caucasian non-Hispanic population, 88.7% graduate from high school, 29.4% achieve a minimum of a Bachelor's degree, and 4.0% have attained less than 9 years of education." By contrast, in individuals from Mexico 25 years or older, 48.6% have not received a high school diploma, 26.6% have graduated from high school, and only 5.2% achieve a minimum of a Bachelor's degree. Aside from specific cognitive protective factors related to education in neuropsychology as postulated by Satz (Satz, 1993), limited or lack of education also interacts with other factors, in some instances leading to increased risk factors in Hispanic populations such as limited economic opportunity, limited knowledge of the impact of preventive medical care or good nutrition, and so on. Therefore, education is an important variable to keep in mind when interpreting neuropsychological test performance and working with Hispanic populations.

Disease and Illness

For specific health problems, illnesses, and diseases, Hispanics living in the U.S. and abroad are most likely associated with impoverished environments, as noted by the World Health Organization (1998), and unfortunately bear a disproportionate burden of disease, injury, morbidity, and mortality when compared with non-Hispanic whites. In addition, the leading causes of death among Hispanics vary from those for non-Hispanic whites in the U.S., information supported by statistical resources kept by the United States Department of Health and Human Services (USDHHS, 2004). For example, the report from the USDHHS indicates that Hispanics of all ethnic backgrounds "experienced more age-adjusted years of potential life lost before age 75 years per 100,000 population than non-Hispanic whites" for mortality associated with "stroke (18% more), chronic liver disease and cirrhosis (62%), diabetes (41%), and human immunodeficiency virus disease (168%)," all with significant implications for neuropsychology and its applied endeavors (cf. Llorente et al., 2000a, 2001).

Occupational Risk Factors

As noted in Chapter 2, the occupational allegiance of Hispanics is not distributed evenly across all occupational categories. In fact, it was noted that large numbers of Hispanics are overrepresented in the farming/forestry industries at rates that sometimes exceed twice the rate of expectation based on U.S. population demographics (cf. Llorente et al., 1999, 2000; Portes and Rumbaut, 1990). Selective recruitment policies and occupational allegiances, particularly in high-risk occupations, have significant implications because such industries may impact large numbers of Hispanics, placing this group of individuals at increased risk for disease or exposure to occupational risk factors and hazards, including but not limited to neurotoxic substances. As a result of this exposure and given the potential impact of these substances on brain functions, individuals may require neuropsychological assessment (see Llorente, 2000). For example, Hispanic populations employed in the farming industries may experience increased risk factors associated with chronic, low-level pesticide exposure (cf. Llorente, 2000), including organophosphates and other pesticides, which impact neurological substrates and neuropsychological functioning (Eskenazi and Maizlish, 1988). Because such exposures impact neuropsychological performance, in some instances they are the reason children and adults are referred for assessment (see Eskenazi and Maizlish, 1988; Llorente, 2000).

Housing and Housing Quality

Although Hispanics have made significant gains in the last few years related to ownership of real estate in the U.S., significant disparities still remain between them and majority groups (Tomás Rivera Policy Institute, 2003). Similarly, quality of housing is often taken for granted by clinicians and researchers alike, despite its health significance, including potentially harmful environmental contaminants that significantly impact brain function (e.g., lead, mercury, organophosphates, and sulfur dioxide) and that are often found in neighborhoods with large Hispanic populations throughout the U.S. Why is it essential and necessary to examine such variables during the course of assessment with Hispanic populations? From a neuropsychological standpoint, it is critical to note that quality of housing may also be associated with other health-related and non-health-related variables, such as environmental deprivation, overcrowding, and added stress, all of which affect neuropsychological functioning.

It is also interesting to note that some of the factors mentioned in Chapter 2, such as geographical affinity of specific Hispanic groups, is not just supported by census or other data examined by Llorente et al. (1999), but they are additionally supported by housing data (Tomás Rivera Policy Institute, 2003).

Religion

Religion, especially organized religion, plays a major role in the life of many Hispanics living in the U.S., and it represents a strong component of their cultural heritage and identity. According to Espinosa, Elizondo, and Miranda (2005), approximately 71% of Hispanics identify themselves as Catholic (Milwaukee Archdiocese, 2005), and about 23% of the 41.3 million Hispanics in the U.S. in 2004 identified themselves as Protestants or other Christians. Complicating this issue, and their cultural identity as well, is the fact that many Hispanics, in addition to practicing Catholicism or other organized religion, additionally may adopt other, less formal religious practices such as "*Santería*." The emphasis placed by Hispanics on religious beliefs and practices dates back to their ancestors and the colonization of the Americas by Spaniards and other western European societies (cf. Dussell, 1992), as well as the introduction of African religious practices into Hispanic cultures, impacting all Hispanics, but particularly those from nations near countries where such practices are highly prevalent (e.g., Dominican Republic and Haiti).

Although some clinicians may argue that these issues are irrelevant to neuropsychological practice, they are important to evaluate because they may significantly impact the conclusions reached about a specific Hispanic patient. For example, from a diagnostic standpoint, a clinician may reach an erroneous diagnostic conclusion because he or she perceives that a client is experiencing hallucinations or other symptoms associated with a psychotic process based on the client's answers to questions during a clinical interview or on a rating scale. In fact, the client may practice Santería and may truly believe that he or she hear voices, but this belief is not subsequent to neuropsychopathology.

Multicultural Diagnostic Considerations

The ever-increasing racial and ethnic diversity of the U.S. population, as noted in Chapter 2, emphasizes the need to account for the role of culture on diagnosis. Groce and Zola (1993) noted, "An individual's culture is not a diagnostic category; no cultural heritage will wholly explain how any given individual will think and act, but it can help health care professionals anticipate and understand how and why families make certain decisions" (p. 1049). Groce and Zola have also emphasized the importance of cultural awareness and its impact on expectations of a client's physical, mental, and psychological development, given the potential for variability in these expectations and a client's experiences within his or her own cultural environment. Cultural awareness and understanding clearly need to be considered an integral part of a clinician's knowledge base when they are called upon to diagnose and provide consultation (Reeve, Groce, Persing, and Magge, 2004). Additionally, Groce and Zola caution that cultural belief systems may be approached in an oversimplified manner, or misinterpreted, which may lead to mislabeling this unique way of responding to the condition or intervention. They further suggest that when faced with a question of whether a behavior is a cultural norm for all patients or unique to that patient with a disability, the practitioner should compare the treatment of the disabled patient with that of nondisabled patient who is matched based on age, gender, socioeconomic, and sociocultural backgrounds. Gannotti and Handwerker (2002) call to adapt and validate standardized measures of health for cross-cultural validation. They examined the Pediatric Evaluation of Disability Inventory (PEDI) and found that without restandardized normative values for use with Puerto Rican children, results would have made this population appear more disabled than expected for their level of impairment or making minimal functional improvements. Results of the study found that cultural, environmental, and accessibility factors needed to be taken into account in order to provide a proper representation of this population.

The *Diagnostic and Statistical Manual of Mental Disorders-Third Edition-Revised* (DSM-III-R, APA, 1987) was the first version of the DSM to acknowledge, albeit simplisticly, the impact of an individual's culture on diagnosis. Subsequent versions of this text (DSM-IV, 1994; DSM-IV-TR, 2000) provide a framework (Appendix) for clinicians to account for the impact of an individual's culture when assessing each of the DSM-IV's axes. This manual also provides a glossary of 25 culture-bound syndromes. According to the DSM-IV, a cultural formulation should supplement the axes and include such factors as the cultural identity of the individual, cultural explanation of the individual's illness, cultural factors related to psychosocial environment and levels of functioning, cultural elements of the relationship between the individual and the clinician, and overall cultural assessment for diagnosis and care (DSM-IV; APA, 2000). Appendix of the DSM-IV provides a glossary of culture-bound syndromes, which are defined as "recurrent, locality-specific patterns of aberrant behavior and troubling experiences that may or may not be linked to a particular DSM-IV diagnostic category" (p. 898).

An example of a culture-bound syndrome found in the Hispanic community, as noted in the Preface, *ataque de nervios*. Guarnaccia, Lewis-Fernandez, and Marano (2003) studied the prevalence of this culture-bound syndrome with a slightly modified Diagnostic Interview Schedule (DIS) in Puerto Rico. They interviewed 912 people, of whom 16% reported having experienced an episode of *ataque de nervios* in their lifetime. *Ataque de nervios* was highly correlated with a range of internalizing disorders. Research on culture-bound syndromes helps close the gap between cultural and clinical knowledge and provides insights into issues of diagnostic universality and cultural specificity (Guarnaccia and Rogler, 1999).

Groce and Zola's (1993) review of the multicultural literature suggests that three recurrent themes emerge: (1) The culturally perceived cause of a chronic illness or disability will play a significant role in determining family and community attitudes toward the individual; (2) the expectations for survival of the individual a chronic illness or disability will affect both the immediate care and future allocation of resources; and (3) the social role(s) deemed appropriate for disabled or chronically ill children and adults will help determine the amount of resources a family and community invest in an individual. In some cultures, even now, illness and disability may be viewed as a form of punishment or retribution – much as they were viewed hundreds of years ago (Groce and Nola, 1993; Reeve, Groce, Persing, and Magge, 2004). For example, the beliefs of witchcraft found in some Caribbean societies (e.g., Dominican Republic) hold that illness or disability may be transmitted through one's associations. Or, if a child has an illness with a rapid onset, some people in Latin American societies believe that the condition is due to the "evil eye" (Groce and Zola, 1993; see also Simpson, Mohr and Redman, 2000). In Manaus, Brazil, an individual may consider cleft lip or cleft palate to result from contagion (e.g.., contracted by sharing eating utensils), personal conduct (e.g.., a pregnant mother looked at an animal with a split mouth or the father cut open the mouth of a fish to remove a hook during his child's pregnancy), or God's will (Reeve, Groce, Persing, and Magge, 2004). In contrast, chronic illness and disability may be seen by some cultures as a unique gift. For example, some Mexican immigrants believe that their child has been singled out by God for the role because of their past kindnesses to a relative or neighbor who was disabled. (Ries et al., 2007)

Consideration should be given to the acculturation of a patient and his or her family as it may have important implications for diagnosis. Groce and Zola (1993) advocate for the assessment of acculturation on an individual basis, particularly an individual or a family's belief system and social structure. The authors note:

> No one can simply assume on the basis of a person's cultural heritage, dress, or language what his or her individual ideas or understandings may be. Nonetheless, it is important to remember that traditional attitudes about disability may hang on long after other cultural beliefs are gone, although more acculturated individuals may be sophisticated enough to know that publicly expressing beliefs, such as the presence of witchcraft, is unacceptable. (p. 1055).

An individual's subjective experience and worldview can play an important role in the assessment and treatment of their presenting problems.

General Perceptions of Ethnic Minority Groups and Immigrants

As mentioned briefly in Chapter 2, the presence of large numbers of immigrant Hispanics in the U.S. makes the issue of immigrant perception and its relation to neuropsychology and neuropsychological assessment deserving of attention. Llorente et al. (2000) noted that "data documenting examiner and patient characteristics capable of biasing an evaluation abounds in the psychological literature." Examiners' expectancy effects (e.g., halo effects) are important to recognize, and if not "kept in check," may infringe upon the validity of the inferences derived from neuropsychological assessment of Hispanics (cf. Donahue and Sattler, 1971; Grossman, 1978; Sattler and Winget, 1970). The patient's history also can significantly impact the manner in which an examiner conducts, scores, and interprets the results of a psychological evaluation (cf. Auffrey and Robertson, 1972). These issues take on greater significance with immigrants since they may possess more pronounced characteristics capable of enhancing the expectancy effects of the examiner, particularly those characteristics that are observable (e.g., anxiety associated with no prior psychological contact [cf. Egeland, 1967]; pronounced accent in speech).

In addition it is critical to note that many negative stereotypes about immigrants and ethnic minorities, including Hispanics, have permeated American society and culture, including television, radio, and other mass media, and these affect lay as well as professional individuals. As noted by Llorente et al. (2000), "these stereotypes are capable of having deleterious impact upon" a neuropsychological evaluation, "despite their unsubstantiated nature and the fact that they have insufficient weight to withstand the rigor of scientific scrutiny." This issue is best exemplified within American society through mainstream perceptions of the immigrant.

Such perceptions historically have been negative, even within the mental health professions (Ødegaard, 1932; Sanua, 1970). As a case in point, during earlier large-scale migrations to the U.S. at the beginning of the last century, a correlation was initially noted between immigrants and innate marginality or psychopathology associated with the process of immigration. Although incorrect, such perceptions were the result of early, inaccurate, and methodologically flawed epidemiological studies indicating the presence of higher incidence of mental illness among immigrants on the basis of hospital admissions (Jarvis, 1866; Rothman, 1971; Sanua, 1970); higher suicide rates among immigrants living in the U.S.; European versus U.S. differential suicide rates in groups of individuals of the same nationality (cf. Faris and Dunham, 1939); and differential patterns and rates of mental disorders in metropolitan areas relative to suburban areas with large immigrant density (Faris and Dunham, 1939). On the basis of these findings, researchers concluded that immigration was associated with mental disorders (Ødegaard, 1932). Unfortunately, these investigations suffered from poor methodology marked by biased samples and similar confounds, and sound research later demonstrated that the effects of objective variables such as age, poverty, and area of residence (Kohn, 1973; Hollingshead and Redlich, 1958; Kessler and Cleary, 1980 ; Srole, Langner, and Mitchell, 1962) accounted for the majority of the differences observed. "Despite the significant shortcomings of the earlier investigations, these findings found their way into mainstream culture and became part of the perception of the immigrant, not just held by lay people but also by mental health providers, regarding the mental abilities" and psychological make-up of the immigrant (Llorente et al., 2000). These stereotypes are capable of biasing the outcome of a neuropsychological examination.

Llorente et al. (2000) noted that "there is no reason to believe, despite our present level of knowledge with regard to which factors affect immigrants and large-scale migrations (e.g., context of immigration, SES of the immigrant, reasons for immigration; cf. Portes and Rumbaut, 1990), that new generations of neuropsychologists will behave differently towards these populations, including Hispanics, relative to past generations of clinicians, unless the former become cognizant of the biases against these populations and the factors capable of encroaching upon their assessments." Although immigration can be one of the greatest stressors that any individual may experience in life, immigration per se is not necessarily responsible for mental illness or the etiology behind abnormal brain-behavior relationships.

Chapter 4
Intellectual Abilities: Theoretical and Applied Assessment Considerations[1]

Christian von Thomsen, Lori Gallup, and Antolin M. Llorente

The assessment of intellectual abilities has held a special place in the history of psychology. Starting with the establishment of the civil service program in China approximately 4,200 years ago, to the Spanish physician Juan Huarte's *Examen de Ingenios* in 1575, the assessment of aptitude, whether valid or invalid throughout the centuries, has attempted to capture the broad range of intellectual abilities noted by Sir Francis Galton in 1869 when he stated that "There is continuity of natural ability reaching from one knows not what height, and descending to one can hardly say what depth" (Galton, 1869).

Although the latter part of the statement made by Galton clearly exemplifies his profound understanding of individual differences in intellectual "gifts," other statements he made have been associated with controversy, as they were adopted by the eugenics movement, and the measurement of intellectual abilities has been far more scrutinized than the measurement of other neuropsychological constructs, in some instances disregarding the importance of the latter. Like no other function of the "mind," intellectual skills seem to include judgment of character and potential in life; intercultural differences in this construct were controversial from early periods (cf. Nell, 2000), most recently in the vernacular literature and in the general public's awareness after publication of Herrnstein's book "The Bell Curve" (Herrnstein and Murray, 1994; Nell, 2000).

It is interesting to note that Spearman chose "g" for "general intelligence" when he partially laid the groundwork for his theories regarding intellectual abilities impacting current assessment. The question whether or not research should and can work with truly general constructs has been addressed in the *emic-etic* paradigm originally defined by Pike (1967, as quoted in Berry, 1999). Pike suggested the term *etic* for an approach that views behavior from an outside perspective, while he proposed the term *emic* for an approach that views behavior from a perspective inside the system in question (Berry, 1999). In cross-cultural psychology, these labels may be used to indicate whether the emphasis of a given study is placed on understanding meaning by utilizing concepts from within the culture in question

---

[1] Portions of this chapter originally appeared in Harris and Llorente (2005).

(emic), or whether "neutral" or "objective" constructs are used to compare and evaluate one culture with another one (etic) (Alegria, Vila, Woo, Canino, Takeuchi, et al., 2004). Spearman's identification of a "general" factor of intelligence thus implied an etic approach to cognitive assessment. Critique of supposedly the generalist approach reportedly led to development of "culture-free" and then "culture-fair" tests (Jones, 1996). Still, in the interest of external validity (generalization), the use of a limited number of cognitive tests for assessment of intelligence is continued in the U.S. (Echemendia and Harris, 2004). Unfortunately, the construct of general intelligence appears to be measured by tests that are strongly correlated with content taught in American schools (Rosselli and Ardila, 2001), particularly those schools with a European heritage, and as noted in Chapters 1 and 3, selected numbers of Hispanics tend to exhibit higher rates of school dropout, lower levels of overall education, and in some instances, an education of poor quality.

In the case of Hispanic populations, experts in the field continue to criticize the etic approach taken by many U.S. practitioners (Artiola i Fortuny, 1998; Artiola i Fortuni et al., 2005). These authors have noted that many neuropsychologists might feel that neurobehavioral principles are "general" or universal and that culture, therefore, requires little consideration (Echemendia and Harris, 2004; Nell, 2000). However, emic measures are few and are difficult to use considering intragroup variance. As LaRue and colleagues (1999) point out, it may be an impossible task to attempt to match a specific client with a suitable norm sample, precisely because "Hispanic" culture encompasses such a wide range of diverse cultural and demographic variables (cf. Pontón, 2001b). Alegria and colleagues (Alegria et al., 2004) demonstrated that the use of both emic and etic concepts can be integrated to develop new assessment instruments for minority individuals.

However, the assessment of intellectual abilities in Hispanics, from an appropriate cross-cultural standpoint, is far more complicated than that suggested by simple arguments for an emic or etic assessment or theoretical approach. The intellectual assessment of Hispanics is not only complicated by a selected number of issues associated with the concept of "Hispanic" or "Latino" as noted above and in Chapters 1 and 2 of this volume, nor by simple issues related to psychometrics, but it is, rather, complicated by several other complex issues. Such complexity includes not just aspects related to tests, including adaptations, test construction, language, standardization samples, and other variables, but also includes factors that could be subsumed under David Wechsler's concept of connative factors (Wechsler, 1950). For example, aside from motivation and other variables that could very well be underscored by Wechsler's concept as connative characteristics, in lieu of cognitive factors, factors such as the prevailing attitudes toward intellectual assessments by Hispanics, cultural interpretations of the concept of IQ or intellectual skills in general, their prevailing cultural perceptions of those who administer the test(s), their prevailing perceptions of tests in general, and the society where they reside, and their perceptions of those who are associated with decision-making processes which they perceive to be outside of their control may also fall under the rubric of connative factors when addressing cross-cultural assessment of intellectual skills with Hispanics. To complicate matters further, other conceptual issues also should play an important role. To understand cross-cultural factors and their implication during the course of intellectual assessment with Hispanics, fields and concepts from sociology, genetics, and anthropology also play important roles. When such factors are included in theoretical frameworks, they lead to comprehensive models of cognitive processes such as the ecocultural framework developed by Berry (2001), which is capable of accounting for cross-cultural mechanisms that are applicable to intellectual variables in Hispanic populations. This perspective includes universalist views of cognition and intellectual abilities related to specific cognitive mechanisms, as espoused by many in the field today (cf. Echemendia and Harris, 2004), as well as the effects of cultural factors on individuals, including Hispanics. Berry (2001) devised a framework in which individual differences, including intellectual skills, emerge within the greater contextual space of universalist factors as a function of sets of variables, including ecological (Eco) and sociopolitical factors, together with other arrays of variables, including culture, genetics, and acculturation, that lead to the emergence of such individual differences. In essence, the model explains individual differences in intellectual abilities as the emergence of general universal psychological mechanisms that are found in all humans (species) that are then infinitely modified through maturation by cultural and other variables as a collection of adaptations to context or ecology. This model clearly adopts concepts from evolutionary theory (Darwin, 1967). It is also consistent with the view noted in Chapter 1 related to the fact that an individual constructs his society and society constructs the individual (cf. Wartofsky, 1983).

Although borrowing from Hebb (1949) regarding what appear to be simple yet important distinctions between intellectual abilities, intelligent behavior and assessed intellect, Sternberg (1984, 1997) also developed a comprehensive theory of intelligence that is capable of incorporating cultural influences in cognition. According to Sternberg's triarchic theory of intelligence, there are three main components that describe mental functioning and, ultimately, how people process information (Sternberg, 1997). The first component includes a contextual piece that considers the unique environment in which individuals reside with regard to intelligence. Within this component, intelligence consists of the individual's ability to adapt, select, and shape his or her environment and make it meaningful to the self. Secondly, the componential subtheory addresses the individual's internal ability to complete mental processes, which consists of encoding, transforming, and comparing information, as well as higher level executive functions consisting of planning, organizing, and monitoring the information (Sternberg). This second part of the triarchic theory is primarily related to information processing. Finally, the third component is referred to as two-facet and describes an individual's intelligence as their ability to work with novel stimuli and their level of automaticity of various cognitive processes (Sternberg).

From a theoretical standpoint, Cattell (1963), Horn (1967; 1979), and Carroll (2005) independently devised theories of intelligence. These theories were then combined and used as the underlying theoretical basis for the development of the *Woodcock-Johnson Tests of Cognitive Abilities - Third Edition* (WJ-III).

Cattell and Horn's theory of cognitive abilities distinguishes between two types of intelligence: fluid intelligence and crystallized intelligence. Fluid intelligence consists of cognitive abilities that are typically thought of as free of cultural influence (even though Berry's [2001] and Sternberg's [1997] models point in a different direction) and includes procedures such as word list recall. According to this theory, fluid intelligence is related to level of maturity and continues to expand until adolescence and young adulthood. Crystallized intelligence is considered to be skills that an individual acquires as a result of residing in a specific culture. Crystallized intelligence is thought to continue to expand and develop throughout one's life as an individual continues to interact with his or her culture and learn over time, and it is therefore much affected by education and other contextual opportunities. Cattell-Horn's theory of intelligence is a hierarchical model that includes all major aspects of intelligence (McGrew and Woodcock, 2001).

John Carroll's three-stratum theory of intelligence is also hierarchical. His theory identifies 69 specific abilities that are narrow in nature and compose Stratum I. Stratum II consists of broader categories of intelligence that group the 69 narrow abilities. Finally, Stratum III incorporates a general intelligence which Carroll refers to as "g." The WJ-III was developed utilizing the theory of cognitive abilities established by Cattell, Horn, and Carroll (CHC theory) as its theoretical foundation (McGrew and Woodcock, 2001). This theory incorporates aspects from two major sources, including Cattell and Horn's work with fluid (Gf) and crystallized (Gc) intellectual abilities and Carroll's hierarchical conceptualization of cognitive abilities that stem from narrow abilities, to broader abilities, and finally to general intelligence, or "g" (McGrew and Woodcock). The application of such a comprehensive framework of intelligence has led to the development of an excellent measure of cognitive abilities.

Although a strong argument has been made for the importance of cultural factors, alternative views should not be excluded. Genetic factors are frequently considered to exert a powerful influence on intelligence (Laosa, 1996), and probably account for a portion of the inter- and intracultural variations (cf. Kwak, 2003). For example, there appears to be evidence for differential onset of certain brain-related conditions in Hispanics (Clark et al., 2005), as well as possible differential cognitive strengths and weaknesses associated with specific cultural and ethnic backgrounds (e.g., Korean versus Hispanic). However, research in the field of molecular genetics makes it seem likely that a complex combination of different genes contributes to variations in cognitive ability and other neuropsychological domains, and that environmental factors may play a crucial role in determining which and when those genes are expressed (cf. Lai et al., 2001; Laosa, 1996).

In summary, one chief problem related to this topic and the process of assessment is that intragroup variance continues to be neglected by clinicians when planning assessments with diverse clients generally (APA, 2001) and Hispanic clients specifically (Artiola i Fortuni et al., 2005; Pontón & León-Correón, 2001).

General Issues Related to Cognitive and Intellectual Assessment

While a number of available cognitive tests seems capable of producing results that are unbiased in select applications for members of ethnic minorities, including Hispanics, a recent review reported that about a third of such measures have been identified in empirical studies of cultural bias to yield biased or mixed results (Valencia, Suzuki, and Salinas, 2001).

In 2004, Echemendia and Harris published data from a 1994 survey of U.S. neuropsychologists regarding the use of tests with Hispanic populations (Echemendia and Harris, 2004). Even though the data were 10 years old at the time of publication, the authors expressed confidence that not much had changed in this time, given a lack of published Spanish tests, as well as their own personal experience. Their sample of 475 responses indicated great variability in the use of tests and norms with Hispanics. In terms of what tests are used with what population, both Hispanic and non-Hispanic clients are most often administered the WAIS for assessment of cognitive capabilities (Echemendia and Harris, 2004). This finding was stable even across different levels of self-perceived competence to work with Hispanic clients, as well as self-perceived language competence (in Spanish).

Regarding test translation, most clinicians (58%) indicated that they used the English WAIS with bilingual clients and the Spanish version with monolingual Spanish speakers, respectively (52%). However, a considerable percentage (20% for the bilingual group and 29% for the monolingual Spanish group) utilized a verbatim translation of the English test items (Echemendia and Harris, 2004). The authors remark that this behavior is highly problematic and can interfere with validity of the measures used (see Chapter 1). When asked what norms are typically employed to compare WAIS test results from bilinguals with the general population, 68% of clinicians stated they used English norms, 4% Spanish norms, and 28% relied on clinical judgment. With monolingual Spanish speakers, 6% of WAIS scores are compared with English norms, 64% with Spanish norms, and 29% by using clinical judgment. The frequent use of clinical judgment rather than norms can be viewed as an appropriate response to lack of suitable norms (Echemendia and Harris, 2004) or as clinicians' tendency to revert to intuitive decision-making processes.

Another important result from this study is data regarding the use of translators. While more frequently reported by neuropsychologists who also endorse lower competence in Spanish fluency and proficiency, reliance on translators is controversial because standardized assessments depend on standardized instructions and interactions (Echemendia and Harris, 2004; Ardila, 2005).

In conclusion, Echemendia and Harris (2004) stated that U.S. neuropsychologists are "not prepared adequately to provide services to Latinos" (Echemendia and Harris, 2004, p. 11). According to them, this is partly due to the fact that bilingual clients are usually administered U.S. normed version of tests, while monolingual Spanish-speaking individuals most often receive a translated version of the same test (Echemendia and Harris, 2004).

As mentioned before, local norms may be required in order to adequately derive scaled scores from assessments (Echemendia and Harris, 2004), at least for a period of time until unbiased intellectual and neuropsychological measures are devised. For example, LaRue and colleagues (1999) report that significant differences have been found between education-matched samples from different South American countries. Furthermore, availability of "norms for Hispanics" may actually keep researchers from investigating demographic and cultural details, since they may feel that they now are in possession of "appropriate" norms for all individuals who speak Spanish. Clearly, intragroup variance remains a considerable problem in this regard.

Recently, cultural fairness of a common instrument has been examined from a psychophysiological point of view (see also Chapter 1 under cultural equivalency). Verney, Granholm, Marshall, Malcarne, and Saccuzzo (2005) built upon recent research showing that pupillary responses can be measured to index mental effort, and found that both Hispanic and non-Hispanic whites displayed similar pupillary changes when exerting mental effort. However, only in non-Hispanic whites did those pupillary responses predict performance on the WAIS-R (Verney et al., 2005). Physiologically based measures of intellectual ability, such as the visual backward-masking task detection accuracy, suggested that Hispanics and non-Hispanic whites did not differ in terms of cognitive capabilities. However, the WAIS-R scores showed the familiar pattern of lower scores in the Hispanic sample. On the basis of these findings, these authors concluded that the WAIS-R may contain cultural factors that result in a test bias favoring non-Hispanic whites, while the more psychophysiological measures used in this study did not share this bias (Verney et al., 2005).

Consistently lower performance on digit-span memory tasks has been reported, and the question has been raised whether this could be related to the fact that Spanish numbers have more syllables than English ones (Olazaran, Jacobs, and Stern, 1996). After varying language content and linguistic characteristics of the task, Olazaran and colleagues (1996) concluded that cultural and educational issues are likely also involved in this performance difference.

Recent research also underscores the profound effects that some of the aforementioned factors can have on performance during the course of intellectual assessment in Hispanic populations. In this regard it is critical to examine the effects of language proficiency on tests of intellectual abilities. With regard to adults, Harris and Llorente (2005) note that it "seems logical to conclude that children acquiring skills in English may not possess sufficient fluency to effectively perform on the more demanding, context reduced" intellectual test, but they question "what about" adult "examinees who appear to be fluent and proficient?" In this regard, a study conducted by Harris and her colleagues (2003), in which "non-native English speaking adults who participated in the WAIS-III standardization," clearly "illustrated the concerns and challenges of determining when an examinee possesses sufficient proficiency for English language intellectual assessment." In that study, a group of adult examinees ($n = 151$) was selected for participation, all of whom reported being born outside of the U.S., yet all reported fluency in English, "criteria corroborated by the standardization test examiner based upon observation of the examinees' conversation before and during the testing session." The sample consisted of individuals representing 37 countries of origin. Individuals from Mexico and Cuba comprised two thirds of the sample. Three variables, obtained from a "demographic questionnaire completed by all study participants, served as proxies for acculturation." The variables included (1) "language preference, derived by weighting reported language preference for speaking, thinking, reading, and writing in English and in the additional spoken language;" (2) "U.S. experience," "calculated by dividing the number of years residing in the U.S. by the total age of the examinee;" and (3) "U.S. education," "calculated by dividing the number of years educated in the U.S. by the total number of years of education attained" by each participant (cf. Harris, Tulsky and Schultheis, 2003). The relationship of these three variables to performance on the WAIS-III and WMS-III factor scores was subsequently analyzed, and all three variables were significant predictors of performance on the various factor scores, with "language preference" essentially "predicting performance on the Verbal Comprehension, Perceptual Organization, Processing Speed, and Visual Memory (using the Visual Reproduction subtest) indices." With regard to children, the impact of language fluency was examined by Harris and Llorente (2005). They investigated the reported differences that usually emerge during the course of assessment of Hispanics relative to mainstream populations in the U.S. Although limited to only one test, they investigated such differences using data from the standardization of the new WISC-IV in 6- to16-year-olds. A cursive examination of initial scores uncontrolled for any demographic characteristics revealed a difference of approximately 10 IQ points in FSIQ between the "Hispanic" and the "Non-Hispanic White" samples. Further analyses controlling for different factors, usually subsumed by the different theoretical models presented above related to demographic characteristics, including age, gender, number of parents living in the household, parental education level, and U.S. region of selection for participation in the standardization sample, reduced the differences in overall intellectual skills (FSIQ) by approximately five points. Subsequent to this finding, the authors questioned whether to assume that the remaining five-point difference represented actual difference found in the standardization sample. After further analyses, it was discovered that a variable could easily account for the remaining five-point difference in overall intellect.

What variable could account for a third of a standard deviation in overall intellect? To investigate this remaining difference and examine the possible influence of English language acquisition and language proficiency on performance, the WISC-IV standardization participants were again matched on age, gender, and parental education level. However, the examinees selected for this analysis also included an important variable, obtained from a comprehensive Family Survey administered to WISC-IV examinees related to language spoken in the home. This variable led to the categorization of the WISC-IV standardization sample into three subgroups, namely a "White non-Hispanic" sample comprised of monolingual "English" speakers," a "Hispanic" sample comprised of monolingual English speakers, and a third "Hispanic" group of children comprised of those who noted that they spoke "Spanish" as their native language in the Family Survey. Subsequent to this analysis, the reduced performance in overall intellect for Hispanic examinees only emerged in the group of Hispanic children whose native language was Spanish. As noted by Harris and Llorente (2005), the "'typical' finding of reduced performance, particularly in verbal indices, for Hispanic examinees" was only evidenced in the sample of Hispanic children whose native language was Spanish. "In fact, although the sample is small, the native English speaking Hispanic children surpass the non-minority examinees in their Processing Speed Index. Such findings are a powerful illustration of the impact of socioeconomic and linguistic variables upon performance." As noted by Harris and Llorente (2005), "What initially appeared to be a large gap between Hispanic and non-Hispanic White children, now appears to be a minimal difference." On the basis of these results Harris and Llorente (2005) also concluded that native language is an important moderating variable and these studies demonstrate the "challenges test developers and clinicians face in determining when a suitable level of language proficiency has been reached" in an individual undergoing assessment (see Table 4.3).

Altogether, these general findings led Harris and Llorente (2005) to address another vital issue often encountered in intellectual assessment (see also the work of Ardila et al. 1994). Harris and Llorente (2005) note that the construct equivalency of a test and its underlying theoretical framework are critical issues to take into account. They more specifically note the importance of conceptual equivalence in the construct and measurement of intelligence and the significance of intellect moderator variables. They note that "differences exist in the conceptualization of intelligence by various theoreticians (cf. Carroll, 2005; Cattell, 1963; Ceci, 1996; Spearman, 1927; Sternberg, 1985, 1997; Thurstone, 1938)," as noted above, yet "Each model has implications for a specific culturally-defined context or question. For example, how is the 'intelligence'" necessary that describes successful adaptation by a child in a metropolitan area in the U.S. "different than the intelligence that describes the successful adaptation of a child to his community in Nicaragua or Zambia? It is certainly not contested that intelligence can be represented differently within different" cultural groups; however, they also note that this is not to say that intelligence "can also be represented similarly when individuals share salient aspects of their cultural and educational backgrounds." In this regard, they note that investigations "concerning the cultural equivalence of the WISC in cross-national studies supports the notion of selected universal cognitive processes across cultures (cf. Georgas et al., 2003a, b)." In addition, the construct structure for specific ethnic or cultural groups that emerges in factor analytic studies "within the U.S. is also generally consistent, although there may be some differences in factor loadings in the lower age ranges due to developmental differences in the acquisition of specific cognitive abilities, such as working memory skills" (Wechsler, 2003). Similar "score comparisons among ethnic groups within a given country also have emerged, and socioeconomic factors have been found to partially account for variability in performance" (Georgas, 2003), and "there is remarkable consistency in the factor structure of the WISC, when translated and adapted into other languages in other countries" (Georgas et al., 2003a, b). When mean score differences have been identified among cross-national samples, these findings have been thought to be attributable to education-related or economic factors (Georgas et al., 2003a, b) Variations in IQ scores across countries have, for example, been found to be related to pupil-teacher ratio for preprimary, primary, and secondary education and to duration of each education level and other factors as noted in Chapters 1 and 3 (Georgas et al., 2003a, b). These investigators also suggested that affluence-related factors, such as the physical quality of the child's living environment, may explain cross-cultural score differences, although "education and affluence are also noted to be highly and positively correlated." Nevertheless, it is clear that construct equivalency is a critical factor when assessing or measuring cognitive skills, and this issue is critical regardless of which skills are being measured, particularly for the development of intellectual tests that attempt to tap into these unique "similarities."

Pediatric Assessment

Gonzalez (2001) identifies a number of tests that are appropriate to use with Hispanic children. He stresses that language cannot be ignored by the assessing clinician, especially given that many Hispanic children are exposed to various levels of English and Spanish. Gonzalez (2001) suggests an in-depth review of language proficiency of each individual client in more than one domain (e.g., home and school) and strongly recommends consultation and cooperation with, if not referral to, a bilingual neuropsychologist.

Bateria III

For cognitive assessment, the *Batería III Woodcock-Muñoz* (Bateria III; Munoz-Sandoval, Woodcock, McGrew, and Mather, 2005) represents a comprehensive resource for clinicians. This is the Spanish version of the Woodcock-Johnson III (WJ-III; Woodcock, McGrew, & Mather, 2001), including cognitive and achievement batteries. Cognitive ability is measured with the *Pruebas de Habilidades Cognitivas* (Bateria-III COG). All tests comprising the Batería have been adapted from the WJ-III. A special characteristic of the Batería is the Language Exposure/Use Questionnaire included as a screening in the beginning of the test. This instrument allows the examiner to verify information about which language is preferred or spoken more proficiently by the client. For example, questions about percentage of time each language is spoken are provided. Likewise, the manual contains a checklist and training exercises for the examiner to ensure proficiency.

Otero (2006) points out that true Spanish proficiency is essential to correctly administer and score the Batería III. She notes several instances where the list of correct answers to given questions does not contain words that are used by residents of certain countries, so that the burden to recognize the answers as correct lies with the examiner (Otero, 2006).

The norming sample consisted of 1,413 individuals who were identified as native Spanish speakers. Of these, 1,134 individuals came from Mexico, Costa Rica, Panama, Argentina, Colombia, Puerto Rico, and Spain. The remaining 279 participants consisted of U.S. residents from nine states, 89 of whom were born in the U.S. The rest were ascertained from a variety of Latin American countries. Spanish language dominance was ensured in the U.S. residents by means of oral language screening and consultation with bilingual experts. Note that not every country of origin was represented by an equal number of participants. Mexico, for example, was overrepresented in relation to Spain, thus impacting comparability of test results (Otero, 2006). On the other hand, a comparison of Batería III data with WJ-III is easily achieved because normative data from the Batería were equated with U.S. norms from the WJ-III. In other words, language proficiency in English and Spanish may be compared using a single score.

Data from the calibration sample, as provided in the manual, indicate generally good reliability for individual subtests ranging from .80 for Word Completion to .93 for Verbal Comprehension. The COG battery offers four clusters with reliabilities ranging from .88 for Auditory Processing to .94 for Verbal Abilities (in the Extended Battery).

The test authors have conducted a confirmatory factor analysis which indicated good fit between the organizational structure of the Batería III and the CHC model of cognitive abilities, and have noted that internal factor structure of the Batería III and the WJ III appeared very similar. However, these factor analyses are the only validity data provided in the manual (Otero, 2006).

Despite a norming sample that might at times suffer from small cell sizes and other weaknesses (e.g., poor sampling for specific groups), the thoughtful and proven organization of this test, together with its comparability with the widely used WJ-III, make it a notable and in some instances a useful tool for the Spanish-speaking clinician who is looking for a well-designed instrument to assess cognitive capabilities. The test also covers many aspects of a neuropsychological battery in a single test.

Wechsler Intelligence Scale for Children - Fourth Edition

The original *Wechsler Intelligence Scale for Children* (WISC) was published in 1949 (Wechsler). The original scale (Wechsler, 1949) has undergone three revisions since its original publication, resulting in the publication of the *Wechsler Intelligence Scale for Children - Revised (*WISC-R; Wechsler, 1974), the *Wechsler Intelligence Scale for Children - Third Edition* (WISC- III; Wechsler, 1991), and the most recent, the *Wechsler Intelligence Scale for Children - Fourth Edition* (WISC-IV; Wechsler, 2003). These revisions have each reflected concomitant advances in theoretical models of intelligence, cognitive theory, information processing paradigms, test construction, and professional practice and assessment guidelines. For example, the most recent WISC-IV manual specifically addresses assessment with diverse populations, including the hearing impaired, reflecting standards and guidelines developed by the American Educational Research Association American Psychological Association, and the National Council on Measurement in Education (APA, 1999). The WISC-IV is an individually administered assessment of intellectual abilities for examinees between 6 and 17 years of age (Wechsler, 2003). The current test (WISC-IV) demonstrates significant progress and growth in theories of cognition, test construction, and more specific guidelines for assessment and use (2003). Through researching the trends of the revisions made to the WISC, a basic observation is that the revision cycles have become shorter. This may be due to numerous factors, including the rapidly changing demographic patterns within the U.S. population as noted in Chapter 2, along with attempts to maintain up-to-date normative data. Over time, if the norms are not reestablished, scores may become obsolete and require specific corrections (cf. Flynn, 1984).

Chief revisions in the WISC-IV involved its standardized scores. The WISC-III traditionally followed prior versions of the Wechsler tests in that a Verbal IQ, Performance IQ, and overall Full Scale IQ could be computed based on the subtest scores. The WISC-IV deviated from this model, in that the primary scores became derivatives of the four-factor-based index scores rather than the traditional IQ scores (Wechsler, 2003). The index scores provided by the WISC-IV include Verbal Comprehension Index (VCI), Perceptual Reasoning Index (PRI), Working Memory Index (WMI), and the Processing Speed Index (PSI) (2003). The WISC-IV maintains some traditional features in that it continues to have a general composite score for the entire scale, which is the Full Scale IQ (Wechsler, 2003).

Through revisions of the WISC-III, two subtests were not included in the core battery of WISC-IV, *Picture Arrangement* and *Object Assembly*. These subtests were eliminated from the core battery due to the tasks' generally low reliability. In addition to eliminating these subtests, the WISC-IV added the following subtests: *Matrix Reasoning, Picture Concepts,* and *Word Reasoning* (Wechsler, 2003). These subtests generally assess greater aspects of fluid reasoning, along with the examinee's ability to reason with knowledge and information that is less crystallized and more novel (Wechsler). *Letter-Number Sequencing* and *Cancellation* subtests were also added to the WISC-IV (Wechsler) as measures of Working Memory. Why is the use of subtests that heavily load on fluid reasoning important? Neuropsychologists, in particular, differentiate between crystallized abilities (i.e., WISC-IV, Vocabulary), which are more influenced by education and opportunity, and fluid abilities (i.e., Wechsler Abbreviated Scale of Intelligence (WASI), Matrix Analogies), which are judged to be less dependent on learning. A large number of the intelligence tests currently in use largely assess crystallized abilities, but do not fully assess, if at all, problem-solving skills that define fluid intelligence (Kaufman and Kaufman, 1990). Children and adults from disadvantaged backgrounds typically score lower on measures of crystallized intelligence, but these differences are not as apparent on tasks of fluid reasoning (Campbell, Dollaghan, Needleman, and Janosky, 1997). It is notable that this lack of differences in scores across majority and minority groups are even apparent when examining the nonverbal reasoning subscales (e.g., Block Design) of the Wechsler scales (Reynolds, Willson, and Ramsey, 1999). Yet tests of fluid reasoning (as opposed to subtests of crystalized reasoning) are less known and, until most recently, less commonly utilized. This state of affairs partially is the result of decisions regarding test utilization to determine diagnostic and differential diagnoses as opposed to patterns of a child's individual strengths and weaknesses (see Chapter 8). Because of ethnic differences in measures of crystallized intelligence, some researchers (Das, Naglieri, and Kirby, 1994) have argued for the exclusion of these measures. Others (Hale, Fiorello, Kavanaugh, Hoeppner, and Gaither, 2001), however, have argued that, from a brain-based perspective, the left hemisphere specializes in processing verbal information and crystallized abilities, and therefore instruments that assess these functions should not be eliminated. They therefore recommend the use of crystallized instruments as well as instruments that assess fluid reasoning and stress the importance of integration and careful interpretation of results.

Within the U.S., the Wechsler scales are frequently administered to minority populations for various reasons, yet the use of tests to assess intellectual ability with minority populations remains controversial in certain circles due to concerns of test bias, particularly when the inappropriate assessment postures noted in previous chapters and above are adopted. A consistently stable scientific finding persists throughout the revisions of the WISC concerning the lower performance of Hispanic children relative to nonminority children in the standardization sample. On average, African-American youth score approximately 15 points lower than European-American youth, and Hispanic youth score somewhere between these two groups (Neisser et al., 1996). In group comparisons of the WISC-IV performance, the Hispanic group generally emerged with a reduced performance of 10 points on the Full Scale IQ (FSIQ), and similar reduced scores appear on the Verbal Comprehension Index (VCI) when compared to white non-Hispanic children (Table 4.1). Differences can be reduced to 5 and 6 points on the FSIQ and VCI, respectively, when subjects are matched on age, gender, region of the country, parental education level, and number of parents living in the household (Table 4.2).

Table 4.1 Mean WISC-IV Scores of Hispanic and White Non-Hispanic Children – Data from Standardization Sample

IQ or index scores	Hispanic	White non-hispanic
FSIQ	93.1	103.2
VCI	91.5	102.9
PRI	95.7	102.8
WMI	94.2	101.3
PSI	97.7	101.4

N = 2080.
Source: Adapted from the WISC-IV: Clinical Use and Interpretation. Reprinted by permission.

Table 4.2 Mean WISC-IV Scores of Hispanic and White Non-Hispanic Children Equated for Age, Gender, Number of Parents Living in the Household, Parental Education Level, and U.S. Region – Data from Standardization Sample

IQ or index score	Hispanic	White non-hispanic
FSIQ	95.2	100.0
VCI	93.7	99.7
PRI	97.7	100.3
WMI	95.7	98.7
PSI	97.9	99.6

$N = 161$.
Source: Adapted from the WISC-IV Clinical Use and Interpretation. Reprinted by permission.

Table 4.3 Matched Sample Mean WISC-IV Scores of Spanish versus English-Speaking Hispanic and White Non-Hispanic English Speaking Children (Equated for Age, Gender, and Parental Education Level) – Data from Standardization sample

IQ index score	Hispanic-spanish	Hispanic-english	Non-nispanic white
FSIQ	93.00 (10.95)	96.58 (12.87)	94.12 (15.58)
VCI	92.31 (9.74)	96.19 (13.02)	94.31 (12.06)
PRI	94.50 (12.24)	97.92 (11.54)	96.69 (15.73)
WMI	93.65 (13.07)	96.27 (15.20)	97.42 (15.04)
PSI	98.31 (11.47)	98.27 (13.84)	91.58 (14.23)

$N = 26$.
Source: Adapted from the WISC-IV Clinical Use and Interpretation. Reprinted by permission.

Through a more thorough evaluation of the standardization sample for those who agreed to complete the "WISC-IV Home Environment Questionnaire," 6% of the children were identified as speaking a native language other than English. Of the Hispanic standardization participants who responded to the survey, 34% indicated that English was not the child's native language and nearly all indicated Spanish as the native tongue. The typical finding of reduced performance, particularly in the verbal indices, for Hispanic examinees is now evident only in the group of Hispanic children who speak Spanish as their native language. In fact, although the sample is small, the native English-speaking Hispanic children surpass the nonminority examinees on their Processing Speed Index (Table 4.3).

The *Differential Ability Scale* (DAS; Elliott, 1990) was developed in the United Kingdom to provide "specific information about children's strengths and weaknesses across a range of cognitive domains" (Elliott, 1990, p. 1). Until recently, there has been no research regarding construct validity of the DAS when used with different ethnicities. Keith, Quirk, Schartzer, and Elliott (1999) conducted a confirmatory factor analysis (CFA) in order to determine if the DAS measures the same construct in White, Black, and Hispanic children of all appropriate ages (DAS ranges from 2 to 17). The authors concluded that this in fact is the case, and that the DAS appears to be an appropriate choice when looking for an intelligence measure that is cross-culturally valid (Keith et al., 1999). However, a word of caution is necessary. The issue was initially discussed in Chapter 1, and care must be exercised in interpreting scores from tests that were originally developed in other cultures than the environment in which the test is being administered, so the findings reported by Keith et al., may not be generalized. Although the DAS was recalibrated in the U.S., its original and predecessor scales were developed in the United Kingdom. Therefore, a careful test interpretation approach should prevail when using this test with American populations, including Hispanics. As a result of this criticism, it is important to ask whether such an issue really makes a difference (see Chapters 1 and 6). Such a query is pivotal because if such an issue has no effects on the psychometric properties of an intellectual test or other procedure used during the course of neuropsychological assessment or the inferences derived from them, it has no real bearing on assessment results. Let's examine this issue with the DAS. A close examination at the correlations coefficients between tests of achievements and the DAS demonstrates that the correlations between the DAS (originally developed abroad) and those tests of achievement are far lower, and as noted by Anastasi and Urbina (1997), are below levels for decision making (<.50) than are those correlations between tests such as the WISC (or other tests originally developed in the U.S). Why is that the case? In order to understand the differences, one has to examine two major factors. First, a close examination of each test protocol is required, which easily demonstrates the significant differences between requirements for reading in the DAS (e.g., Word Reading) versus tests developed in the U.S., showing that reading tests for the DAS are far more difficult than reading achievement tests developed in the U.S., predominantly for early levels of academic achievement. The second factor is related to differences in the educational systems of the two countries, particularly during early periods of instruction, and the reader is independently invited to examine such issues. Nevertheless, this example underscores the importance of paying attention to such factors when foreign tests, including tests of intellect developed abroad, are applied with American children, but particularly Hispanic children living in the U.S.

Escala de Inteligencia Revisada para el Nivel Escolar (WISC-RM)

Another procedure that deserves mention is a version of the Wechsler Intelligence Scale for Children adapted and published in Mexico (Escala de Inteligencia Revisada para el Nivel Escolar, WISC-RM; Palacio M., Padilla, and Roll, 1984). This scale was devised to be used with Mexican children and adolescents 6.5 to 16.5 years of age after researchers in Mexico noted that the normative sample curve that emerged from the WISC in the Mexican sample was distinct to the curve that emerged from the American sample (Padilla et al., 1982). The test represents an adaptation of the WISC rather than a translation, with changes in the scales that are representative of Mexican society such as changes in the Information subtest. Overall, the scale parallels the original WISC, including its subtests. The WISC-RM consists of 10 primary subtests, including Information, Picture Completion, Similarities, Picture Arrangement, Arithmetic, Block Design, Vocabulary, Object Assembly, Comprehension, and Coding and two supplementary subtests (Digit Span and Mazes). The statistical properties of the WISC-RM are acceptable, and it is a preferential test to administer to Mexican children born and raised in Mexico, who have recently immigrated to the U.S. from Mexico, or who are monolingual Spanish speakers or most fluent in Spanish. Inferences derived from the test with appropriate populations tend to posses high validity and reliability. Subtest correlations with the Verbal, Performance, and FSIQ indices varied from .65 to .85 and .58 to .76 at the group level, respectively. Correlations between the Verbal and Performance Indices and FSIQ are high (.89 and .88, respectively). Finally, the scale has received wide application in Mexico, and in that sense local norms are sometimes available. The scale may sometimes be used with Hispanic children from Central American regions, particularly those who have resided in Mexico with significant acculturation or whose culture and region is extremely close to Mexican culture. In these cases, nevertheless, caution should be exercised in test interpretation.

The *Naglieri Nonverbal Ability Test* (NNAT; Naglieri, 1997) is a general cognitive ability test that was designed to assess children from grade level K to 12. No reading, writing, or speaking is required by the children; rather, the children respond by pointing to or selecting from complex matrix items. The NNAT was evaluated with regard to differences between ethnic groups (Naglieri and Ronning, 2000). The NNAT was administered to 2,306 "Black" children, 1,176 "White," and 1,176 "Hispanic" children, and only small intergroup differences were found. Naglieri, Booth, and Winsler (2004) investigated whether significant differences in performance could be found between Hispanic children with and without limited English proficiency (LEP). This study analyzed data from a sample of 296 Hispanic children that consisted of two matched groups with 148 LEP children and 148 proficient English speakers. The differences between the two groups were small (effect size $d = 0.1$), indicating that the NNAT can contribute to assessment of bilingual children with scores that will be minimally influenced by language similar to the sample evaluated (Naglieri et al., 2004). Furthermore, good correlations with tests of achievement emerged in this study (Naglieri et al., 2004). However, as pointed out earlier in this chapter, other cultural factors such as the ones identified by Berry (2001) or Sternberg (1997) might still contribute to differential response patterns in Hispanics or other members of minorities.

Other Pediatric/Adolescent/Adult Assessment Measures

The Wechsler Abbreviated Scale of Intelligence

The *Wechsler Abbreviated Scale of Intelligence* (WASI) was published in 1999 and is similar to the traditional Wechsler tests in that it yields a Verbal IQ, Performance IQ, and Full Scale IQ (The Psychological Corporation). The WASI differs from the other Wechsler tests in that it consists of four subtests that provide an estimated assessment of cognitive functioning (The Psychological Corporation, 1999). The Verbal scale consists of two subtests; the *Vocabulary* and *Similarities* subtests; whereas the Performance scale is comprised of *Matrix Reasoning* and *Block Design* subtests (The Psychological Corporation). Administration of the four subtests usually takes approximately 30 minutes to complete and the shortened two-subtest version takes approximately 15 minutes to complete (The Psychological Corporation). The two-subtest version consists of the *Vocabulary* and *Matrix Analogies* (The Psychological Corporation). The WASI is individually administered to examinees from 6 through 89 years of age (The Psychological Corporation). The WASI manual states that this assessment instrument's primary use should be for screening purposes or to evaluate cognitive functioning (The Psychological Corporation). In addition in most instances the WASI should not be utilized for legal or forensic purposes or when a comprehensive assessment of cognitive functioning is required (The Psychological Corporation).

The WASI standardization sample consisted of 2,245 individuals between the ages of 6 to 89 and was considered to be representative of the U.S. English-speaking population (The Psychological Corporation, 1999). However, the normative data appear to be more representative of race than education in the 1997 census data (Salvia and Ysseldyke, 2001). Similar to the WAIS-III and the WISC-IV, the normative sample was not standardized for use with modifications, thus if modifications are utilized they must be noted on the protocol and in the psychological report (The Psychological Corporation).

Some studies demonstrated that the WASI correlates highly with other Wechsler tests, including the WAIS-III and the WISC-III; however, in one study, when the WASI was administered prior to the WAIS-III, the WASI IQs were not predictive of the WAIS-III IQ scores (Axelrod, 2002). Similar findings were found in a study that assessed 72 male patients at a Veterans Affairs Medical Center (Ryan et al., 2003). Finally, the WASI poses difficulties for clinicians, as some subtests responses are inaccurate for adults but given credit by the test publisher because young children provided such answers in the standardization sample (e.g., see responses in Vocabulary [alligator]).

Kaufman Brief Intelligence Test and Kaufman Adolescent and Adult Intelligence Test

The *Kaufman Brief Intelligence Test* (K-BIT) is a short cognitive assessment that takes approximately 20 to 30 minutes to administer (Kaufman and Kaufman, 1990). The K-BIT consists of three subtests, *Expressive Vocabulary* and *Definitions*, which combine to form a Vocabulary standard score and *Matrices*, which forms a different standard score (1990). The K-BIT utilizes the same normative sample as other Kaufman cognitive instruments, including the *Kaufman Adolescent and Adult Intelligence Test* (KAIT) (Kaufman and Kaufman, 1993). The K-BIT can be individually administered to individuals 11 through 85 years of age (Kaufman and Kaufman, 1990).

The KAIT is considered to be a comprehensive assessment of cognitive functioning for adolescents and adults aged 11 through 85 (Kaufman and Kaufman, 1993). The KAIT consists of 10 subtests, with 6 subtests in the core battery and four supplemental subtests (Kaufman and Kaufman).

Stanford-Binet Intelligence Scales, Fifth Edition

The *Stanford-Binet Intelligence Scales, Fifth Edition* (SB5), maintains some aspects of the prior editions, including the rotating assessment of different kinds of abilities through difficulty levels (Roid, 2003). The SB5 differs from its predecessors in that the battery is organized into five factor-related domains consisting of Fluid Reasoning, Knowledge, Quantitative Reasoning, Visual-Spatial Processing, and Working Memory (Roid). Each of these domains consists of a verbal and a nonverbal subtest (Roid). The examiner begins with a verbal subtest *Vocabulary* and a nonverbal subtest *Matrices* (Roid). The examinee's performance on these two subtests directs the examiner on how to proceed with the assessment (Roid). The SB5 provides a Full Scale IQ, Verbal IQ, and Performance IQ scores (Roid). The SB5 is an individually administered assessment of cognitive functioning that can be utilized with examinees between the ages of 2 through 85+ (Roid). The SB5 normative population consisted of 4,800 individuals between the ages of 2 through 85+ (Roid). The normative population matched the 2001 United States Census Bureau in terms of age and demographic region (Roid).

The Wechsler Adult Intelligence Scale - Third Edition

The *Wechsler Adult Intelligence - Third Edition* (WAIS-III) was published in 1997 by the Psychological Corporation (Wechsler). The current WAIS began in 1939 with the publication of the *Wechsler-Bellevue Intelligence Scale* (Wechsler, 1997). After revisions were made to this initial assessment instrument, it was then renamed the *Wechsler Adult Intelligence Scale* and was published in 1955 (1997). Revisions to the WAIS in 1981 resulted in the publication of the WAIS-R. The current WAIS-III is utilized for the assessment of intellectual ability. The WAIS-III is individually administered to adults aged 16 through 89 years (Wechsler).

Upon administration and scoring of the WAIS-III, the traditional three composite IQ scores are generated: Verbal, Performance, and Full Scale (Wechsler, 1997). In addition to these three IQ scores, four index scores can be calculated: Verbal Comprehension, Perceptual Organization, Working Memory, and Processing Speed (Wechsler). The four index scores were an enhancement that was added to the WAIS-III based on revisions of the WAIS-R (Tulskee, Saklofske, Wilkens, and Weiss, 2001). Throughout the WAIS-III manual, equal weight was provided to the IQ and the index scores (Tulskee et al., 2001). The WAIS-III consists of 14 subtests, 11 of which came from the WAIS-R, and three new subtests: *Symbol Search, Matrix Reasoning*, and *Letter-Number Sequencing* (Wechsler, 1997).

Hispanic individuals whose primary language spoken is not English may be at a disadvantage on the Verbal subtests of the WAIS-III, thus obtaining deflated intellectual quotients (Wechsler, 1997). This low performance may be an underestimate of the examinee's actual cognitive abilities and may be attributed to differences in language (Wechsler). According to the WAIS-III manual, some individuals may require modifications of the test procedures; however, the WAIS-III was not standardized for use with modifications (Wechsler). When modifications are necessary, the examiner should be informed of and follow the general principle of test use that has been established by the *Standards for Educational and Psychological Testing* (American Psychological Association, 1985):

> When a test user makes a substantial change in test format, mode of administration, instructions, language, or content the user should revalidate the use of the test for changed conditions or have a rationale supporting the claim that additional validation is not necessary or possible. (Standard 6.2, p 41).

This standard applies to the assessment of the Hispanic population when their primary mode of communication is not English or when they are deemed as not proficient in English. When modifications are utilized, including translation of tasks to Spanish or modified instructions, they may affect the test scores, which may then raise questions about the validity of the scores. If modifications are utilized, it is then important to note them on the record form and again in the psychological report (Wechsler 1997).

The WAIS-III normative data was collected on individuals who speak English fluently (Wechsler, 1997). The standardization sample for the WAIS-III consisted of 2,450 adults 16 through 89 years of age (Kaplan and Saccuzzo, 1997). These individuals were then broken down into 13 different groups based on age: 16 to 17, 18 to 19, 20 to 24, 25 to 29, 30 to 34, 35 to 44, 45 to 54, 55 to 64, 65 to 69, 70 to 74, 75 to 79, 80 to 84, and 85 to 89 (Kaplan and Saccuzzo). All of the specific aged groups consisted of 200 participants with the exception of two groups aged 80 to 84 and 85 to 89 that were comprised of 150 and 100 subjects, respectively (Kaplan and Saccuzzo, 1997). The sample was selected to correspond well to the U.S. Census in terms of gender (Kaplan and Saccuzzo, 1997). If the WAIS-III is translated to the examinee's native language, this may invalidate the normative information (Wechsler, 1997). The WAIS-III manual states that in situations similar to that described above "use your clinical judgment to evaluate performance in circumstances where translation of directions is necessary for completion of a given task" (Wechsler, 1997, p 34).

Geriatric Population

Since persons of Hispanic heritage form the most rapidly growing minority group in the U.S., the geriatric segment of the overall population is also experiencing a significant diversification (LaRue, Romero, Ortiz, Liang, and Lindeman, 1999). One of the main tasks in geriatric neuropsychology is to distinguish normal from abnormal aging processes (Rosselli and Ardila, 2001), especially for differential diagnoses or rule-outs of dementias such as Alzheimer's disease (AD) with other conditions such as mood disturbances. Compared with non-Hispanic Whites, Hispanics who live in the U.S. have been found to show a mean onset of AD symptoms more than 6 years earlier, even if matched for education, gender, and location (Clark et al., 2005). At this point, it is unclear if a similar prevalence or incidence rate of AD can be expected in the Hispanic population (LaRue et al., 1999).

As Lopez and Taussig (1991) point out, the conflict between emic and etic approaches to assessment becomes evident in testing of elderly populations. Older Hispanic clients, foreign or U.S. born, are more often less fluent in English, adhere more closely to a culturally different worldview, and frequently have not been exposed to extensive education, which mediates differences in cognitive development.

Clinicians face the choice of using etic instruments such as the WAIS for assessment, which carries with it the risk of underestimating cognitive performance in elderly Hispanics, and emic instruments such as the EIWA (Wechsler, 1968). Lopez and Taussig (1991)'s study demonstrated that emic measures tend to overestimate performance in elderly Hispanics much as the etic instruments biases results in the other direction. Additionally, both tests did not cause over- or underestimation across different samples and tasks but instead exhibited more pronounced errors in certain subgroups and subtests. Thus, the authors conclude that assessment must not rely on scores from one test but should draw upon multiple data sources, including history, behavioral observation, and a variety of tests. Furthermore, clinicians must be aware of each instrument's inherent flaws regarding certain populations and refrain from simply administering a standard battery to all clients – another example of how aspirational ethics influence neuropsychological assessment with Hispanic clients (cf. Ardila, 2005; APA, 2001; Artiola i Fortuny and Mullaney, 1998).

Cultural standards influence the definition of what is "normal" and useful for assessment of Hispanic clients. While utilization of an etic test might be useful to gain information about placement options in specific elderly programs or legal stipulations, classification of what is impaired cognitive functioning may be much more dependent on emic cultural standards.

Norms for elderly Hispanic populations are still lacking (LaRue et al, 1999; Rosselli and Ardila, 2001) but are currently being developed (e.g., Mungas et al., 2005). LaRue and colleagues (1999) provide preliminary norms for a neuropsychological battery suitable for assessing the cognitive decline typically observed in AD in Hispanics, including the Digit Forward Task, the Fuld Object Memory Test (Fuld, 1981), Verbal Fluency, Clock Drawing, and Color Trails 1 and 2. Rosselli and Ardila (2001) offer an overview of tests that have been used with the elderly Hispanic population.

Cognitive Status

Instruments to determine mental status are among the most frequently used to screen for dementia. While these instruments tend to be short and typically do not contain complex items, they usually have been translated into Spanish without extensive back-translation or more advanced procedures used in test adaptation. Furthermore, clinicians tend to prefer a version they have used for a while, which has led to some variability regarding exactly what questions are asked (Mejia, Gutierrez, Villa, and Ostrosky-Solis, 2004).

A Spanish version of the Minimental Status Exam was examined by this group of researchers because the original version (Folstein, Folstein, and McHugh, 1975) is one of the most frequently used instruments for detection of dementia (Mejia et al., 2004). When administered to a sample of Spanish-speaking elderly that had previously been categorized as normal, mild cognitive impairment (MCI), or dementia patients, the MMSE mean of the normal group was 20, which is below the established impairment cutoff point of 23. Level of education was found to function as an important moderator in this study (Mejia et al., 2004), so that clinicians relying on the MMSE will misdiagnose individuals with low education as demented. As Rosselli and Ardila point out, low academic achievement is more likely a result of economic factors when found in Hispanics, and less likely associated with failure to adapt to the academic environment, than with non-Hispanic Whites (Rosselli and Ardila, 2001). They also note that one typical item from mental status exams, "What season is it?," might be of less relevance for orientation in Hispanics from tropical or subtropical countries (Rosselli and Ardila, 2001).

One approach to dealing with the many cultural influences on neuropsychological measures is to employ functional measures instead (Rosselli and Ardila, 2001). However, even this is a poor solution, since many functional skills may be viewed by Hispanic elderly as limited to (for example) one gender, such as cooking or managing money (Rosselli and Ardila, 2001).

Summary and Conclusions

After providing a brief overview of the historical roots (see Sattler 2001 for a more comprehensive review) of cognitive assessment, classic theories of intelligence were reviewed, including those of Carroll, Cattell, Horn, Spearman, and Sternberg. Special emphasis was placed on the role of cultural factors in these influential theories. Emic and etic approaches were described, and recent attempts to integrate these were introduced. The literature relevant to these questions seems to indicate that complete generality and equivalence of a "g" factor cannot be assumed across all cultures. More complex and modern models of intelligence, such as those proposed by Sternberg and Berry, are more comprehensive and better account for cultural factors. Also, specific models of influences on cognitive functioning in Hispanics have been suggested by researchers, including variables such as acculturation, language proficiency, and immigration patterns, as noted in previous chapters in this volume and as elucidated above.

Recent data regarding the use of tests with Hispanic populations were reported. Even though research suggests that language proficiency and cultural status strongly influence performance on cognitive and neuropsychological tests, many clinicians reportedly continue to utilize tests in a way that may yield biased results. The use of appropriate norms is an important problem in this regard, but difficult challenges emerge as a result of the heterogeneity of the Hispanic population.

A broad range of assessment instruments was briefly reviewed, as were their applicability to Hispanic children, adolescents, and adults and specific instruments suitable for the elderly Hispanic population. Although significant advances have been made in instrumentation in the last decade, a great deal of work remains ahead. In particular, advances in instrumentation with established, appropriate norms and psychometric properties remain to be constructed that will lead to valid and reliable inferences with Hispanics.

In conclusion, a review of the extant literature supports a view of intellectual assessment with Hispanics that is complex, dynamic, and challenging to clinicians and researchers alike. Despite greater understanding of such factors, the range of variables that influence performance on tests of cognitive abilities has continued to grow in recent years, while the development of instruments that take these variables into account has lagged behind despite best efforts by test developers and publishers. However, it is encouraging to see the recent publications of sophisticated assessment instruments and up-to-date norms.

Chapter 5
Language: Development, Bilingualism, and Abnormal States

Christine French and Antolin M. Llorente

Language is a common denominator in all settings, including social relationships, education, and professional interactions. According to Warner and Nelson (2000), "a language is built through orderly combinations of linguistic symbols into words, sentences, and discourse." Language is what truly sets humans apart from other animals in that we have a pattern of vocalizations that produce effects on the listener and allow individuals to interpret their world through verbal means. In this regard, the outstanding social sciences philosopher D. C. Dennett (1978) has brilliantly noted that it is linguistic skills that allow humans to "generate" and "test" hypotheses inside their brains without the need to expose their organisms to situations that may represent peril, unlike animals without language. In other words, presupposing the absence of executive dysfunction, language allows for the formulation of testable hypotheses inside our minds without the need of exposure to dangerous circumstances, providing for species preservation, consistent with evolutionary theory (cf. Darwin, 1967). Our experiences are richer and fuller due to the capacity we have to communicate and understand language. In some instances, individuals with language difficulties are less able to effectively share their experiences or do not learn new skills nearly as efficiently as individuals without such difficulties. Whether language develops normally with intact hearing and speech processes, or with a significant hearing deficit that induces parents to teach their child sign language, verbal and nonverbal language continues to be the means by which experiences are predominantly shared between individuals. Finally, as we saw in Chapters 1 and 2, language is a critical issue for Hispanic populations and is at the core of cultural differences in these individuals.

This chapter will encompass important aspects of language development, including general markers and milestones for the various stages of language development. Information regarding the specific nuances of monolingual and bilingual language development also will be briefly discussed. A section of this chapter will be devoted to discussing language disorders, their related impairments, and the underlying brain structures that may have been affected. This chapter will include a discussion about the different types of language disorders, with specific content covering the more common aphasias and less well-known disorders. Lastly, it will examine common language evaluation practices and diagnostic procedures, including a review of some of the commonly used and psychometrically sound measures that will be helpful to clinicians evaluating specific language impairments in Hispanic populations in the U.S. and abroad.

Language Development

The development of language during maturation is a fascinating time in a young child's life. Parents might observe their child having an extreme burst of language development during a short period of time, often around their first birthday. Other times, their child might appear stagnant in the attainment of language skills, yet normal language development emerges. Language development is often a yardstick used by parents, pediatricians, physicians and teachers to decide whether or not an adult or a child is suffering from a language disturbance or developing language appropriately. As a result of its overt nature, it is not surprising, then, that a majority of neuropsychological evaluation referrals of adults and children, regardless of culture, are due to concerns with language functions or its development.

Although there is a relatively narrow developmental window in which language acquisition takes place (Comrie, 2000), there is tremendous variability in the language development of very young children (Warner and Nelson, 2000), and such variability may be considered the result of the dynamic interaction between the child and her environment (Evans, 2001). Although the first birthday is the traditional marker for single word usage, late development (e.g., 14 months) should in no way be the diagnostic criterion for the diagnosis of a language delay or impairment.

There are many distinct aspects to any spoken language. Language incorporates rules of morphology, phonology, syntax, semantics, and pragmatics (Bates, Thal, Finlay, and Clancy, 2003; Eisenson, 1984; Warner and Nelson, 2000). All of these rules are combined and overplayed on general language learning. Although children are not cognizant of the fact that learning to raise their voices at the end of a question is a rule of morphology, most often they will nevertheless learn to engage in conversation that fits each of these rules, particularly for their specific language, and in this way are impacted by their culture. In fact, Warner and Nelson (2000) note that only when each of these rules is mastered can a person fully appreciate all of the nuances of language.

Language development, to the lay person, is a mysterious and seemingly simple pattern of a child hearing words and being able to emulate them after some successive approximations of the words. However, under that crop of unruly hair, there is tremendous growth and maturation occurring in the child's brain. As most readers of this chapter will already know, there is a remarkable level of activity occurring in a child's brain that aids in the development of language (Bates, Thal, Finlay, and Clancy, 2003). Even before birth, cells are generated and incoming sensory pathways are developed, although outgoing connections are still undergoing development at birth and thereafter (Bates, Thal, Finlay, and Clancy, 2003). The brain is engaging in continuous activity of cell division and migration. Following birth, neuronal migration, synaptogenesis, proliferation, apoptosis, and synapse elimination are primary activities. Neuronal axons and dendrites simultaneously extend outward to connect different areas in the brain. Also, glial cells form a fatty sheath (i.e., myelin) to insulate these connections (Mushi, 2002), which facilitates efficient processing. During this flurry of brain development, a child is undergoing significant and observable development in many areas, including language development, motor development, and general association to their environment; however, this development does not necessarily directly coincide or result from neural events (Bates, Thal, Finlay, and Clancy, 2003). For language development to progress, there is an underlying assumption that there must be a functional connection between neurons in the language centers of the brain (Evans, 2001). In fact, neuronal development and connectivity may be the underlying factor influencing the differences between individual language development, even among monozygotic twins. Furthermore, much of neuronal development and connectivity is largely influenced by environmental factors, again accounting for differences in individual language development. As there are many texts that provide a very inclusive description of the physiological changes in the brain regarding cell division, migration, myelination, and neuro-chemical development, this chapter will not attempt to expound in this area. Rather, the interested reader is directed to peruse these texts (cf. Kolb and Fantie, 1997).

After discussing the processes of neuronal growth and development, it is imperative to highlight other important broader functions and variables that facilitate language development. These functions include the development of motor, perceptual, and symbolic abilities (Kolb and Fantie, 1997). At the same time, language development is impacted not only by neuronal growth and development, but by general development of the temporal and frontal cortices, which house language centers and circuits in the brain, including the perisylvian language arc (Kaufman, 2001). In reviewing the important functions that facilitate successful language development, the first process that should be noted is motor development. The ability to form words by controlling the facial and oral musculature is a complex process. Being able to move the tongue to control air volume and have appropriate placement behind the teeth to say "da da" is taken for granted by those with appropriate language development.

A second function that clearly affects language development is the maturation of perceptual skills. Without identifying words and phrases as meaningful combinations of sounds and syllables, it would be impossible to comprehend and express meaningful language. The development of formulating and understanding sounds as a means of information communication necessitates a child understanding them as symbols. To identify and then be able to understand the group of sounds as meaningful depend significantly on a child's ability to perceive and make sense of his or her environment. These perceptual skills are just as important as motor development in the facilitation of language. In fact, a person may never develop the motor capacities to have appropriate expression of language via verbal means; nevertheless, this person may still have developed the necessary perceptual skills and abilities to be able to comprehend what others say and to express their thoughts, although perhaps through alternative means (i.e., sign language, writing).

After reviewing the specific biological functions that must develop in order for language development to occur, it is necessary to review a vital variable that can significantly impact a brain's capacity for language development, namely environmental factors and their effects on the biological processes previously listed. The nature versus nurture argument is centuries old and continues today. Many take the position that all development is determined by the genetic and biological makeup of the individual. Others take the position that an individual's development is open to tremendous influence by external factors, such as sensory stimulation and nutrition, among many others. However, external factors work in combination with general biological factors and likely have a cumulative effect on an individual's development. Kolb and Fantie (1997) suggest that environmental stimulation has a significant effect on the biological substrates of language, including neuronal development. Poor environmental stimulation might delay myelination or decrease dendritic connections. These differences will likely cause a delay or impairment in general development, including that of language.

As can be seen, the processes necessary for a child to begin to attain language skills are complex regardless of cultural or ethnic background. Beginning very early on, neurons begin their migration and proliferation to the areas of the brain for which they are destined. Pruning, apoptosis, and myelination further facilitate the language development process, while making the necessary connections between the language centers of the brain. While these microscopic changes are made, further growth of the cortices occurs, providing the child with the necessary building blocks on which language skills rely.

Developmental Milestones and Language Acquisition

After perusing many texts that expound on the development of language, one might perceive language development to be incremental in nature, occurring in discrete stages. However, this simplification of the language development process does not take into consideration the fluidity and complex process of expressive and receptive language development. Nevertheless, a discussion of language development as an increasingly complex and cumulative process will facilitate a greater understanding of its course and progression. Readers of this section should be reminded that language development is divided into stages based on age only for ease of discussion and that allowances should be made for individual variability. In fact, individual variability of language acquisition can range over many months (Bates, Thal, Finlay, and Clancy, 2003); therefore, the following text should not be construed as diagnostic criteria, but rather as a simple guideline to understand general language development. Table 5.1 should be used as a quick reference guide to general developmental milestone expectations.

Neonates are not known for their conversational proficiency; however, this is not to say that they do not communicate with their environment. Many students of language development agree that infants are born into the world prepared to acquire language (e.g., Bates, Thal, Finlay, and Clancy, 2003; Chomsky, 1991; Stuart, 2002; Tager-Flusberg and Sullivan, 1998). In fact, infants are very adept at influencing and

Table 5.1 Early Language Developmental Expectations

Approximate age of onset	Language function/behavior
Birth	–Reflexive vocalizations tied to diffuse feeling states
	–Vegetative sounds
	–Emotional-prosodic in quality
6 weeks	–Cooing and pleasure noises
	–Differentiated cries
	–Responds to voice
2 months	–Defined babbling with oral-motor exploration
	–Distinguishes different speech sounds
3 months	–Orients head to voice
	–Vocal response to speech
	–Vocalizes two different vowel sounds
4 months	–Cries reflect specific feeling states
	–Increased frequency of imitative babbling
	–Imitates tone
	–Varies pitch of vocalizations
6 months	–Babbling with consonant use
	–Laughs out loud
	–Prosodic imitations of speech
8 months	–Canonical babbling with temporal-sequential properties imitative of true speech
	–Production of word-like sounds
	–Vocalizes three different vowel sounds
	–Inhibition of nonnative language sounds
	–Defined pitch, tone, and prosody
	–Comprehension of simple words and commands
11–13 months	–True production of words
	–Vocalizes four different vowel-consonant combinations
	–Gestures accompany word production
	–Comprehends some gestures
	–Follows simple one-step commands
	–Points to objects when asked "show me"
18–20 months	–Two-word phrases
	–Naming explosion
	–Increased use of different type of words (nouns, verbs, adjectives)
24 months	–Increased verbal fluency
	–Use of more complex phrases using nouns and other word types
	–Understands and responds to yes/no and wh- questions
28 months	–Three-word phrases
	–Increase in grammatically correct utterances
36 months	–Development of egocentric speech
	–Production of 3- to 4-word phrases
	–Uses pronouns
	–Understands concept of "one"
	–Understands two prepositions
	–Follows two-step commands

Adapted from Bates, Thal, Finlay, and Clancy (2003); Bayley (1993); Eisenson, 1984; Kolb and Fantie (1997); Sattler (1998); and Warner and Nelson (2003).

being influenced by their surroundings, to which new parents can readily attest (Taylor, 1999). Nevertheless, much of their communication is reflexive. That is, vocalizations made by very young infants (birth to approximately three months of age) are reflexive and occur as a result of diffuse feeling states (Bates, Thal, Finlay, and Clancy, 2003; Eisenson, 1984). Their physical being is uncomfortable in some way, whether this lack of comfort is represented by hunger pangs or elevated temperature. They reflexively verbalize their lack of homeostasis by crying or making another similar verbalization. As stated by Joseph (1996), these random vocalizations typically are "emotional-prosodic in quality and mediated by limbic and brainstem nuclei" (p. 128). Neonates have very little awareness of their surroundings unless they somehow infringe on their homeostasis. If a blanket covers the eyes, a diaper is wet, or if the child is startled, the child reflexively vocalizes in order to have the uncomfortable stimuli removed. As such, the attitudes of accepting or rejecting are the only feeling states an infant under one month of age experiences and reacts in an attempt to return to homeostasis by removing the uncomfortable stimuli in favor of pleasing stimuli (Joseph, 1996). Undifferentiated cries and other vocalizations, commonly referred to as *coos* (Kolb and Fantie, 1997) characterize this prespeech period, or prelocutionary stage (Stuart, 2002), and are precursors to an infant's development of more accurate and differentiated speech sounds (Tager-Flusberg and Sullivan, 1998).

By two to three months of age, infants continue to engage in much random vocalization in response to their individual needs (Joseph, 1996). However, more defined babbling begins to emerge, although it is better explained by accidental motor activity and positively reinforcing activity rather than purposeful approximations of speech (Joseph, 1996). This early babbling could be construed as a means of "testing the waters" as infants experiment with the sounds they can make with their tongue, lips, and mouth (Bates, Thal, Finlay, and Clayson, 2003). It is an "important developmental precursor to meaningful speech" (Oller, 1986), and it is "strongly influenced by biological mechanisms underlying the language-articulatory system" (Oller, Eilers, Steffens, Lynch, and Urbano, 1994). According to Sattler (1998), infants should be able to vocalize two separate vowel sounds by three months of age. Again, these vowel sounds, although they may sound like words to eager parents, are little more than accidental verbalizations produced by the interplay between an infant's random oral motor activity.

After the first several months of a child's life, a distinct change in the vocalizations of the infant occurs. Although much of an infant's vocalizations continue to be random and reflexive, they begin to reflect certain feeling states instead of a general lack of homeostasis (Joseph, 1996). In fact, many parents report that they can decipher the differences between their child's cries at this stage. Distinct cries and vocalizations serve different purposes, such as relating causes of discomfort (i.e., hunger, wetness, tiredness), requesting a goal or desired object, and interacting with others (Tager-Flusberg and Sullivan, 1998). As these vocalizations are more tied to specific stimuli, they begin to interact with their world in a qualitatively different manner. In fact, being able to influence and interact with their environment is a significant motivating factor in language learning (Bates, Thal, Finlay, and Clancy, 2003; Tager-Flusberg and Sullivan, 1998).

Not only do the vocalizations of a three- to four-month-old infant begin to represent specific feelings, they also begin to take on a quality of imitation. That is, their attempts at verbalization are successive approximations of what is said to them and they imitate the sound patterns of the child's native language (Bates, Thal, Finlay, and Clancy, 2003; Eisenson, 1984; Dronkers, Pinker, and Damasio, 2000). There is likely to be a rapid change in the number and type of verbalizations that an infant of this age expresses (Kolb and Fantie, 1997). As this exploration of oral-motor capabilities continues to increase through about 12 months of age, children become more aware of how their verbalizations impact the environment and their caregivers' responses to their verbalizations. However, they continue to respond to the emotional qualities of their caregivers' verbalizations rather than the content (Joseph, 1996).

As Bates and colleagues (Bates, Thal, Finlay, and Clancy, 2003) describe it, the time period from 8 to 10 months of age is a type of "watershed." They noted that this time period is marked by quantitative and qualitative change in phonological development, canonical babbling, clear and purposeful inhibition of nonnative language sounds, and language comprehension. At the same time that an infant's vocalizations increase to more closely approximate the speech sounds they hear, they are also inhibiting speech sounds that are not in their native language (Bates, Thal, Finlay, and Clancy, 2003; Dronkers, Pinker, and Damasio, 2000). It becomes apparent to caregivers that as the quantity of verbalizations continues to increase during this stage, the quality of an infant's vocalizations also changes. The pitch, tone, and prosody also take on a more definitive quality (Bates, Thal, Finlay, and Clancy, 2003; Kolb and Fantie, 1997). Some babbling, according to Joseph (1996), becomes more than simply reflexive and emotional, carrying possible meaning and changing to "temporal-sequential language" (p. 130). Stuart (2002) identified this period as the beginning of the illocutionary stage. These distinct changes in vocalization are related to significant growth and development of the major language pathways in the left hemisphere. The major language pathways lie in and around the perisylvian arc; the arcuate fasciculus links the two major language centers, Broca's area and Wernicke's area (Damasio and Damasio, 2000; Dronkers, Pinker, and Damasio, 2000). These connections are made possible by rapidly developing dendritic growth and myelination throughout the cortices.

This time period also involves a tremendous increase in word comprehension (Bates, Thal, Finlay, and Clancy, 2003). It is during this stage that children recognize and respond to their own name, understand when a parent says "no," and can engage in simple actions, such as "patty cake" and "high five," or for Hispanic children, "la viejita," upon command. After the initial comprehension of words, a child's comprehension of language develops about three months ahead of a child's expression of language (Warner and Nelson, 2000).

Language learning and imitation assumes that fact that a child is remembering or recalling what was previously heard. Although memory is not typically thought of as necessary for language development, Bates and colleagues point out that language learning is facilitated by memory (Bates, Thal, Finlay, and Clancy, 2003). The process of hearing and then storing, encoding, and recalling verbalizations in their correct context is very dependent on the memory process. Not only do a child's verbalizations depend on memory, a child's comprehension of spoken language also relies on memory processes. In order to truly comprehend what is said to them, they must be able to adeptly recall the meaning or categorization of the word or words presented to them.

Somewhere between a child's first birthday and 18 months of age, their vocalizations and verbalizations begin to mimic what might otherwise be called "true speech" or "anticipatory language" (Bates, Thal, Finlay, and Clancy, 2003; Eisenson, 1984; Kolb and Fantie, 1997). Words are no longer secondary to gestures, but become primary in a child's communication repertoire. This is the beginning of the locutionary stage (Stuart, 2002). At this time, a "naming explosion" typically occurs in which there is rapid growth in the quantity of words produced (Tager-Flusberg and Sullivan, 1998; Warner and Nelson, 2000). According to Bates and colleagues, the naming explosion, also known as a vocabulary burst, occurs when a child has attained about 50 words (Bates, Thal, Finlay, and Clancy, 2003). At first, a child is able to name numerous concrete objects, including their parents, siblings, and common play toys. Their interaction with the world becomes more heavily based on language compared to their previous use of gestures and other vocalizations. As previously noted, about three months prior to their ability to express their first words, children are typically able to comprehend simple words (Warner and Nelson, 2000).

Around 18 months of age, a child's utterances become slightly more complex, typically increasing in length of utterance from single words to two-word utterances (Tager-Flusberg and Sullivan, 1998). There is also a notable increase of types of words. When a child utters his or her first word, it is typically a noun, some kind of concrete object, and such a finding may be cross-cultural. However, at this point, children increase their vocabulary to include other words, including verbs, adjectives, and relational terms (Bates, Thal, Finlay, and Clancy, 2003). This qualitative change incorporates several different facets of language development, including phrase complexity and fluency. Two-word phrases typically emerge slightly before a child's second birthday, but some research has shown that children begin to combine words when their vocabulary exceeds 50 words (Bates, Thal, Finlay, and Clancy, 2003; Tager-Flusberg and Sullivan, 1998). Rapid advances in word fluency and semantic development are also noted (Bates, Thal, Finlay, and Clancy, 2003; Stuart, 2002).

This process of quickly acquiring a greater quantity and quality of speech production and comprehension continues to occur through a child's second birthday and beyond. According to Warner and Nelson (2000), an 18-month-old child engages in approximately two communicative acts per minute, adding about five words per day until age six. This communication frequency quickly increases to approximately five communicative acts per minute by 24 months of age, and children of this age are typically able to produce any where from 150 to over 300 words (Bates, Thal, Finlay, and Clancy, 2003). Interestingly, about three-quarters of what a child says at two years of age can be understood by caregivers and other adults (Warner and Nelson, 2000). Children at this stage are able to produce correct phonemes and can frequently engage in conversation, albeit simple, with peers and adults.

More complex speech development typically begins occurring sometime after a child's second birthday and involves increases in syntax and pragmatics (Eisenson,

1984). Although they continue to make significant gains in the quantity of words they are able to produce, children in this stage also make significant gains in the quality of their communication. By two and a half years of age, children typically have about 500 words in their lexicon from which to draw, many of which are nouns and concrete objects. An increasing percentage of other words, such as verbs, prepositions, and the like, are used on a more frequent basis (Bates, Thal, Finlay, and Clancy, 2003; Fenson et al., 1994; Warner and Nelson, 2000).

After children acquire the foundational skills for language by three years of age, they begin engaging in what could be termed "true language." According to Joseph (1996), true language incorporates verbal language production of words, including concrete nouns and more abstract relational terms, adjectives, and prepositions. True language at this age involves thinking words out loud, which coincides with the development of egocentric speech. This type of "thinking out loud" is also known as "egocentric speech" and usually involves "self-directed self-explanatory monologue" (Joseph, 1996). Many a caregiver has unobtrusively observed a child playing alone, dictating his actions out loud. As the child matures, this egocentric speech turns inward and develops into thought (Joseph, 1996).

By entrance into these early childhood years, often signified by enrollment in preschool, children begin to use their language skills to categorize and control their environment (Kolb and Fantie, 1997). Now that the young child is exposed to adults and same-age peers, even further language development occurs. They begin to experience the importance of knowing and being sensitive to their listener (Bates, Thal, Finlay, and Clancy, 2003; Tager-Flusberg and Sullivan, 1998). Three-year-old children learn the rules of communication, which involved turn-taking and pragmatics (Tager-Flusberg and Sullivan, 1998; Warner and Nelson, 2000). As they are exposed to more formal educational practices and cultural experiences children of this age typically are viewed as making rapid strides in grammar, semantics, and syntax (Bates, Thal, Finlay, and Clancy, 2003; Tager-Flusberg and Sullivan, 1998; Warner and Nelson, 2000).

Beyond the preschool years, children continue to make significant strides in language development. However, many of the changes made are likely to be much less apparent to caregivers. By age six, children typically have access to approximately 14,000 words. However, the way they combine the words and the length of their utterances may continue to grow quite significantly through the early school years. Formal training in grammar (morphology and syntax), semantics, and pragmatics further increase language development and conversational efficiency (Bates, Thal, Finlay, and Clancy, 2003).

Bilingualism and Variations in Language Acquisition

As some may assume, all developmental markers of language acquisition are not necessarily exactly the same among different languages and cultures or ethnic groups. Therefore, Table 5.1, indicating specific language developmental milestones may not be applicable to all languages and many clinicians and researchers assert that language milestones vary in nature and timing depending on the language being acquired (Bates, Thal, Finlay, and Clancy, 2003; Choi, 1999; Crago and Allen, 1999). However, others have indicated that the language milestones and developmental trajectories should be considered similar for different languages (Bedore, 1999; Fortin and Crago, 1999; Shonkoff and Phillips, 2000) and for achievement of language developmental milestones during simultaneous language acquisition (Petitto and Holowka, 2002). Prelinguistic language markers may be similar between languages, especially between English and Spanish (Bedore, 1999). However, general babbling may have wide variations depending on the child's native language. For instance, children learning Spanish and Italian meet certain language developmental milestones sooner because the phonological system is less complex than the English phonological system (Holm, Dodd, Stow, and Pert, 1999; Leonard, 1999; Rhodes, Kayser, and Hess, 2000). Different languages also have other factors that affect language development, including morphology, inflection, word order, grammar, syntax, honorifics, and tone (Bedore, 1999; Fortin and Crago, 1999; Leonard, 1999). All of these factors are also influenced by a child's exposure to a second or third language (Leonard, 1999; Rhodes, Kayser, and Hess, 2000). (For efficiency and ease of discussion, Spanish is used to denote a second language.)

Bilingualism is a special case of language development. Multiple languages can be learned simultaneously or sequentially. Regardless of the inherent benefits of being bilingual, many individuals, including those that have frequent contact with limited English-proficient students, have erroneous beliefs and negative perceptions of limited English-proficient and bilingual individuals. It is clear that there are many individuals in the nation's schools and workplaces who have limited proficiency in English or are bilingual. In fact, in the mid-1990s, 7% of students enrolled in schools in the United States (Taylor, 1999) and in excess of 18% of individuals in the workplace had limited English proficiency.

Just as it is assumed that an infant is born into the world prepared for language development (Comrie, 2000), it also must be understood that the brain is not limited to the acquisition of only one language. The "single space theory" contends that there is not enough "room" in the brain for more than one language. This argument leads to further assumptions that learning more than one language will actually compromise or crowd other abilities at the cost of multiple language acquisition and development (Mushi, 2002).

Acquisition of a second language does not differ significantly from development of language in general (Hamayan and Damico, 1991; Krashen, 1982); however, some distinguish between language acquisition and language learning, indicating that the latter occurs due to a conscious effort of learning the rules of a second language, whether by implicit or explicit means (Krashen, 1982; Rosa and Leow, 2004). As with infants who approximate speech sounds by mimicking others, second language learners form habits based on what they hear others say. Students in high school Spanish classes can often be heard repeating over and over, "¿Como está? Bien, gracias. ¿Y tu?" (How are you? Fine, thank you. And you?). This automatic habit formation is the foundation for language learning (Hamayan and

Damico, 1991). Second language acquisition also involves conscious rule learning (Rosa and Leow, 2004), similar to what toddlers and preschool age children learn in their interactions with peers and adults and through formal instruction. Individuals learning a second language learn proper grammar and phonology through active learning (S.H. Ochoa, personal communication, 2000). Through social interactions with peers, there also is a phase of natural acquisition of meaningful language. As Krashen (1982) noted, children learn a new language by doing. Therefore, single words will increase to phrases, even though there will be developmental errors and the interference of verbal habits from the first language (S.H. Ochoa, personal communication, 2000). The more an individual engages in any skill, the more proficient he or she will become.

The definition of a bilingual individual has many different facets which are important to understand, especially when interacting with or teaching bilingual individuals. A person can be bilingual through sequential (coordinate) or simultaneous (compound) means (Mushi, 2002; Quinn, 2001). Simultaneous bilinguals grow up learning two languages at once. Simultaneous bilinguals could have grown up in homes where one parent spoke English and the other parent spoke Spanish to the child (Mushi, 2002). They could have been exposed to both languages by one parent. Either way, simultaneous language learners develop two languages simultaneously (Mushi, 2002). Contrary to what many lay individuals might assume, simultaneous acquisition of two languages does not differ significantly from single language development and there is little evidence of negative effects (Krashen, 1982). However, simultaneous bilingual development is typically four to five months behind monolingual language development, at least until the early school years when the child is able to catch up to their single-language-learning peers (Hamayan and Damico, 1991). Simultaneous language learners will tend to outperform their sequential language-learning peers (Collier, 1995). However, it is important to note that the individual must reach a certain level of proficiency in both languages before positive effects can be observed (Cummins, 1979; Cascallar and Arnold, 2001).

Sequential, or successive, language learners vary greatly in the reasons and contexts in which they learn a second language. Some second language learners "elect" to learn the language for purposes of upward mobility and the need to belong or to meet academic expectations or educational programming criteria (cf. Mushi, 2002). Individuals in these categories may decide to enroll in an English-as-a-second-language class as an adolescent or adult. In contrast, circumstantial language learners have to learn the second language in order to achieve minimum expectancies for success in a society ("to survive") or to meet purposes other than those their native language can serve (cf. Mushi, 2002). This is the case for many groups that have been displaced from their home country for whatever reason, or groups of immigrants as noted in Chapter 2.

The rate and means at which individuals learn a second language also vary greatly. Although children might be exposed to English during classroom instruction, they may continue to use their native language during recess or lunch, thereby reducing their exposure to the second language. As Quinn (2001) notes, this has a significant impact on the time it takes a child to become proficient in a second language. Research also has shown the individuals acquiring a second language in a sequential manner follow a different grammatical sequence of learning compared to development of their native language (Quinn, 2001). Although many individuals may hold a false hypothesis that children quickly learn a new language when immersed in an environment that requires use of a second language, research has shown that this is not the case. Collier (1995) discovered that children who had no formal schooling in their native language prior to enrolling in an English-speaking school required 7 to 10 years to reach the same level of language competence in English. Children who had previous education in their native language and then enrolled in an English immersion setting required 5 to 7 years to attain second language proficiency (Collier, 1005; Cummins, 1981).

There are multiple factors that affect proficiency in a second language (Cascallar and Arnold, 2001; Hamayan and Damico, 1991; Taylor, 1999). At the very basic level, cognitive ability and learning style will greatly affect an individual's ability to learn a second language. As can be assumed, an individual's affect and personality, including their attitude toward the second language and their motivation to learn it, has significant implications for learning a second language. These attitudes might also include the perceived social distance between the two linguistic communities (Collier, 1995). In addition, the individual's proficiency in their first language will significantly determine the extent to which they can become proficient in the second language. In fact, McLaughlin's (Cascallar and Arnold, 2001) interdependence hypothesis indicates that as proficiency in an individual's first language increases, it will also increase in a second language. To many, this idea is counterintuitive. In fact, many schools have adopted a "sink or swim" attitude and support the practices of immersion classrooms. The placement of 93% of nonproficient or limited English-proficient students in monolingual English classrooms is a false and extremely detrimental practice (Petitto and Holowka, 2002). There are other factors that further affect second language acquisition, including level of formal schooling in the native language prior to immersion in a second language setting, parental and community attitudes, integration patterns (i.e., assimilation, adaptation, preservation), social identity, and the level of literacy in the home (Cascallar and Arnold, 2001; Collier, 1995; Hamayan and Damico, 1991).

Centeno and Obler (2001) describe bilingualism as "the alternate use of two languages by the same individual" (p. 76). However, there are several different types and levels of proficiency for bilingual individuals (Paul, 1996). Balanced bilinguals have an equivalent level of comfort and proficiency in both languages in all situations, including reading, writing, speaking, and listening (Centeno and Obler, 2001; Hamayan and Damico, 1991). Very few people attain this level of proficiency in all aspects of both languages and may find themselves using each language for different functions (i.e., social relationships or professional interactions). It is far more likely for individuals to have a higher proficiency level in one language. These individuals are known as nonbalanced bilinguals. Their skills are better developed in the four areas (reading, writing, speaking, listening) in one language (Hamayan and Damico, 1991). Another rather common type of bilingualism is the mixed bilingual individual. In this particular type of bilingualism, the individual is dominant in a particular skill in one language (i.e., speaking), but has better skills in other areas in another language (Hamayan and Damico, 1991). A specific type of mixed bilingualism is receptive bilingualism, in which a person can understand spoken and written language in the second language, but is unable to write or speak the second language (Centeno and Obler, 2001).

As previously inferred, placing a non-English-proficient or limited English-proficient student into a regular English-speaking classroom can have detrimental effects on many areas of functioning, including cognitive, emotional, social, academic, and linguistic development (Petitto and Holowka, 2002). In subtractive bilingualism, the development of a second language has detrimental effects on the maintenance and further development of the first language (Cummins, 1981; Hamayan and Damico, 1991). If a child has not yet gained full proficiency in the first language and is subsequently placed in an environment where they are expected to learn a second language, the development of the first language will likely slow down and perhaps even stop altogether (Collier, 1995). This occurs when early exposure to both languages is provided but with no adequate training, resulting in semi- or a-lingualism (Hamayan and Damico, 1991; Mushi, 2002; Petitto and Holowka, 2002; Piper, 1993). A semilingual's language skills in the two languages are not equivalent to the skills of a monolingual speaker of either language (Centeno and Obler, 2001). To overcome semilingualism, Hamayan and Damico (1991) state that the first language must be valued and developed. As can be seen, the extent to which a child learns the first language prior to exposure to a second language is highly correlated to how well a second language can be learned (Collier, 1995).

Before reviewing the benefits of being bilingual, it is important to review the negative perceptions and erroneous beliefs held by lay people about bilingual individuals. First, some contend that individuals who are bilingual have a smaller vocabulary and are therefore at a disadvantage. In fact, some may believe and propose that these individuals (with smaller vocabularies) are at risk for developing a language delay or disorder (Mushi, 2002; Petitto and Holowka, 2002). Another misconception about bilingual individuals is that they cannot think of the proper word or get confused when they code switch, or when they use both languages simultaneously, and that it reflects poor bilingual and cognitive ability (Mushi, 2002; Petitto and Holowka, 2002; Rhodes, Kayser, and Hess, 2000).

Another misperception of bilingual individuals, especially of non-English-proficient children entering into school in the United States for the first time, is the appearance of rapid increases in English during the first few weeks or months (Petitto and Holowka, 2002). Many teachers perceive the child to be picking up the language very quickly and automatically assume that the child is as fluent in English as their monolingual counterparts. However, this linguistic façade will lead to erroneous beliefs by the teacher. This rapid learning of English is only surface fluency and is described by Cummins (1979, 1984; Paul, 1996; Woodcock and Muñoz-Sandoval, 1993a, 1993b) as Basic Interpersonal Communication Skills

(BICS), or communicative proficiency. This is the type of language necessary to carry on social conversation and is gained within the first two or three years of exposure to a second language. Although it is the first type of language proficiency a non-English-proficient individual will gain, it is not the level of proficiency needed to perform successfully in the classroom or other demanding environments.

Cummins (1984) further described another type of language proficiency: Cognitive Academic Language Proficiency (CALP). There are five levels of CALP, and they are listed as follows: Level 5, Advanced Spanish or English; Level 4, Fluent Spanish or English; Level 3, Limited Spanish or English; Level 2, Very Limited Spanish or English; and Level 1, Negligible Spanish or English (Woodcock and Muñoz-Sandoval, 1993b). CALP takes approximately five to seven years to acquire and is an instrumental competency in order to succeed in cognitively demanding environments such as school. With this in mind, a monolingual child who is five years old is just beginning to truly acquire the full range of language proficiency. As we consider six–year-old non-English-proficient children who are placed in English-speaking classrooms, they are at a loss because they have not yet developed CALP in their first language, not to mention they have yet to develop even the basic requirements for BICS in their second language. This places them at serious risk for becoming semilingual (Piper 1993).

Research (Cummins, 1979) indicates that the best way to achieve CALP in the second language is to first acquire CALP in the first language. If the child does not have a minimum threshold level in the first language, it will be detrimental to instruct only in the second language. When considering bilingual education programs, two-way/dual language or maintenance programs would be best suited for non-English-speaking children who are enrolled in schools in the United States (Collier, 1995; Mushi, 2002; for a review of bilingual education programs, visit the National Association for Bilingual Education).

The benefits of being bilingual far outweigh the limitations, assuming that an individual has attained more than semilingual proficiency. With regard to the issue of code switching, it is not engaged in because the individual does not know the word, but because the Spanish word better reflects the meaning that they are trying to convey. In fact, some believe that code switching is a strength, not a deficit. Hamayan and Damico (1991) states, "the main reason for switching is not inability to come up with the right word or phrase in one language: rather, code switching is a skill that evolves through high levels of proficiency in both languages. Switching takes place so that the speaker may be better able to convey meaning. …" Code switching is a sign of adaptability and may be the result of social perception in an attempt to alter the conversation to better suit the listener (Crystal, 1987; Seymour and Roeper, 1999).

Many bilingual communities encourage the use of code switching (Rhodes, Kayser, and Hess, 2000). Because an individual has two languages from which to pull, their vocabulary is twice as large and they have more words to convey a tremendous depth and breadth of meaning. In fact, Peal and Lambert (1962) argue that when individuals switch linguistic codes, it gives them flexibility while performing cognitive tasks that monolinguals do not have available to them. Even very young bilingual children engage in code switching, although the nature of code switching in young children is qualitatively different than code switching in older children and adults (Rhodes, Kayser, and Hess, 2000). For example, young children tend to insert single words to express meaning ("I like perros [dogs]"). By the time a child is about three years old, Rhodes, Kayser, and Hess (2000) state that children of this age code switch by making a complete statement in both languages, and this is often observed in Hispanic children living in the U.S. For example, a child would say, "Quiero una manzana. I want an apple." This method is used to "resolve ambiguities, clarify statements, and attract attention." By eight years of age, a child's code-switching activities are used for emphasizing statements, making commands, and elaborating upon previous statements. For example, a child might state, "Quiero un lápiz" (I want a pencil). These examples are types of intrasentential code-switching activities (Hamayan and Damico, 1991). By nine or ten years old, code switching takes on a different nature, occurring at the phrase and sentence levels, and is known as intersentential code switching (Hamayan and Damico, 1991). A child may say one sentence in English, and say the next sentence in Spanish. As can be seen, the practice of code switching enriches a bilingual's verbal expressions and increases their cognitive flexibility (Hamayan and Damico, 1991).

There are additional benefits to being bilingual. According to Cummins and Gultusan (1975) and Mushi (2002), children who are bilingual become more knowledgeable about language and are therefore able to think about language in an abstract way. In other words, they are better suited for objectification of language and metacognition. Furthermore, bilingual speakers are typically more aware of language, especially as the contexts and situations for each language vary throughout a typical day. From this assumption arises the verbal mediation hypothesis (Hakuta, Ferdman, and Diaz, 1987). This hypothesis purports that bilingual individuals use language more efficiently because they are more aware of language. Based on this review of the limitations and benefits of bilingual individuals, it is evident that the benefits of being bilingual clearly outweigh the limitations that are surreptitiously placed on those that are bilingual.

In summary, it is clear that bilingual individuals, especially those that are simultaneous language learners, have an advantage over monolinguals. It is especially important for teachers and others who have frequent contact with sequential language learners to understand that they do not develop the level of language proficiency that would allow them to be successful in academic environments until many years after their exposure to the second language. Fallacies about bilingual children being unable to succeed in academic environments are compounded by the lack of knowledge regarding simultaneous versus sequential language learning. The importance of understanding the many facets of bilingualism has been clearly addressed in this section. In addition, new research (Harris and Llorente, 2005) points to the importance of addressing multiple language issues when considering differences in performance on measures of cognitive ability (see Chapter 4), and this is a vital issue because when developing norms for neuropsychological procedures and tests, it is common not to include individuals in the standardization sample who are not fluent in English, although those who speak English as a second language are commonly included. However as noted by Harris and Llorente (2005), "Realistically," "very little is known about the language abilities of these individuals and the degree to which they are [really] bilingual." In addition, Harris and Llorente note that "language preference is not synonymous with language proficiency, yet it is usually self-reported preferred language that enters as a "key variable for planning assessment strategies and for other decision making, such as inclusion in normative studies." Furthermore, as previously noted, the degree of proficiency can vary widely among individuals from ethnic with minority status, which is not the case for the vast majority of nonminority White examinees. According to Harris and Llorente (2005), "Within various ethnic groups, such as Hispanic, American Indian, and Alaskan Native, not only does this imply heterogeneity of English receptive and expressive abilities, but the very concept of bilingualism signifies more than a simple characterization of two languages for many of these groups."

Bilingualism and Brain Trauma

Although a detailed examination addressing bilingualism and brain insults is beyond the scope of this chapter, before discussing various language disorders, it is proper to introduce the reader to the impact of injury on language in bilinguals, within the context of ethnicity and cultural factors, particularly given the fact that many individuals from such minority backgrounds may possess complete or partial fluency in more than one language. Therefore, a concise exposure will be provided to obtain a hint of the complexity associated with this issue by briefly examining the effects of traumatic brain injury in language in bilinguals and polyglots.

Although the literature predominantly presents single case studies and small samples, it provides cohesive data suggesting that multilinguals may show unique patterns of language recovery after brain trauma (cf. Paradis, 1995). In this regard, differential levels of improvement in one language versus the other, even after rehabilitation, have been noted in multilingual individuals who have sustained strokes (Junque, Vendrell, and Vendrell, 1995). In some instances, partial recovery of one and complete recovery of another language, complete loss of one language but not the other, and other patterns of recovery after injury and rehabilitation have been evidenced among populations, including bilingual Hispanics (cf. Paradis, 1995). Although several modulating and moderating factors have emerged in the literature as critical in recovery, including the language under investigation (e.g., Spanish), the first language learned (English versus Spanish), age at the time of language acquisition, most frequently used language, and other factors including type of injury (TBI vs. stroke), specific patterns of recovery are complicated and many unanswered questions remain, including issues associated with language localization and representation in multilinguals (cf. Hernandez, Dapretto, Mazziotta, and Bookheimer, 2001). It should also be noted that languages do not depend on the same mechanisms of representation. While some languages predominantly depend on phonemes, others depend on pictorial representations, and this issue also may impact recovery after injury during rehabilitation in multilinguals from ethnic minority backgrounds, including Hispanics (Paradis, 1995).

Nevertheless, attending to language factors during the course of neurocognitive rehabilitation in bilinguals is important. Not just because it is the ethical posture to adopt, but because erroneous assumptions and attributions may be used in explaining the impact of the insult and subsequent recovery of specific language functions in multilingual individuals from ethnic minority backgrounds during the course of rehabilitation.

The Relationship Between Language Proficiency, Bilingualism, and Cognitive Performance

The relationship of language proficiency and bilingualism to cognitive performance has vital and direct impacts on the performance discrepancies observed for some ethnic minority (e.g., Hispanic), versus nonminority groups. Early studies concluded that bilingualism was a cognitive and academic learning liability. This conclusion was reached on the basis of flawed research methodologies, such as failure to control for socioeconomic and other confounding variables as noted in Chapters 1 and 3, the heterogeneity in the samples designated as "bilingual," and failure to measure abilities in both the stronger and the weaker language (cf. Hamers and Blanc, 1989; Romaine, 1995). As noted by Harris and Llorente "The social and political context of emerging bilingualism and acceptance of the acquisition of two languages is also a critical factor in the perceived advantages or disadvantages of speaking two languages." In other words, social expectations and support for bilingualism are essential to the acquisition of and development of proficiency in a second language as much as other factors, such as individual differences in ability to learn a second language (Ardila, 1998; Ardila, 2003; Centeno & Obler, 2001).

Support may not exist until a language has been officially sanctioned by governmental policies (e.g., Canada's Official Language Act of 1968-1969 and similar European laws) (cf. Centeno & Obler, 2001) or when the norm for bilingualism is otherwise ingrained in the societal and educational structure of a nation. Unfortunately, unlike most countries in Europe, some in South America, and Canada, in the "U.S. preserving the native language has always been viewed as incompatible with learning the English language and indeed bilingual education has a controversial and poorly understood history" (Harris and Llorente, 2005). The reader is now referred to Chapter 4 to examine the specific impact of this variable on a test of intellect (see also Harris and Llorente, 2005).

A Brief Survey of Language Disorders

There are a variety of reasons an individual may experience a language disorder. Crowley (1992) and Law (1992) described some of the factors associated with language impairment, including gender, sensory impairments, environment, social/

family issues, behavior, and language dominance. Some of the more common reasons for acquired language disorders include cerebral vascular accidents, acquired traumatic brain injury, epilepsy, tumors, and hypoxic or anoxic events that affect the language centers and circuits of the brain, specifically the perisylvian arc (Kaufman, 2001). However, some individuals have congenital language disorders as a result of genetic or other etiology and struggle with language expression and reception from birth. Whether a language disorder is acquired or congenital, an individual's functioning is clearly affected. When one thinks about the daily inter-actions with individuals at school, work, or home, one can begin to realize how dependent society is on communication. With language delays or disorders, indi-viduals have greater difficulty facilitating connections with those around them. In fact, many children with congenital language disorders have a tendency to with-draw from social interactions because of their reduced or limited ability to compre-hend information or express their thoughts and needs. It becomes clear that language is important not only for the exchange of information between individu-als, but for social connectedness as well. From a clinical standpoint, in Hispanics as well as other groups, the course of language disorders may also provide impor-tant diagnostic information because it is related to the "natural history" of a specific condition affecting language skills. Therefore, the course observed in children with autism in which proper, initial language development is followed by rapid declines in these skills (APA, 2000) may provide important diagnostic information when working with Hispanic children.

Language disorders are commonly believed to affect the expression of language. However, language disorders may also impact an individual's capacity to understand. Language disorders are also different from speech disorders. Speech disorders affect the oral-motor output of language and do not impact the actual language code that is being verbalized. Children who stutter or have poor articulation are thought to have a speech disorder and not a language disorder, unless there are other impairments. Speech and linguistic disorders, although different, can occur simultaneously. This section will focus mainly on language disorders with regard to understanding the differences between the many different forms of aphasia.

Before entering into a discussion of specific linguistic disorders, it is important to lay the foundation for understanding how a language disorder is defined. According to the American Speech-Language-Hearing Association (1982) a language disorder is:

> the impairment or deviant development of comprehension and/or use of a spoken, written, and/or other symbol system. The disorder may involve (1) the form of language (phonologic, morphologic, and syntactic systems), (2) the content of language (semantic system), and/or (3) the function of language in communication (pragmatic system) in any combina-tion" (p. 949).

The Diagnostic and Statistical Manual of Mental Disorders – Fourth Edition (DSM-IV; APA, 2000) delineates several requirements for determining an Expressive Language Disorder (315.31) or a Mixed Receptive-Expressive Language Disorder (315.32). The first requirement indicates that a language disorder cannot be diagnosed unless scores on standardized individually administered measures of language development are significantly below scores obtained on standardized measures of nonverbal intelligence. The second requirement necessitates the interference of language difficulties with academic achievement, social communication, or occupational achievement. Other than Expressive Language Disorder and Mixed Receptive-Expressive Language Disorder, the DSM-IV details several other Communication Disorders, including Phonological Disorder (315.39), Stuttering (307.0), and Communication Disorder, Not Otherwise Specified (307.9).

The International Classification of Diseases – Ninth Revision Clinical Modification (ICD-9-CM; Hart and Hopkins, 2002) includes many different language and speech disorders, including stammering/stuttering (307.0), lisping (307.9), elective mutism (309.83, 313.23), developmental language disorder/developmental aphasia/word deafness (315.31), developmental articulation disorder/dyslalia (315.39), acquired aphasia (784.3), voice disturbance (784.4), and dysarthria/dysphasia/slurred speech (784.5). As can be seen, there is much overlap between the DSM-IV and the ICD-9 classification systems.

Language is the understanding and expression of meaningful information from one person to another. As mentioned previously, language is also the capacity to understand and comprehend what another individual says. However, language is not always verbal. American Sign Language is one example of nonverbal language. Although words may not be verbalized, hand movements express the thoughts of one individual to another. Furthermore, language includes being able to read and write information. These clarifications are necessary to understand prior to discussing the particularities of each of the language disorders.

There are a large number of language disorders, many of which will be discussed in detail in this section. The disorders that will be discussed include the many different types of acquired aphasia (Broca's, Wernicke's, anomic, conduction, expressive, global, sensory, mixed) and several other types of language disorders, including word blindness, word deafness, other transcortical/extrasylvian aphasias (motor, supplementary motor, subcortical), and single modality disturbances (alexia, optic aphasia, aphemia). Although some sources separate acquired aphasia from other congenital and developmental language disorders, this section will not attempt to make a notable demarcation between these two general areas.

According to the definition, aphasia is a neurologic disorder associated with the impairment of language due to brain damage (Bates, Thal, Finlay, and Clancy, 2003; Benson, 1993; Damasio and Damasio, 2000; Kalat, 1998). Different aspects of language can be affected, including fluency, articulation, word finding, repetition, comprehension, syntax and grammar, reading, and writing. The skills affected are related to the anatomical structures involved and the language pathways affected by injury (Goodglass and Kaplan, 1983b). These different aspects include gestural, prosodic, semantic, syntactic, and pragmatic language skills (Benson, 1993). Benson (1993) strongly urges that aphasia is an acquired disorder due to injury or damage to the brain and should not be interchanged with slow language development. Although this is an important distinction to make, acquired expressive language aphasia does not differ significantly from a developmental expressive language disorder in its diagnostic criteria. Furthermore, discussions of language impairments are often clouded by the numerous terms to describe the same set of symptomatology. A brief

Table 5.2 Language Disorders and Their Pseudonyms, Related Pathology, and Subsequent Neurologic Disturbances

	Pseudonym	Related pathology	Neurologic disturbances
Broca's aphasia	Nonfluent aphasia, Motor aphasia, Expressive aphasia	Left frontal lobe adjacent to primary motor cortex	Contralateral hemiparesis, sensory loss, or visual-field cut
Conduction aphasia		Arcuate fasciculus and/or supramarginal gyrus of the left hemisphere, disconnection between Broca's area, inferior parietal lobule, and Wernicke's area	Possible depending on location and extent of lesion
Expressive aphasia		Left frontal cortex	Contralateral hemiparesis of upper extremity
Global aphasia		Global left hemisphere involvement of the language axis, middle cerebral artery	Contralateral hemiparesis, sensory loss, or visual-field cut
Wernicke's aphasia	Fluent aphasia, Receptive aphasia, Sensory aphasia, Jargon aphasia, (Non-pure) word deafness	Left superior temporal cortex, extending from the auditory association cortex toward the inferior parietal lobule	Contralateral upper extremity hemiparesis
Word blindness		Left temporal superior lobe and angular gyrus of parietal cortex, white matter beneath the supramarginal gyrus	Ideomotor apraxia in buccofacial and extremity activities
Word deafness	Cortical deafness	Primary auditory area in the superior temporal lobe (Heschl's gyrus), disconnection between Wernicke's area and the pathways from the medial geniculate nucleus, bilateral involvement of the superior temporal gyrus	Possible depending on location and extent of lesion
Anomic aphasia		Lesion or abnormality in any part of the language cortex	Possible depending on location and extent of lesion

(continued)

Table 5.2 (continued)

	Pseudonym	Related pathology	Neurologic disturbances
Mixed aphasia		Anterior and posterior cortical areas, left internal carotid artery	Possible but not consistent
Motor aphasia	Transcortical aphasia	Frontal/prefrontal regions of the left hemisphere, anterior-superior to Broca's area and disconnected from the supplementary motor area	Possible depending on location and extent of lesion
Sensory aphasia		Left temporal-parietal regions posterior to perisylvian region	Possible depending on location and extent of lesion
Subcortical aphasia		Basal ganglia and thalamus, occasionally lesion in language cortex	Possible depending on location and extent of lesion
Supplementary motor aphasia		Left hemisphere medial frontal areas, including the cingulate cortex and supplementary motor area	Hemiparesis of contralateral lower extremity and shoulder, possible sensory impairment

Adapted from Benson (1993); Joseph (1996); Kalat (1998); and Lezak (1995).

perusal of Tables 5.2, 5.3, and 5.4 will help the reader familiarize themselves with the primary names of the numerous language disorders, their pseudonyms, probable related anatomical pathology, and associated neurologic deficits.

Broca's Aphasia

Broca's aphasia, also known as nonfluent, expressive, or motor aphasia, is probably one the most well-known types of acquired language impairment (Kaufman, 2001). As noted by one of the senior author's lecturers, Professor D. Frank Benson at UCLA, this is likely a result of Broca's aphasia being one, if not the first, official language impairment recognized and well documented in the literature (cf. Benson, 1993). The diagnostic usage of Broca's aphasia developed after Paul Broca, a French surgeon, completed an autopsy on a man he had previously treated for gangrene. The man had been mute for the last three decades of his life. When Dr. Broca reportedly completed the autopsy, he discovered a small lesion in the area now

Table 5.3 Neurocognitive Skills Impaired by Language Disorders

	Spoken language comprehension	Written language comprehension	Verbal fluency	Writing	Reading	Repetition	Naming/word finding	Artic.	Prosody	Grammar
Anomic aphasia			X				X			
Broca's aphasia			X		X	X	X	X		X
Conduction aphasia				X*	X**	X	X			
Expressive aphasia			X	X	X**	X		X	X	X
Global aphasia	X	X	X	X	X	X	X			
Mixed aphasia	X	X	X	X	X		X			
Sensory aphasia	X	X		X	X		X			
Wernicke's aphasia	X	X		X	X	X	X			
Word blindness	X	X								
Word deafness	X					X				

Note: X = major dysfunction; x = minor dysfunction; *write to dictation; **read out loud.
Adapted from Benson (1993); Joseph (1996); Kalat (1998); and Lezak (1995).

Table 5.4 Characteristics of Selected Language Disorders

	Circumlocution	Conversation	Difficulty with prepositions	Echolalia	Neologisms	Omission of nouns/verbs	Paraphasias	Short utterances	Substitutions
Anomic aphasia	X						x		X
Broca's aphasia			X			X			
Conduction aphasia	X	X					X	x	X
Expressive aphasia			X				X	X	X
Global aphasia	X	X	X		X	X	X	X	X
Mixed aphasia				X			X		
Sensory aphasia				X			X		
Wernicke's aphasia	X	X	X		X	X	X		

Note. X = major dysfunction; x = minor dysfunction
Adapted from Benson (1993); Joseph (1996); Kalat (1998); and Lezak (1995).

known as Broca's area (cf. Kalat, 1998), which is a small area in the left, lateral frontal cortex adjacent to the primary motor cortex – areas 44, 45, and 46 in Broadmann's map. After following up on this discovery during autopsy of several more language-impaired patients, Broca discovered strong similarities in the presenting problems (i.e., nonfluent verbal output, reduction in grammatical complexity, intact language comprehension) and the affected physiological structure of the brain (Bates, Thal, Finlay, and Clancy, 2003; Kalat, 1998). Although there likely was damage to other cortical and subcortical structures to cause such chronic and severe language impairments with these patients, as damage only to Broca's area would only cause limited language impairment, Broca had made an important discovery in finding the anatomical structure related to language functioning (cf. Benson, 1993; Kalat, 1998).

Limited or impaired language production is the main characteristic of Broca's aphasia. Even individuals with Broca's aphasia who use American Sign Language to communicate have impaired expressive language, even though they can use their upper extremities and hands to perform other non-language-related tasks. Although impaired expressive language ability appears to be easily described at the outset, there are many components that make up language production and output. An individual's language impairment may be so severe that they can only produce noises instead of words. This significantly limits an individual's ability to communicate.

As previously noted, individuals with Broca's aphasia may also be known as nonfluent aphasics; that is, the ease with which individuals with Broca's aphasia produce expressive language is hindered (Benson, 1993). Broca's aphasia also affects an individual's ability to name objects, although his or her performance can typically be improved with phonetic or contextual cues (Benson, 1993). Another difficulty that individuals with Broca's aphasia encounter is the impaired ability to repeat words and phrases (Benson, 1993). Furthermore, these individuals experience significant difficulty using words that are not nouns or verbs. They may omit word endings, prepositional phrases, conjunctions, and modifiers in their expressive language. When the meaning of their communication is dependent upon these types of words, their output is very much impaired.

Individuals with Broca's aphasia have difficulty with the pronunciation and meaning of language, while their comprehension of language remains fairly intact (Benson, 1993), and these problems are discernable during bedside visits. It is critical to note that this is quite applicable to Hispanic patients, and these individuals are able to comprehend most of what is said or written in Spanish, if monolingual, and English and Spanish if bilingual. However, they also have difficulty understanding the connector words in sentences; that is, they understand nouns and verbs much better than they comprehend pragmatic language, prepositional phrases, and conjunctions (Bates, Thal, Finlay, and Clancy, 2003; Kalat, 1998). Basically, the comprehension of individuals with Broca's aphasia "resembles that of normal people who are greatly distracted" (p. 390). Just as they have difficulty using these words, they have difficulty comprehending them.

With regard to the identifiable anatomical correlates of Broca's aphasia, the specific area that is responsible for the fluency expression of language is in the left frontal cortex directly adjacent to the primary motor area as noted above. According to Joseph (1996), information from the posterior language axis converges via the arcuate fasciculus in Broca's area and receives the "final sequential (syntactical, grammatical) imprint so as to become organized and expressed as temporally ordered motoric linguistic articulations" (p. 134). This area also is responsible for the musculature of the mouth and face and the right hand (Joseph, 1996). Because of this close relationship with the primary motor cortex, individuals with Broca's aphasia may also suffer from hemiparesis of their right upper extremities, in addition to sensory loss or visual-field disturbance (cf. Benson, 1993).

According to Professor Benson (1993), there are two subtypes of Broca's aphasia: Big Broca's aphasia and Little Broca's aphasia. Big Broca's aphasia results after injury to the brain, leaving the individual with severe total aphasia and contralateral hemiparesis. As healing and restorative processes occur in the brain, the symptoms ameliorate, leaving the individual with some of the aforementioned characteristics (i.e., nonfluent output, dysnomia, impaired repetition, impaired use of modifiers and connectors). Reportedly, this pattern of impairment is indicative of injury to the dominant, typically left, hemisphere's frontal opercular region, with an associated lesion in the basal ganglia. On the other hand, Little Broca's aphasia begins with the basic aphasic symptoms, which improve to feature hesitant output and mild agrammatism. This pattern of impairment is indicative of damage to the left hemisphere's frontal opercular region without extending lesions into subcortical structures.

As can be seen, there are variations in the presentation of Broca's aphasia (Bates, Thal, Finlay, and Clancy, 2003; Benson, 1993). The characteristic symptoms differ not only as a result of injury, but also as a result of gender differences. Joseph (1996) contends that Broca's area is not as well developed in men compared to women. He indicates that because the anterior regions of the female brain are more responsible for expressive and emotional speech, women are likely to become more severely aphasic with left frontal injuries compared to their male counterparts. Conversely, the left parietal region is argued to house more of a man's expressive and emotional speech capacity, therefore putting men at risk for Broca's aphasia with left parietal injuries.

Wernicke's Aphasia

Karl Wernicke was a contemporary of Paul Broca and had a career as a German neurologist and psychiatrist. Through his work, Wernicke discovered an area of the brain that was responsible for language output in the left superior temporal cortex, extending from the auditory association area of the first temporal gyrus toward the inferior parietal lobe (Benson, 1993; Joseph, 1996; Kalat, 1998) – posterior area 22 in Broadmann's map. It is closely tied to Broca's area and is connected by the arcuate fasciculus. As a result of this close connection, the distinction between Broca's aphasia and Wernicke's aphasia is often muddy, and the two language impairments share many of the same deficits. Nevertheless, damage to Wernicke's area is known to affect comprehension of semantics (Bates, Thal, Finlay, and Clancy, 2003). Joseph (1996) indicated that the area known as Wernicke's area is responsible for decoding and encoding "auditory-linguistic information … to extract or impart temporal-sequential order and related linguistic features" (p. 139) from language expressed verbally or via written means. Joseph also related that Wernicke's area is responsible for providing meaning and labels for information expressed by others. Because of the physiological structures of the brain affected in individuals with Wernicke's aphasia, they might also experienced hemiparesis of their contralateral upper extremity.

Although it is best known as Wernicke's aphasia, this acquired language disorder has many other pseudonyms. Some of these alternate names include fluent aphasia, receptive aphasia, sensory aphasia, jargon aphasia, and non-pure-word deafness. These additional names will become clear when the specific symptoms of Wernicke's aphasia are discussed.

The basic characteristics of Wernicke's aphasia or fluent aphasia include difficulty understanding spoken and written language (Joseph, 1996; Lezak, 1995). Expressive language (speaking and writing) is typically intact unless there are concomitant injuries in language pathways or other language centers. Also, the motor production and fluency of speech is typically undamaged (Bates, Thal, Finlay, and Clancy, 2003; Benson, 1993; Joseph, 1996; Kalat, 1998; Lezak, 1995). Interestingly, Kalat (1998) indicated that deaf individuals are still able to understand sign language even if they have Wernicke's aphasia. However, those that communicate through verbal means have difficulty comprehending what is being said to them. Joseph (1996) contended that individuals suffering from Wernicke's aphasia cannot distinguish between the separate units of speech and their temporal order. They will typically be able to decipher and understand more familiar and commonly used words, such as family member names. However, their comprehension of less commonly used words, in addition to prepositional phrases, possessives, or verb tense changes, is very limited. As a result, what an individual with Wernicke's aphasia likely hears is a blur of verbal output that carries absolutely no meaning. Nevertheless, it has been shown that their comprehension can be improved if the sounds are separated by long intervals so they can decipher the individual sounds (Joseph, 1996).

In his lectures, Benson (1993) made a clear differentiation between severity level of comprehension between the two modalities of receptive language – spoken and written language. Individuals with relatively weaker comprehension of spoken language compared to comprehension of written language are known as word deaf. When this pattern emerges, Benson argues that there is likely pathology deep in the connections of the first temporal and Heschl's gyrus. On the other hand, when individuals experience more greatly impaired comprehension of written language, they are known to have word blindness, which is associated with involvement of the angular gyrus.

Besides difficulty in receptive language and comprehension, individuals with Wernicke's aphasia often have some difficulties with expressive language, including reading and writing. In fact, Joseph (1996) purports that the writing of an individual with Wernicke's aphasia will likely be unintelligible. Because they have difficulty initially understanding language, these individuals have select difficulties repeating words and phrases (Bates, Thal, Finlay, and Clancy, 2003; Joseph, 1996). Wernicke's sufferers also have significant difficulty with anomia and often omit nouns and verbs in their expressive language (Joseph, 1996; Kalat, 1998). Their naming ability is not typically aided by cueing (Benson, 1993). Although their speech is usually fluent, they may experience nonfluency and articulation problems when they pause to think of the name of something. As a result, these individuals use circumlocution to express their ideas. Also, speech is often empty because of the omission of nouns and verbs (Joseph, 1996). Instead, the language of Wernicke's patients often contains paraphasic errors and neologistic distortions (Benson, 1993; Joseph, 1996) to replace the lack of content. As a result, these individuals may first appear to a mental health professional as evidencing psychotic thought processes because of these errors. These individuals also typically omit pauses and sentence endings, so that their verbal output may sound like a foreign language (Joseph, 1996). This pattern of expressive language difficulties in Wernicke's sufferers is a direct result of damage to the respective language area, in that "Wernicke's area also acts to code linguistic stimuli for expression prior to its transmission to Broca's area" (Joseph, 1996, p. 140). Furthermore, these individuals, including Hispanic patients, may perpetuate others' belief that they are indeed psychotic because they do not have any awareness that what they are saying is meaningless, and anosognosia is quite common in Wernicke's aphasia (Joseph, 1996).

Anomic Aphasia

Anomic aphasia is considered one of the several transcortical, or extrasylvian, aphasias (Benson, 1993). It is a severe word-finding difficulty and usually involves the greatly impaired naming of tangible objects or description of pictures, which cannot be aided by providing categorical or phonetic cues and hints. Anomia affects the ability to name nouns more commonly than verbs and other words (Joseph, 1996). Anomia can be caused by damage to any area of the language cortex or pathways (Benson, 1993; Joseph, 1996; Lezak, 1995). According to Kay and Ellis (1987), anomia can also be caused by a deficit in activating the correct phonological-sound-word patterns. Interestingly, depending on the interconnectedness between different language and other processing centers within the brain, it is possible for anomic individuals to be able to give the proper name for an object if they are allowed to hold it or if the object is described to them by another person (Joseph, 1996).

Joseph (1996) indicated that children may experience forms of anomia because the development of their language centers and related pathways and axonal connections, especially within the inferior parietal lobe, are still not fully developed. However, because of the development of the interconnections between areas of the brain, children will most likely outgrow word-finding difficulties. As can be surmised, because of the many possibilities of damage to the language cortex, neurological disturbances (i.e., hemiparesis) vary, as they are dependent upon the location and extent of the lesion.

A concomitant deficit of individuals with anomia is dysfluent and empty speech (Joseph, 1996; Lezak, 1995). Anomic individuals may pause to try to think of the word, causing disruptions in the flow of conversation. They also use circumlocution as an aide to describe the word they are trying to say (Benson, 1993; Joseph, 1996). As a result, their utterances are typically quite lengthy, simply because they have to use many words to describe the object they are trying to say (Benson, 1993). As a result of trying to come up with the proper word, they often experience paraphasias and substitutions (Joseph, 1996). Even though they could not come up with the proper word at will (confrontation naming; Lezak, 1995), anomics typically retain the ability to repeat words (Benson, 1993).

Dysnomia typically refers to a less severe form of word-finding difficulty. It is a very common occurrence in many individuals who have experienced some type of brain injury. Even individuals who have dysnomia may have no other language deficits and typically can demonstrate fluent speech and good comprehension (Benson, 1993; Joseph, 1996). Because it may be an isolated difficulty, individuals with dysnomia or others close to them may attribute mild-to-moderate word-finding difficulties to impaired memory retrieval (Joseph, 1996).

Conduction Aphasia

One of the most difficult types of aphasia to observe at the patient's bedside, partially because it may only be observed for a period of time during the acute phase of rehabilitation, conduction aphasia results from lesions within the arcuate fasciculus and the white matter of the supramarginal gyrus, as well as lesions in the posterior perisylvian region of the dominant hemisphere (Bates, Thal, Finlay, and Clancy, 2003; Benson, 1993). With such lesions, the three main areas of the language center, namely Broca's area, Wernicke's area, and the inferior parietal lobe, become disconnected (Joseph, 1996). Based on the location and extent of the lesion, neurological disturbances vary; however, Benson argued that individuals with conduction aphasia commonly experience "ideomotor apraxia that involves buccofacial and limb activities" (p. 26).

Individuals with conduction aphasia are similar to those with Wernicke's aphasia in many respects. They typically have good articulation and fluent output, but experience different levels of anomia circumlocution and are unable to repeat what others say (Benson, 1993; Kalat, 1998). They also have difficulty maintaining conversations and make paraphasic errors and word substitutions.

Although individuals with conduction aphasia have several characteristics that resemble the language deficits of individuals with Wernicke's aphasia, they typically have better comprehension of written and verbal language (Benson, 1993; Joseph, 1996; Kalat, 1998). Also, individuals with conduction aphasia are not as likely to experience anosognosia; that is, they are aware of their language deficits (Joseph, 1996). As a result, they engage in much circumlocutional speech in attempts to come up with the proper words through successive approximations. Regardless, Joseph (1996) indicated that these individuals have shorter, unrelated utterances than those with Wernicke's aphasia. Those suffering from conduction aphasia also have notable difficulty in reading out loud or writing to dictation (Joseph, 1996).

Expressive Aphasia

Expressive aphasia is another language impairment that results from damage to the language center of the brain, typically the left frontal convexity (Joseph, 1996). Because of the localization of pathology in individuals with expressive aphasia, they may experience hemiparesis of the contralateral upper extremity. Expressive aphasia typically limits an individual's capacity to speak, which impacts their ability to repeat what others say, articulate words, or provide more than one- or two-word utterances. Comprehension of language is usually spared in these individuals, as is the ability to copy words by writing, silent reading comprehension, and verbalization of semantically meaningful words or statements (Joseph, 1996). In many cases, these individuals may be able make emotional statements or sing words that they are unable to say (Joseph, 1996). Although reading is intact, the ability to write, even to dictation, is significantly impacted. According to Joseph (1996), individuals with expressive aphasia have major deficits in grammar, prosody, naming, fluency, and syntax, and often evidence paraphasias, substitutions, and omissions of relational words.

Global Aphasia

One of the most devastating events in a Hispanic patient's life, as the name suggests, global aphasia results in dysfunction in all the aspects of language (Benson, 1993). It typically results from damage to the left middle cerebral artery, secondary to cerebrovascular disease and related cerebrovascular accidents (Benson, 1993; Joseph, 1996). As a result, there are typically several neurological disturbances associated with global aphasia, including contralateral hemiparesis of the upper and lower extremities, sensory loss, and even visual-field cuts. Not only is comprehension of language affected in spoken and written modalities, expression of language is also significantly impacted. Individuals who have suffered from cerebrovascular accidents have language skills that are compromised in areas of speaking, writing, and repeating (Benson, 1993; Joseph, 1996). In addition, their speech, if present at all, is severely nonfluent (Benson, 1993; Kaufman, 2001). They may have difficulty maintaining conversation and have brief utterances.

Sensory Aphasia

Sensory aphasia is one of several types of extrasyvlian transcortical aphasia, in that the lesions that cause its characteristics lie posterior to the perisylvian region in the temporal-parietal area (Benson, 1993). Depending on the location and extent of the injury, neurological disturbances are possible, but may vary widely. Individuals with sensory aphasia experience impaired comprehension of spoken and written language. Also, their ability to read, write, and name objects is often affected (Benson, 1993). Although an individual's ability to repeat is intact, it may become deleterious in that the individual may begin repeating much of what they hear, evidencing echolalia. They also may not understand the words they are repeating (Benson, 1993). Furthermore, individuals with sensory aphasia have fluent speech, although it is often replete with paraphasias and jargon. As a result, Benson (1993) purported that, like individuals with Wernicke's aphasia, mental health professionals may initially believe that the individual with sensory aphasia is suffering from impaired psychotic thought processes.

Mixed Aphasia

Pathology in the anterior and posterior cortical areas may result in mixed transcortical (extrasylvian) aphasia (Benson, 1993). It shares the characteristics of motor and sensory aphasia, in addition to global aphasia; however, an individual's ability to repeat words or phrases is typically spared in mixed aphasia. Mixed aphasia can be caused by several different events, including occlusions within the internal carotid artery or the residual effects of hypoxic events or edema (Benson, 1993). Although neurological disturbances are likely, there are no consistent findings, which reflect the true "mixed" features of this type of aphasia. Although repletion is intact, individuals with mixed aphasia experience many other difficulties, including poor comprehension of spoken and written language, reading, naming, fluency, and use of paraphasias (Benson, 1993).

Pure Word Blindness and Pure Word Deafness

As previously mentioned in the section discussing Wernicke's aphasia, word blindness and word deafness might be considered subtypes of receptive aphasia, especially if the individual's impaired comprehension is not complete lack of comprehension. In other words, individuals having difficulty, but not a complete lack, of comprehension of either spoken or written language would likely be better described as suffering from Wernicke's aphasia. To make this distinction, word blindness and word deafness are referred to here as "pure," denoting their complete inability to comprehend the respective language modality (Benson, 1993).

At this point, it is worth discussing these two subtypes in slightly more detail in order to illuminate their specific characteristics. First, pure word blindness involves damage to the left superior temporal area, the angular gyrus, and the white matter beneath the supramarginal gyrus (Benson, 1993). The main feature of pure word blindness is impaired comprehension of written language and is often associated with neurological disturbances in ideomotor apraxia in buccofacial and extremity activities.

Pure word deafness, also known as cortical deafness, is associated with the inability to comprehend spoken language, even in the presence of normal hearing acuity and reading ability (Benson, 1993; Joseph, 1996; Kalat, 1998). Joseph (1996) purported that individuals with pure word deafness also have deficits in being able to discriminate between sound loudness and localization. Pure word deafness is distinct from receptive aphasia in that individuals suffering from pure word deafness have the ability to read and write (Joseph, 1996). Pure word deafness occurs when there is injury to the primary auditory area in the superior temporal lobe, including Heschl's gyrus (Benson, 1993). There also may be bilateral involvement of the superior temporal gyrus. Often, the connections between Wernicke's area and the medial geniculate nucleus have been disrupted in some way. Based on this information, it is difficult to provide the exact neurological signs that may accompany pure word deafness, as they vary depending on the location and depth of the lesion. For the most part, individuals suffering from pure word deafness have no other aphasic symptoms besides the inability to repeat what is said to them (Benson, 1993; Joseph, 1996). Pure word deafness has characteristics of global auditory agnosia, in which these individuals are unable to perceive and identify linguistic and nonlinguistic sounds (Joseph, 1996). Based on this hypothesis, it could be argued that the level of comprehension may increase if the rate of speech is slowed down (Joseph, 1996). They are able to understand nonverbal communication and their expressive language is within normal limits (Joseph, 1996), possibly demonstrating paraphasic errors for a brief time after the injury (Benson, 1993).

Other Extrasylvian Aphasias

There are several other types of extrasylvian, or transcortical aphasias. Though they are not as common as the perisylvian aphasias (e.g., Broca's aphasia, Wernicke's aphasia, global aphasia), a brief review of them is in order. The ability to repeat words and phrases is typically spared in individuals with any of the extrasylvian aphasias. Besides extrasylvian motor and mixed aphasias, the other three transcortical aphasias include motor, supplementary motor, and subcortical aphasia.

Extrasylvian motor aphasia occurs when there is injury anterior and superior to Broca's area, in the frontal area of the language cortex, resulting in a disconnection between Broca's area and the supplementary motor area (Benson, 1993). Neurological disturbances vary depending on the injury. For the most part, individuals with motor aphasia experience nonfluent speech and echolalia, even though their ability to repeat is intact. Furthermore, these individuals' ability to comprehend spoken and written language remains largely intact.

Individuals with extrasylvian supplementary motor aphasia often present with mutism immediately following injury. According to Benson (1993), these individuals experience hypophonic expressive language that improves with practice. To create this pattern of symptoms, there is likely injury to the cingulated gyrus and supplementary motor area, resulting in neurological impairment of the contralateral side. These disturnces may include weakness in the lower extremity, in addition to sensory impairments (Benson, 1993).

Extrasylvian subcortical aphasia may result from injury to the language cortex; however, most occurrences of subcortical aphasia result from injury to subcortical structures, namely the basal ganglia and thalamus, although other subcortical structures may be involved as well (Benson, 1993). Depending on the location and extent of the injury, there may be neurological disturbances on the ipsalateral or contralateral side. It is important to note that if the injury involves subcortical structures as well as the language areas, the level of impairment is likely to be greater than if the injury were confined to small subcortical structures; otherwise, the characteristics of subcortical aphasia are likely to quickly ameliorate (Benson, 1993). Similar to supplementary motor aphasia, individuals with subcortical aphasia initially present with mutism, which develops into a "hypophonic, slow, and poorly articulated output...contaminated with paraphasias which disappear when asked to repeat spoken language" (Benson, 1993, p. 31).

Single-Modality Disturbances

There are several language impairments in the category of single-modality disturbances. The three that will be discussed briefly here are alexia, optic aphasia, and aphemia. Although they have a low incidence of occurrence, it is important to be familiar with them in the context of the other language impairments already described in this section.

Many individuals are familiar with dyslexia, which is a type of reading disability. Many people associate it with the tendency to switch letters and words around. A better description of dyslexia is a specific neurological learning deficit that hinders a person's ability to read and is characterized by difficulties with word recognition, decoding, spelling, and general phonological awareness (International Dyslexia Association, 2000). Along the same lines, alexia is a type of reading disability. However, alexia is described by Kalat (1998) as the complete loss of the ability to read. Therefore, based on this definition, it cannot be classified as a developmental learning disability, simply because there has to be a loss of ability, rather than simply the incomplete or lack of development of reading. Its only characteristic is the loss of ability to read, even in the presence of normal comprehension of spoken language. It is similar to pure word blindness as Benson (1993) described it; however, pure word blindness is the lack of comprehension of written language. Even though the individual with pure word blindness is not able to comprehend any written language, they have the ability to read. Individuals with alexia cannot even read written language.

Optic aphasia is another type of single-modality disturbance. Like alexia, it affects the ability to read. However, optic aphasia limits the individual's ability to read fluently because he or she can only read one letter at a time (Kalat, 1998). Therefore, the ability to integrate the letters to form a word with meaning will also be impacted, which in turn impacts comprehension.

Aphemia is the third single-modality disturbance. It is also known as pure word dumbness, or anarthria (Benson, 1993). Injury directly to or inferior to Broca's area may result in aphemia. As with subcortical aphasia and supplementary motor aphasia, individuals with aphemia initially present with mutism, gradually developing into hypophonic, dsyprosodic, and slow speech. Although it also shares some similarities with Little Broca's aphasia, aphemia does not impact grammar in either speech or writing (Benson, 1993). Also, the ability to understand spoken language and express language in verbal and written modalities remain intact (Benson, 1993).

This section is concluded by addressing aspects of bilingualism affected by specific pathologies sometimes observed in Hispanic populations. Case studies, and more recently, neuroimaging and neurosurgical studies, have elucidated important data regarding bilingualism in individuals who have sustained neurovascular trauma. For example, the research literature suggests that there are usually different levels of recovery in each language (e.g., Catalan v. Spanish) after strokes affecting substrates in the brain subserving language functions. In these cases, is not unusual for an individual to exhibit almost complete recovery in the language learned first, with greater loss in the language most recently learned (Junque, Vendrell, and Vendrell, 1995; Paradis, 1977). Although open to alternate interpretation (Hines, 1996), such findings, coupled with recent neuroimaging studies, have suggested the presence of a clear neuroanatomical dissociative representation in the brains of bilinguals for each language (cf. Gomez-Tortosa et al., 1995).

An Introduction to the Evaluation of Language Functions

There are several different aspects of language that are evaluated during assessment. A thorough language evaluation involves an assessment of an individual's ability to understand "what is said to them" (i.e., receptive language) and their ability to "express their thoughts" (i.e., expressive language). Beyond these two main areas of language evaluation, there is much variability between the language evaluation batteries on which individual evaluators rely. Professionals completing language evaluations may include an evaluation of other abilities, including articulation, prosody, naming, fluency, pragmatics, grammar and syntax, length of utterance, repetition, and rate. This section will describe methods in which language skills and abilities are measured, using formal and informal assessment tools. It is important to recognize that care must be exercised in the use of these measures, partially because of the problems and shortcoming noted previously. For example, although many of these measures may have "Spanish' versions, they do not have normative data for Hispanic populations, particularly for monolingual Spanish-speaking Hispanics born abroad. Therefore, it is left to the clinician to exercise careful judgment when using these measures. Finally, a subsection is provided below describing tests that can be used with monolingual and bilingual Hispanic patients.

Formal Evaluation Measures

There is a vast array of standardized evaluation measures that are used to evaluation different aspects of language. Although a review of every language measure is not warranted here, the more commonly used evaluation tools will be discussed. This summary will give the reader an awareness of some of the more commonly used tools used by practitioners in the field at the current time. Please refer to other assessment texts for a more comprehensive review of language measures (cf. Baron, 2004; Lezak, 1995; Spreen and Strauss, 1998). In addition, coverage of tests that could possibly be used with bilingual Spanish-speakers follows this section.

Vocabulary

Perhaps one of the most well-known measures utilized in a formal language evaluation battery is the Boston Naming Test (Kaplan, Goodglass, and Weintraub, 1983). The Boston Naming Test was originally created in an attempt to focus on the naming abilities and general expressive language skills of individuals with aphasia (Johnstone, Holland, and Larimore, 2000; Spreen and Strauss, 1998). The test consists of 60 black and white drawings of objects, ranging from everyday objects (e.g., chair) to less common objects (e.g., xylophone). Individuals are requested to name the object presented to them. If they are unable to provide the name of the object, a prompt may be provided, giving the individual information regarding the use or purpose of the object. If the individual is still unable to name the object, the examiner provides a phonetic cue, giving them the first phoneme of the word. This method of providing the individual with category and phonetic cues allows the examiner to differentiate lack of exposure or knowledge of the object to dysnomia that may possibly be associated with other concomitant language deficits.

The Peabody Picture Vocabulary Test – Third Edition (PPVT-III; Dunn and Dunn, 1997) is a commonly used measure to assess receptive vocabulary for individuals aged 2 years, 6 months, through 90 years of age. According to Anastasi and Urbina (1997), vocabulary measures such as the Peabody Picture Vocabulary Test – Third Edition (PPVT-III; Dunn and Dunn, 1997) are useful to assess "use" vocabulary. This test consists of 204 test plates, each consisting of four numbered pictures. As each test plate is shown to the individual, the examiner provides the stimulus word orally. According to the test directions (Dunn and Dunn, 1997), the examinee is required to indicate the correct picture by pointing to or stating the number of the picture that best represents the meaning of the word. For each age group, certain blocks of items are administered until the individual obtains eight errors in a block, at which time the test is discontinued.

Other measures of expressive and receptive vocabulary include the Expressive One-Word Picture Vocabulary Test – 2000 Edition (EOWPVT-2000; Gardner, 2000), the Receptive One-Word Picture Vocabulary Test – 2000 Edition (ROWPVT-2000; Gardner, 2000), and the Beery Picture Vocabulary Test (BPVT; Beery and Taheri, 1992). The Test of Word Finding (TWF; German, 1986) contains a group of tasks that assess an individual's verbal abilities similar to the Evaluation of Language Fundamentals Preschool – Second Edition (CELF-II Preschool; Wiig, Secord, and Semel, 2004) both of have which Expressive Vocabulary subtests.

Rapid/Speeded Naming

Rapid or speeded naming techniques can be traced back to Norman Geschwind and his identification of a disconnection syndrome (Baron, 2004). These tasks draw upon language and executive functioning, as a person has to quickly "call to mind" the verbal labels for visual stimuli. Rapid naming tasks have been created using a variety of stimuli, including blocks of color, color words, numbers, letters, and simple objects.

There are several examples of rapid naming measures. The Clinical Evaluation of Language Fundamentals – Fourth Edition Rapid Automatic Naming subtest (CELF-IV; Semel, Wiig, and Secord, 2003) is a criterion-referenced measure used to assess an individual's ability to rapidly name shapes, colors, and color-shape combinations. The NEPSY Developmental Neuropsychological Assessment has the Speeded Naming subtest (NEPSY; Korkman, Kirk, and Kemp, 1998), which requires the child to rapidly identify the size, color, and shape of objects presented to them (e.g., small, blue triangle). The Comprehensive Test of Phonological Processing Rapid Naming subtests (CTOPP; Wagner, Torgesen, and Rashotte, 1999) incorporate some of the aforementioned tasks, and include the rapid naming of colors, numbers, letters, and objects. The Delis-Kaplan Tests of Executive Function (D-KEFS; Delis, Kaplan, and Kramer, 2001) have provided for a new and unique way to measure speeded naming ability. The Delis-Kaplan Tests of

Executive Function Color-Word Interference Test (D-KEFS; Delis, Kaplan, and Kramer, 2001) begins with typical color naming and color word reading tasks; however, the test authors combine the rapid naming tasks with a Stroop-like task, thereby using the more basic rapid naming measures to rule out basic skills that may interfere with an individual's performance on higher-order tasks such as the Inhibition and Inhibition/Switching tasks.

Verbal Fluency

Verbal fluency has long been evaluated by use of the FAS or other means of Controlled Oral Word Association tasks (Baron, 2004; Johnstone, Holland, and Larimore, 2000). FAS, as it is commonly known, requires individuals to provide the examiner with as many words as they can that begin with those letters, and allows 60 seconds for each letter. The individual is instructed not to use names of people, places, or numbers. Similar to FAS, category verbal fluency is often used. Common category prompts include animals, food, fruits, and names (Spreen and Strauss, 1998). Other evaluation measures also include a verbal fluency subtest within their battery. Examples of these include the NEPSY Developmental Neuropsychological Assessment Verbal Fluency subtest (Korkman, Kirk, and Kemp, 1998) and the D-KEFS Verbal Fluency Test (Delis, Kaplan, and Kramer, 2001). The CELF-IV Word Associations subtest (CELF-IV; Semel, Wiig, and Secord, 2003) is a criterion-referenced verbal fluency measure. Pontón and his colleagues (1996) provide normative data on a verbal fluency task that have been stratified by age and educational levels for Hispanics ascertained from the Los Angeles, California, metropolitan areas with their specific cultural and ethnic factors as noted in Chapter 2.

Phonological Processing

Phonological processing is an essential component to oral language; however, phonological processing also contributes to appropriate reading and writing skills. The Comprehensive Test of Phonological Processing (CTOPP; Wagner, Torgesen, and Rashotte, 1999) was created as a tool to measure several different aspects of phonological processing, including phonological awareness and phonological memory. Tasks involved in the assessment of phonological awareness and memory on the Comprehensive Test of Phonological Processing (CTOPP; Wagner, Torgesen, and Rashotte, 1999) include elision, blending words and nonwords, sound matching, segmenting nonwords, and reversal of phonemes. Other tasks that assess phonological awareness are included in larger assessment measures, including the Clinical Evaluation of Language Fundamentals – Fourth Edition Phonological Awareness subtest (CELF-IV; Semel, Wiig, and Secord, 2003) and the Clinical Evaluation of Language Fundamentals Preschool – Second Edition Phonological Awareness subtest (CELF-II Preschool; Wiig, Secord, and Semel,

2004), which are criterion-referenced measures. The NEPSY Developmental Neuropsychological Assessment (Korkman, Kirk, and Kemp, 1998) also has a Phonological Processing subtest.

Broad Language Evaluation

There are an increasingly greater number of evaluation tools designed to measure general language abilities. As noted before, this chapter will not attempt to delineate every language evaluation tool. However, specific measures will be detailed here in an attempt to allow the reader insight into the more commonly used measures in pediatric and adult language evaluation.

Among the evaluation measures used with pediatric populations, possibly the most commonly used is the Clinical Evaluation of Language Fundamental – Fourth Edition (CELF-IV; Semel, Wiig, and Secord, 2003). The CELF-IV is an assessment tool that covers a range of abilities, including expressive language, receptive language, language memory, language content, and working memory. It can be used with children, adolescents, and young adults ranging in age from 5 through 21 years of age.

The Preschool Language Scales – Fourth Edition (PLS-4; Zimmerman, Steiner, and Pond, 2002) and the Clinical Evaluation of Language Fundamentals Preschool – Second Edition (CELF-II Preschool; Wiig, Secord, and Semel, 2004) are two more pediatric language evaluation tools used for children ranging in age from birth to six years, seven months of age, and three years to six years of age, respectively. The Preschool Language Scales – Fourth Edition measures the ability areas of auditory comprehension and expressive communication. It also has two ratings that the examiner can complete, including a screening of articulation and a listing of language samples. The Clinical Evaluation of Language Fundamentals Preschool – Second Edition (CELF-II Preschool; Wiig, Secord, and Semel, 2004) provides broad scores for several key areas, including core (broad) language, receptive language, expressive language, knowledge of language content, and knowledge of language structure. It is worthwhile to note that the CELF-II possesses a version in Spanish, yet care must be exercised in its interpretation because of its limited norms.

There are many other broad evaluation tools that incorporate language measures into their batteries. Some of the tools for very young children include the Bayley Scales of Infant Development – Second Edition (BSID-2; Bayley, 1993) and the Mullen Scales of Early Learning (Mullen, 1995). The BISD-2 can be used with children from birth through 42 months of age. The Mullen can be used with children from birth to 68 months of age. Another pediatric measure that includes an evaluation of language abilities is the NEPSY Developmental Neuropsychological Assessment (Korkman, Kirk, and Kemp, 1998).

Like the availability of numerous measures of pediatric language evaluation, there is a wide array of adult language assessment batteries. Lezak (1995) and Spreen and Strauss (1998) are excellent resources to review the details of these batteries. Some of the more common language evaluation measures available include the Boston Diagnostic Aphasia Examination (BDAE; Goodglass and Kaplan, 1983a) and the Multilingual Aphasia Examination – Third Edition (MAE-3; Benton, Hamsher, Rey, and Sivian, 1994). The Boston Diagnostic Aphasia Examination (BDAE; Goodglass and Kaplan, 1983a) covers many areas of language functioning, including auditory comprehension, oral expression, written comprehension, and written expression (Goodglass and Kaplan, 1983b). The Multilingual Aphasia Examination – Third Edition (MAE-3; Benton, Hamsher, Rey, and Sivian, 1994) evaluates a range of language skills, including oral expression, spelling, oral verbal understanding, and reading; it also has observational rating scales in which to rate an individual's articulation and praxic features of writing (Spreen and Strauss, 1998). Another broad language evaluation measure, and possibly one of the most famous, is the Halstead-Wepman Aphasia Screening Test (Halstead and Wepman, 1959).

Caregiver Evaluation of Language

In addition to the various language evaluation measures that can be administered directly to the individual, there are a variety of rating scales that can be used with caregivers of individuals who are undergoing evaluation. The Vineland Adaptive Behavior Scales Interview Edition (Sparrow, Balla, and Cicchetti, 1984) and the Adaptive Behavior Assessment System – Second Edition (Harrison and Oakland, 2003) are broad measures of an individual's level of adaptive behavior. Within the scope of the ratings, however, they provide information related to the individual's functional language abilities, including expressive and receptive abilities, as perceived by their caregivers. The Clinical Evaluation of Language Fundamentals – Fourth Edition (Semel, Wiig, and Secord, 2003) and the Clinical Evaluation of Language Fundamentals Preschool – Second Edition (CELF-II Preschool; Wiig, Secord, and Semel, 2004) both provide a brief measure for caregiver ratings on an individual's pragmatic language. This rating scale covers several areas of pragmatic language, including rituals and conversational skills; asking for, giving, and responding to information; and nonverbal communication skills. Other caregiver rating scales that have a language component include the Scale of Independent Behavior – Revised (SIB-R; Bruininks, Woodcock, Weatherman, and Hill, 1996), the AAMR Adaptive Behavior Scale – School Second Edition (Lambert, Nihira, and Leland, 1993), and the Preschool Language Scales – Fourth Edition (Zimmerman, Steiner, and Pond, 2002).

Informal Evaluation Methods

After a perusal of the previous section regarding formal evaluation measures, it is clear that practitioners can occupy their time using standardized assessment tools.

However, relying only on these tools may leave out qualitative information about an individual's language abilities. Simply allowing an individual to tell a story may allow the practitioner exceptional insight into the individual's ability to maintain conversation appropriately, express the information in a grammatically correct fashion, and pronounce words in articulately.

Lezak (1995) noted several aspects of speech that are important to assess during language evaluations. These aspects include prosody, fluency, and articulation, which are not always amenable to formal language evaluation. Rhodes and colleagues (Rhodes, Kayser, and Hess, 2000) also noted that linguistic complexity is another important aspect to evaluate, especially in individuals who are multilingual.

Lezak (1995) and others (Damico, 1985, 1991; Johnston, 1982; Warner and Nelson, 2000) detail informal techniques used to identify discourse abilities by means of language sampling techniques. Johnston (1982) and Damico (1985, 1991) modified this type of descriptive assessment of language abilities for use with limited English-proficient students; however, the technique also can be used to gain additional insights into the specific language abilities of an individual. The informal language assessment is meant to be descriptive and not based on norm-based standards of evaluation. The informal language assessment consists of two parts: the oral monologic assessment and the oral dialogic assessment.

The Oral Monologic Assessment is an assessment of language abilities based on "communication that is preplanned" based on visual or verbal cues (p. 183, Damico, 1991). Oral Monologic assessment evaluates skills in three main areas: static tasks (object description, giving directions), dynamic tasks (story reformulation, narrative analysis), and abstract tasks (opinion-expressing) (Damico, 1991). On the contrary, the Oral Dialogic Assessment is spontaneous and unplanned communication that is typically embedded within conversation. The individual must be able to modify his or her dialogue based on the thoughts and ideas expressed by another person. Based on an analysis of the information conveyed by the speaker, information is gained regarding fluency, clarity of expression, and comprehension. Damico (1991) details four main categories in which language can be analyzed, including quantity, quality, relation, and manner.

Evaluation of Multilingual Individuals

As can be seen, clinicians may spend much time in formal and information evaluation of individuals with language impairments. However, with the ever-changing needs of the population of the United States, clinicians will likely encounter individuals with language impairments that are bilingual, multilingual, or with limited English proficiency. As a result, it is important to understand the intricacies of evaluation with this special group of individuals. Even two decades ago, research was touting the importance of second-language proficiency in school psychologists in order to effectively evaluate children who were linguistically different (Figueroa,

Sandoval, and Merino, 1984; Kamphaus, 1993). At the same time, psychologists are encouraged to use instruments appropriate to evaluate a child's language abilities in their first and second (or third) language (Figueroa, Sandoval, and Merino, 1984; Ochoa, Rivera, and Ford, 1997). In order to gain an accurate picture of a multilingual individual's language level of impairment (if any), there must be a valid assessment of skills in both languages, using information from a variety of sources, including formal and informal evaluation, as well as observational data.

Centeno and Obler (2001) detail two main concerns when working with multi-lingual individuals. They indicate that the clinician's initial responsibility is to evaluate the level of language balance or dominance in order to determine the most appropriate evaluation measures. Second, Centeno and Obler strongly assert that neuropsychological and other deficits may be falsely exaggerated by impaired language proficiency. This pattern of impaired language proficiency, if not fully examined, may indeed mimic a language impairment. For instance, semilingualism, when two languages are not equivalent to the skills of a monolingual speaker of either language (Centeno and Obler, 2001), may be the result of a language impair-ment or the mode of instruction (S.H. Ochoa, personal communication, 2000). If an individual's semilingualism is falsely attributed to a language impairment, inappro-priate goals and intervention strategies may be employed to remediate the impairment, rather than supplement the lack of proficiency in either language.

Some of the more commonly used measures designed to assess language profi-ciency in English and Spanish include the Woodcock Language Proficiency Battery – Revised English and Spanish Form (WLPB-R; Woodcock, 1991), the Woodcock Language Proficiency Battery – Revised Spanish Form (WLPB-R; Woodcock and Muñoz-Sandoval, 1995), the Woodcock-Muñoz Language Survey English Form (WMLS; Woodcock and Muñoz-Sandoval, 1993a), and the Woodcock-Muñoz Language Survey Spanish Form (WMLS; Woodcock and Muñoz-Sandoval, 1993b), which can be used with individuals ages 2 through 90. The Woodcock Language Proficiency Battery – Revised English and Spanish Form (WLPB-R; Woodcock, 1991) and the Woodcock Language Proficiency Battery – Revised Spanish Form (WLPB-R; Woodcock and Muñoz-Sandoval, 1995) provide the following scores: Oral Language, Broad Reading, Basic Reading Skills, Reading Comprehension, Broad Written Language, Basic Writing Skills, Written Expression, and Broad Ability. In addition to these broad ability areas, the Woodcock Language Proficiency Battery – Revised Spanish Form (WLPB-R; Woodcock and Muñoz-Sandoval, 1995), the Woodcock-Muñoz Language Survey English Form (WMLS; Woodcock and Muñoz-Sandoval, 1993a), and the Woodcock-Muñoz Language Survey Spanish Form (WMLS; Woodcock and Muñoz-Sandoval, 1993b) also provide a score detailing the individual's level of Cognitive Academic Language Proficiency (CALP; Cummins, 1984).

The Bilingual Verbal Abilities Test (BVAT; Muñoz-Sandoval, Cummins, Alvarado, and Ruef, 1998) is designed to assess the level of language proficiency in English and another language. It is comprised of three tests from the Woodcock-Johnson Tests of Cognitive Ability – Revised (WJ-R Cognitive; Woodcock and Johnson, 1989), namely the Picture Vocabulary, Oral Vocabulary, and Verbal

Analogies subtests. The Bilingual Verbal Abilities Test (BVAT; Muñoz-Sandoval, Cummins, Alvarado, and Ruef, 1998) has been adapted into 18 other languages, including Spanish, Arabic, Chinese, Hmong, and Navaho, and can be used with individuals aged five years old through adulthood. The benefit of using the Bilingual Verbal Abilities Test (BVAT; Muñoz-Sandoval, Cummins, Alvarado, and Ruef, 1998) is that it provides an estimate of the individual's verbal ability based on the use of the native and secondary language, thereby yielding what is likely to be a better estimate of language skills compared to the assessment in only one language.

There are several other language measures commonly used during evaluation of Spanish speakers. These include the Test de Vocabulario en Imagenes Peabody (TVIP; Dunn, Padilla, Lugo, and Dunn, 1986), the Expressive One-Word Picture Vocabulary Test – Revised Spanish Edition (Gardner, 1990b), the IDEA Oral Language Proficiency Test Pre-IPT – Spanish (Ballard, Tighe, and Dalton, 1989), the IDEA Oral Language Proficiency Test IPT 1 – Spanish (Ballard, Tighe, and Dalton, 1996a), and the IDEA Oral Language Proficiency Test IPT 1 – Spanish (Ballard, Tighe, and Dalton, 1996b) . The Test de Vocabulario en Imagenes Peabody (TVIP; Dunn, Padilla, Lugo, and Dunn, 1986) is the "Spanish-language, Hispanic-American adaptation" of the Peabody Picture Vocabulary Test – Revised (PPVT-R; Dunn and Dunn, 1981), which was described earlier. The Expressive One-Word Picture Vocabulary Test – Revised Spanish Edition (Gardner, 1990b) is the Spanish version of the Expressive One-Word Picture Vocabulary Test – Revised (Gardner, 1990a). The Expressive One-Word Picture Vocabulary Test – Spanish Bilingual Edition (EOWPVT-SBE; Brownell, 2001) is a relatively new measure somewhat similar to the Bilingual Verbal Abilities Test (BVAT; Muñoz-Sandoval, Cummins, Alvarado, and Ruef, 1998) in that it allows the individual to respond in either English or Spanish. Therefore, the score obtained is a measure of the individual's total acquired vocabulary. The Expressive One-Word Picture Vocabulary Test – Spanish Bilingual Edition (EOWPVT-SBE; Brownell, 2001) can be used for individuals aged 4 years, 0 months, to 12 years, 11 months of age. The IDEA Oral Language Proficiency Test Pre-IPT Spanish (Ballard, Tighe, and Dalton, 1989), the IDEA Oral Language Proficiency Test IPT 1 – Spanish (Ballard, Tighe, and Dalton, 1996a), and the IDEA Oral Language Proficiency Test IPT II – Spanish (Ballard, Tighe, and Dalton, 1996b) were designed to assess the oral Spanish language proficiency of children whose first language is Spanish. The Spanish versions of the tests were developed along the same lines as the English version of the tests, and may be used with children who are 3 to 5 years of age (Pre-IPT), children in kindergarten through 6th grade (IPT I), and children in grades 7 through 12 (IPT II). The test covers four basic areas of oral language proficiency, including vocabulary, comprehension, syntax, and verbal expression. Pontón and his colleagues (1996) provide normative data for an experimental measure, a modified Boston Naming Test.

There are two additional and prominent measures that are designed for Spanish speakers. For individuals who are proficient in Spanish, they allow the clinician to get an accurate measure of a person's cognitive functioning and level of academic achievement for individuals aged two to adulthood. Namely, these measures are the Batería Woodcock-Muñoz Pruebas de habilidad cognitiva – III (Tests of Cognitive Ability; Woodcock, Muñoz-Sandoval, McGrew, Mather, and Schrank, 2004a) and the Batería Woodcock-Muñoz Pruebas de aprovechamiento – III (Tests of Achievement; Woodcock, Muñoz-Sandoval, McGrew, Mather, and Schrank, 2004b).

Summary

Language is a fascinating area of investigation and clinical practice, especially when consideration is given to the effects of the environment and exposure to other languages and how they contribute to cognitive outcomes. This chapter has provided a thorough overview of language development in monolingual and bilingual individuals. At this point, the reader should be well informed of the myths and fallacies promoted by individuals who are unaware of the research being conducted on children and adults who sequentially acquire a second language. A lack of understanding of these very important issues will only promulgate further misconceptions regarding linguistic minorities, including a select number of individuals in the Hispanic population, and should be rectified through self-study and the offering of education to less informed individuals and groups.

Information was also provided regarding specific language disorders and the physiological correlates that are associated with each disorder through brain-behavior relationships. It is important to remember that injury and insult to the brain are often diffuse, thereby resulting in mixed language difficulties, rather than what ideally might be expected based on a very focal injury, such as a gunshot wound or other focal head injury. With this in mind, it is important for the reader to be aware of the variability that is likely in an individual's demonstration of their neurocognitive and linguistic skills, particularly individuals who are bilingual.

Finally, the reader was exposed to a number of assessment methods that are used in the evaluation of language skills. It is evident that there are many evaluation tools available to the practitioner, including instruments for Hispanics who are monolingual English-speakers and monolingual Spanish-speakers. Above all, the clinician should be careful in choosing methods that have demonstrated adequate psychometric properties. Also, neuropsychologists must rely on sound clinical judgment in ascertaining skill level based on qualitative information, in addition to information obtained via quantitative methods.

In summation, it is evident that language is critical for the survival of the species, and that this particular function differentiates *Homo sapiens* from other animals in the animal kingdom, providing software used by the brain to generate and test hypotheses without the need for exposure to dangerous conditions. Language acquisition is not a simple process, regardless of cultural and linguistic context or background, and this is true for Spanish. Many factors affect the way children develop their native language or other languages they may be exposed to during developmental periods. However, these issues are extremely important to understand, especially when there is concern regarding the possibility of a language disorder. From an applied and tangible standpoint, if individuals exhibit deficits in their secondary language, but such deficits are absent in the native or primary language, it should lead the clinician to take a conservative inferential posture suggesting the presence of language impediments. It may thus be surmised that there may not be a "true" language disorder but rather difficulties in the acquisition of another language, or other factor, and these possibilities are indeed applicable to Hispanics living in the U.S. However, if a bilingual Hispanic individual displays deficits in both languages, it may be surmised that a language disorder is present, which hopefully will be classified as such and delineated with a degree of accuracy that leads to appropriate intervention and treatment.

Chapter 6
The Neuropsychological Assessment
of the Hispanic Client

Antolin M. Llorente and Deborah Weber

The senior author remembers eagerly reading the book *The Art of Loving* (Fromm, 1956) for the first time as a teenager. In its Foreword, Dr. Fromm notes in its first sentence that "reading of this book would be a disappointing experience for anyone who expects easy instruction in the art of loving." Unfortunately, the same disappointment is applicable to this chapter, in that the reader will quickly surmise the complexity involved in the neuropsychological assessment of the Hispanic client. This chapter, or this entire volume for that matter, is incapable of providing "easy instruction" in such an art.

Such complexity is the result of the potential, synergistic impact of all the factors so far discussed. For example, level of education, specific cultural background, and other demographic variables (e.g., age and geographical region within the U.S.), in conjunction with language fluency and proficiency (English, Spanish, both, neither for valid assessment purposes), coupled with the limited availability of tests and norms from which valid and reliable inferences can be generated interact to create the aforementioned complexity.[1] Therefore, detailed examples will be provided below in an attempt to show potential strategies or elucidate plausible courses of action to address such issues. However, before providing applied examples, there are a few theoretical issues regarding neuropsychological assessment not covered thus far that should be addressed.

Traditional psychological evaluation approaches often focus on identifying the diagnosis (e.g., depression, mental deficiency, learning disability) used to determine

---

[1] The authors firmly believe that such complexity is also commonly encountered daily in unique individuals in American society from other ethnic groups that would be qualified by the U.S. Census Bureau as part of a "majority" group if due attention and weight are given to important demographic characteristics. In this regard, and for ridiculously obvious reasons, the reader is asked to consider the following patients: A "White" individual from an Amish background from Lancaster, Pennsylvania, who received a fifth grade education and predominantly speaks "Pennsylvania Dutch"; a "White" child from a "Cajun" background from Lafayette, Louisiana, who only speaks standard English at school; and a highly educated "White" adult from an Orthodox Jewish background from inner city New York who predominantly speaks Hebrew. Clearly, even ethnic minority is a relative term, and more important, race should never be confounded with culture or ethnicity.

placement, rehabilitation, or other appropriate services or treatments (cf. Sheridan and Gutkin, 2000, in the case of children, and Lezak et al., 2004, in the case of adults). Such an assessment posture fails to take into account specific individual strengths and weaknesses and often places Hispanic clients, be they children or adults, at a distinct disadvantage, leading to inappropriate placement of youths and to an overrepresentation in special education programs (Committee on Minority Representation in Special Education, 2002; Losen and Orfield, 2002; Office of Special Education Programs, 2001) in the case of children and/or misdiagnosis in the case of adults (cf. Lu, Lim and Mezzich, 1995). This leads in some instances to negative repercussions in many applied settings, including career, vocational, and judicial settings. Adopting a neuropsychological assessment perspective with Hispanics requires not just a comprehensive functional assessment capable of delineating areas of strengths as well as areas of cognitive weaknesses, but it additionally requires a different, holistic "mind set," particularly regarding perceptions of the client. A neuropsychological examination with such a perspective permits a better determination and comprehensive neurocognitive and neurobehavioral assessment and a greater degree of delineation and tailoring of interventions, rehabilitative programs (see Chapter 8), and treatments for the client that includes his or her cultural and ethnic fabric. Adopting a theoretical perspective based on a science of brain-behavior relationships incorporating cultural and ethnic variables allows a potential shift in focus from the identification or labeling of the Hispanic client to interventions truly based on the client's unique and idiographic patterns of cognitive assets and liabilities in information processing. Hence, adopting an integrative and comprehensive neuropsychological approach to assessment significantly enhances multicultural assessment and treatment of Hispanic adults and children.

A Comprehensive Neuropsychological Perspective of Assessment

Neuropsychology focuses on studying complex relationships between behaviors and brain functions. From a clinical standpoint, a neuropsychological approach to assessment involves an understanding of these relationships subsequent to clinical assessment of specific domains. Using a nomothetic approach, cognitive functions and behaviors within this framework are evaluated via the use of standardized instruments; test performance is then expressed in the form of a score (Lezak et al., 2004). Understanding of brain-behavior relationships occurs as a result of interpreting patterns of performance and models of cultural and neural development through assessing an individual's assets and limitations in specific domains of functioning.

The ultimate goal of most neuropsychological evaluations is to answer referral questions while considering cognition, behavior, genetic, medical, psychosocial, and specific environmental factors (cf. Lezak et al., 2004; Teeter and Semrud-Clikeman, 1997), including cultural variables (cf. Wong et al., 2000). In addition, within a developmental framework we would like to add, even in the case of adults when possible, developing hypotheses related to brain functions responsible for comportment. To achieve such a lofty goal, the astute and ethical neuropsychologist depends on a variety of collateral sources of information, including the patients' verbal report, past personal and family history, school, vocational and other records (e.g., military), and cross-informant reports (e.g., caretaker, partner, teacher). In addition, the neuropsychologist depends on information related to current and past over-the-counter and prescribed medication use, as well as current and past use of complementary therapy and controlled substances, cross-diagnostic data including laboratory reports (e.g., blood work, metabolic block), results from past audiological, medical, neuropsychological, ophthalmologic, and psychological evaluations and data from structural and functional neuroimaging, in addition to an armamentarium of psychometric instruments, clinical interviewing, and behavioral observations. A comprehensive and integrated neuropsychological approach to the assessment of the Hispanic client also is concerned with the functional and/or practical conceptualization of the condition afflicting the individual, if any, at various levels within different contexts. In the forensic arena, such evaluations also require the use of assessment techniques to examine response bias and feigned symptoms (cf. Rogers, 1997). It is also involved with the determination of disruptive mechanisms and their rehabilitation (cf. Lezak et al., 2004; Rourke, Fisk, and Strong, 1986).

Given the various and numerous issues discussed thus far, in conjunction with the factors presented in Chapters 1–5, it is clear that the major obstacle during the course of assessment of Hispanic patients becomes the ability to obtain reliable and valid results. Nevertheless, state of the art, comprehensive, and integrated neuropsychological evaluations examine brain-behavior relationships by assessing more specific domains than general intellect and psychological assessment in the Hispanic patient. The evaluations are often supplemented by the assessment of other domains in order to address the specific referral question. Assessment typically includes multiple domains of functioning (e.g., intelligence, academic achievement, attention, executive functions, information processing, perception and perceptual organization, learning and memory, language, motor skills, and personality factors to name a few), and in some instances, when valid and prudent, includes assessment of premorbid functioning through the use of methods or tests that permit such estimations. Although only provided as guideline, Table 6.1 shows some of these domains with tests that could potentially be used with Hispanics.

Theoretical Assessment Approaches

Several theoretical assessment approaches to neuropsychological assessment are now discussed. One method relies on assessment and conceptualization using a standardized battery approach (e.g., Halstead-Reitan Neuropsychological Test Battery for adults or children, Reitan and Davison, 1974; SENAS, Mungas et al., 2004). A standard battery uses a quantitative approach that infers brain functioning based on measures of behavior that have been validated on individuals with brain

Table 6.1 Assessment Domains, Sample Procedures Utilized in Evaluations, and Potential Functions Screened**

Domains	Tests and procedures	Function(s)
Developmental	Bayley Scales of Infant Development –II (BSID-II)*	Emerging cognitive and behavioral development
	Mullen Scales of Early Learning	Multiple Intelligences
Intelligence	Wechsler Intelligence Tests	
	WAIS-III*	
	WISC-IV	
	WISC-IV in Spanish*	
	WISC-RM*	
	Woodcock-Johnson-Third Edition (WJ-III)	Crystallized and Fluid Intelligence
	Kaufman Assessment Battery for Children (K-ABC)-Revised	Simultaneous and sequential processing skills
	Batería Woodcock-Muñoz Pruebas de Habilidades Cognitivas-Third Edition (Batería-III)*.^	
Nonverbal Function	Test of Nonverbal Intelligence, Second Edition (TONI-2)*	Nonverbal Intelligence
	Comprehensive Test of Nonverbal Intelligence (C-TONI)	
	Universal Nonverbal Intelligence Test (UNIT)	
	Naglieri Nonverbal Intelligence Test	
Achievement	Woodcock-Johnson, Tests of Achievement (WJ-III ACH)	Intracognitive & achievement
	Kaufman Test of Educational Achievement (K-TEA)	Achievement (ability-achievement discrepancies)
	Batería Woodcock-Muñoz Pruebas de Aprovechamiento-Third Edition (Batería-III)*.^	
Motor Functions		
Speed	Grooved Pegboard Test	Finger dexterity
Strength	Hand Dynamometer (Grip Strength Test)	Hand strength
Coordination	Finger Tapping Test	Index finger speed and coordination
	Hand Movements (K-ABC)*	go-no-go processes
	McCarthy Scales of Children's Abilities (Motor Scale)	Gross and fine motor skills
Visual-Motor	Block Design (WAIS; WASI; WISC)*	Analysis and synthesis of abstract designs*

Category	Test	Function
	Object Assembly (WAIS; WASI; WISC)*	Synthesis of concrete parts into meaningful wholes*
	Coding (WAIS; WASI; WISC)*	Processing speed/Visual motor dexterity*
	Developmental Test of Visual-Motor Integration (VMI)*	Visual-motor integration
	Rey-Osterrieth Complex Figure Test (RCFT),* Copy	Complex visual-motor integration*
Language/Communication	Peabody Picture Vocabulary Test-Third Edition	Emerging reception/auditory comprehension
	Expressive One Word Vocabulary Test	Emerging expression/expressive language
	Tests of Written Language	Written language
	Boston Naming Test (BNT)	Confrontational naming task
	Controlled Oral-Word Association (COWA)*	Verbal fluency
	Token Test	Verbal comprehension
	Clinical Evaluation of Language Fundamentals – III (CELF-III)	Receptive & expressive language
	Preschool Language Scale – IV (PLS-IV)	Receptive & expressive language
	Test de Vocabulario en Imagines Peabody	
Sensory-Perceptual		
Visual	Motor-Free Visual Perception Test discrimination	Spatial relations, visual closure, & figure- ground
Auditory	Wepman's Auditory Discrimination Test	
Tactile-Kinesthetic	Tactile Perception Test	Attention, tactile localization
	Fingertip Number-Writing Test	Complex tactile perception
Perceptual Organization	Hooper Visual Organization Test	Perceptual organization
	Rey-Osterrieth Complex Figure Test (RCFT),* Copy	
Information Processing	Clock Drawing	Visuo-spatial and executive functions
Learning and Memory	Benton Visual Retention Test – Revised	Memory
	Rey-Osterrieth Complex Figure Test (RCFT),* Recall	Visual learning and memory
	Children's Auditory Verbal Learning Test-Second edition (CAVLT-2)	Auditory rote learning & memory
	Test of Memory and Learning (TOMAL)	Learning and memory
	Children Memory Scale	Verbal and visual learning & memory
	Wide Range Assessment of Memory and Learning (WRAML)	Verbal and visual information

(continued)

Table 6.1 (continued)

Domains	Tests and procedures	Function(s)
Attention & Concentration Visual	Test of Variables of Attention (TOVA)	Vigilance, impulsivity, attention, reaction time
	D2 Test: Concentration Endurance Test	Sustained attention, visual scanning
	Leiter International Performance Scale – Revised (Attention Sustained Only)	Sustained attention
	Color Trails 1 & 2 and Children Color Trails 1 & 2*	Alternating attention, concentration, Planning, measure of inhibition
Auditory	Digit Span*	Immediate simple auditory recall
	Test of Variables of Attention (Auditory)	Vigilance, attention, reaction time
Executive Function(s)	Behavior Rating Inventory of Executive Functioning (BRIEF)	Report of emerging executive skills
	Design Fluency Test	Production of novel designs, planning
	Symbol Digit Modalities Test (SDMT)	Visual scanning and tracking, inhibition
	Color Trails 2 and Children's Color Trails 2*	Inhibition, mental flexibility
	Children's Category Test	Abstraction, mental flexibility, learning
	Stroop Interference Test	Attention, cognitive flexibility, inhibition
	Wisconsin Card Sorting Test (WCST)	Problem solving, concept formation, shifting and maintaining set
Psychosocial Functioning	Behavior Assessment System for Children (BASC)*	Adaptive & clinical behaviors, multimethod, multidimensional (Validity Scales)
	Clinical Interview	
	Millon (MACI)	
	Minnesota Multiphasic Personality Inventory–Adolescent	
	Sentence Completion Tests	
	Adaptive Behavior Assessment System (ABAS)	Report of adaptive behavior

* These procedures are available in Spanish. Norms also may be available (e.g., Pontón et al., 1996).

** Some procedures may not assess the domain purported to be under scrutiny as a result of injury to the CNS.

^ Identifies batteries with good subtests capable of being independently administered to assess specific domains such as language. In those cases, to guard against circularity, it is recommended that another test be administered to investigate overall cognition. See Chapter 5 for additional procedures.

damage, thus supporting the premise that behavior is controlled by the brain. Based on the premise that there is an organic basis to behavior, performances on behavioral measures are used to assess brain functioning. This approach is designed to draw on a broad range of abilities and functions of Hispanic patients, regardless of the referral question. Obvious limitations include cost-effectiveness, limited flexibility in assessment, and emphasis on differential diagnosis instead of interventions. A strength of the method is the large number of normative and standardized bases of many of these tests, not to mention the ability to develop batteries of tests with very high internal consistencies and so on.

Similarly, the Luria-Nebraska Neuropsychological Battery (Christensen, 1975; Golden, 1986) has a strong focus on process and is based on the application of the theories and procedures developed by A.R. Luria. Luria's theory of higher cortical function viewed information processing as involving "simultaneous" and "successive" mental processes. This model involved the transitional interaction of various regions and zones in the brain, which thus produces complex behavior. This approach matches corresponding neurological strengths with methods of acquiring and presenting information that capitalize on an individual's strengths.

Another approach, the Boston Process Approach, also involves the integration of qualitative and quantitative methods to analysis and interpretation of test results. According to Kaplan (1996), evaluations to assess cognitive function are often scored as right or wrong en route to a total score designed to identify global achievement. However, this type of assessment approach does not assess strategies that may be employed when an individual scores a right or wrong answer. This achievement-oriented approach fails to take into consideration the multitude of diverse processes (and systems) that an individual may use or engage to arrive at a final solution. Employing a process-oriented approach enables analysis of a person's unique problem-solving behavior and compensatory strategies. Final assessment of clinical limits is possible with alternative formats of various available traditional tests, and formal assessment of the clinical limits provides relevant diagnostic information regarding strategies an individual employs to compensate for cognitive difficulties or subtle cognitive dysfunction. Although the Boston Process Approach allows great flexibility in addressing specific referral questions, research addressing the validity of the approach is limited, and it is possible for the clinician to overdiagnose and overinterpret pathology (cf. Reynolds and Mayfield, 1999).

Another major approach is the integrative flexible battery approach (combination of traditional, educational, psychological, and developmental tests). This approach focuses on the individual and is designed to address specific referral questions. The flexible battery approach lends itself to the needs of the individual in addition to being sensitive to a wide range of patient variables, including gender, language, familial history of handedness, handedness, age, educational background, family structure, individual and family medical, psychiatric, and neurological history, etiology of dysfunction, and premorbid functioning. This approach provides an analysis of an individual's strengths and weaknesses instead of focusing on a specific localization of impairment. It employs both an ideographic and nomothetic approach to assessment (cf. Fennell and Bauer, 1989). As with other approaches, this method suffers from inherent weaknesses, including the fact that the test battery created has not been validated for the purpose used in most instances.

Despite the emphasis of neuropsychology on brain functioning, and the resulting interpretation of assessment results within this context, other environmental factors and their interactions and potential influences on the outcomes of neuropsychological assessment should not be ignored. These variables include immigration patterns, culture, socioeconomic status, educational attainment, acculturation, and a client's primary language.

Applied Examples and Integration

Although brief, truncated, and limited by space considerations, an example of how to integrate all these issues follows. Although it is impossible to cover all variables discussed thus far, an attempt will be made to cover a broad scope of issues presented throughout this book, with emphasis on specific, important, and intricate considerations of subtle details.

Regardless of theoretical orientation, or developmental stage of the individual, the evaluation of the Hispanic patient begins long before the start of the actual examination. It begins with information gathering and review of existing records related to past adaptation, birth, employment, military, school, vocational, and other records; results from past audiological, medical, neurological, neuropsychological, ophthalmological, psychiatric, and psychological evaluations; and surgical interventions and data and reports from past structural and/or functional neuroimaging or any other functional procedures (e.g., EEG), if available. In addition, review of past laboratory results (e.g., metabolic workup) is essential. It also begins with gathering of demographic characteristics of the patient by intake personnel, the specific reason for referral (not a general referral question such as "testing"), as is the case for all other patients. However, unlike clients for whom cultural and ethnic issues are not as important,[2] such issues begin to play a preeminent role at this point for Hispanic patients. For example, in Chapters 1, 2, and 3, and above, we attempted to note the importance of critical issues to be considered during the course of neuropsychological assessment of the Hispanic patient. Now, let us examine how such information and data inform the evaluative process and their critical relevance to assessment decisions.

Above it was noted that level of education, specific cultural background, and other demographic variables in conjunction with language fluency and the availability of specific tests and norms interacted to create a complex evaluative situation and decision-making process. Therefore, let us examine these factors and

---

[2] It should be clear from the previous footnote that from the authors' vantage point, such patients are few, particularly in the U.S.

some of the decisions regarding how best to evaluate an adult "Hispanic" client, a 55-year-old, right-handed, married, Hispanic female from Illinois with an undergraduate degree in accounting from the University of Chicago (she recently resigned from her position as a result of "memory" difficulties), who reports to be bilingual (English- and Spanish-speaker), referred for neuropsychological assessment to "rule-out the onset of Alzheimer's disease" (Alzheimer-type dementia, AD). In this case, as we refer to the initial discussion in this chapter, the patient described is a Hispanic woman whose education took place in the U.S. in a quality institution and is equal to or greater than 16 years (i.e., ≥16 years). Because the panethnic term *Hispanic* is meaningless, upon further scrutiny of her cultural and ethnic identity, it was determined that her specific cultural background was that of a second-generation "Latina" who identified herself as "Mexican-American" from a family background whose ancestors immigrated to Mexico from Spain at the turn of the 19th century. In addition, both of her parents came from similar backgrounds and spoke only Spanish and were without formal exposure to any aboriginal language, although they were exposed informally in social situations while growing up in Mexico. Her parents had immigrated to Illinois during the late 1920s, both with advanced educational backgrounds (undergraduate and graduate degrees). The client grew up in the Chicago metropolitan area (North Central U.S. region) and resided there all her life. Concerns related to poor nutrition, probable exposure to environmental toxins, or similar factors did not emerge, and she has experienced a benign medical history thus far. When asked by intake staff, she reported she was bilingual, but she "predominantly uses English," except at "home when visiting her parents," where "she constantly speaks Spanish." This information was supported by the intake coordinator, as she sometimes spoke in Spanish during the intake interview.

How should a comprehensive, integrated, and culturally competent neuropsychological assessment be conducted with this client? How would it assess this client's skills in an effort to rule out AD? At first glance, an examination of the information collected and presented above would not appear important, particularly because the client appears to be fully fluent in English. However, a closer examination of her demographic characteristics, history, and language fluencies, coupled with the availability of specific tests available and, more important, normative data, reveal a more complex picture.

Before getting into details addressing one of neuropsychologists' favorite subjects, namely test selection, let us examine other vital assessment components. During the course of evaluation, the collection and review of collateral sources of information, including the patient's verbal report, past personal and family history, and cross-informant reports (e.g., husband, former supervisor, sibling) are critical. In this particular case, the information emphasizes declines in global or overall functioning and recent or acute cognitive changes (e.g., "memory" difficulties noted); changes or alterations in her psychosocial and recent (as well as immediate past) vocational histories (with specific emphasis on her recent resignation as a result of memory problems); significant changes in self-care and emotional functioning, beyond what would be expected from normal aging and her personal and family cultural phenomenology, including alterations in "personality," judgment, and abstraction – particularly given concerns about the early detection of AD. A thorough evaluation of past family history of dementia, particularly AD, should also be included. Marital issues, stress, and other factors, including leisure time and time spent socializing, should be examined. A good example of such a historical questionnaire can be found in Spreen and Strauss (1998) for adults (cf. Baron, 2004, for children). In addition, current and past histories of over-the-counter and prescribed medication use, as well as current and past use of complementary therapy and controlled substances and alcohol, are explicitly covered. Neuroimaging records, if available, also should be examined to determine if they provide information consistent with the brain-behavior relationships usually observed in individuals with dementias in general and more specifically with AD, a prototypical cortical dementia.

With regard to some of the factors discussed in Chapter 3, a large number of those variables additionally can be examined in detail during the course of the clinical interview with the client to determine their potential impact. For example, nutritional history (including on the day of evaluation); current and past medical care; socioeconomic status (growing up and current); and other important factors should be examined. The reader is referred to Spreen and Strauss (1998) and Baron (2004) for examples of information obtained before the assessment in the form of a questionnaire. At this point it is fundamental to note that such information is again explored in detail during the course of the clinical interview in children and adults, and the clinical interview in large part serves as an excellent conduit, not just to establish good rapport with the Hispanic patient but to obtain critical historical information leading to a better understanding of their degree of acculturation, cultural and ethnic background, as well as a host of other factors (e.g., mastery and language fluency). It also is vital to recognize, as for all clients, the importance of a good clinical interview (cf. Baron, 2004; Lezak et al., 2004). Such information serves as an interpretative backdrop for all subsequent results from psychometric instruments.

To further illustrate an integrative, cross-culturally sound, neuropsychological assessment, consider the 55-year-old Hispanic woman referred to above with concerns related to AD. Specifically, difficulties associated with a dementia include problems in memory (as reported by the client), yet a dementia could be mimicked by a host of other conditions, including a severe depressive episode or a medical condition such as hypothyroidism, to name a few. Such conditions also must be ruled out through the use of test data, in addition to review of medical, historical, and laboratory reports. Aside from underscoring the importance of the clinical interview, behavioral observations and review of medical records (including an examination of a medical workup and laboratory results such as metabolic assays) should be used to assist in ruling out a metabolic condition such as hypothyroidism. The evaluation should also use formal indices of mood, in addition to verbal report and behavioral observations, to rule out alterations in mood (see below).

Subsequent to the clinical interview, the client's linguistic skills should be investigated. In this regard, it was noted that Pontón and León-Carreón (2001) has provided a flowchart that can be helpful if this determination if required. Additionally, tests of academic achievement can be used to ascertain a client's level of reading and written language arts in the language he or she reports to be most fluent. All this information is used in conjunction with the linguistic preference reported by the client to determine which language to use during the course of assessment and test selection. Although in the example above, such an assessment would have most probably been easy to accomplish, and test data may have supported such a finding (see Chapters 1 and 3), care must be taken not to assume a specific level of linguistic fluency from "simple" conversational interactions or other contextually rich interactions with the client during the course of the clinical interview. A formal assessment posture is recommended because clients, for whatever reason (e.g., dementia), may not accurately report their level of fluency or linguistic mastery. This is particularly true regarding issues discussed in Chapter 5 related to deep linguistic structures in Hispanics who report themselves to be bilingual or who appear to have achieved a certain level of "social" linguistic mastery in English – particularly adults and children who immigrated to the U.S. and who have spent less than five to seven years in residence with significant acculturation, who were monolingual Spanish speakers, or who are suspected of possessing "surface structure but not deep structure' in English (or the language of choice for assessment). Finally, even though the client is predominantly an English speaker, the interpretation of her test scores strongly suggests considering the fact that she spoke Spanish at home as she grew up and as an adult when she lived with and visited her parents (language spoken in the home; cf. Harris and Llorente, 2005).

The linguistic component of the evaluation is followed or preceded by an investigation, preferably formal, of level of acculturation if required and/or necessary. This assessment component can be accomplished through the use of existing scales as noted before (e.g., Franco, 1983; Marin et al., 1984). If formal assessment is not possible or necessary, an informal assessment should be conducted addressing the same topics found in formal measures. This component of the assessment also should examine the role culture currently plays, and has played, in the client's life, as well as the role of her ethnic self-identification. Within this context her own perception of her present situation, including having to undergo the current evaluation (see Chapter 8), should be included. All this information is then used during the assessment process to make important decisions about linguistic and test use throughout the process and during the interpretative phase when making inferences about specific test performance. In the case above, it is possible that an informal assessment could have addressed such an issue, but acculturation and its assessment frequently involves a more complex assessment posture during the course of assessments with Hispanics.

With regard to test selection, it is critical to note that despite the fact that practitioners are left with some options regarding appropriate test instruments to use with Hispanic populations, they are often faced with making decisions regarding instrumentation based on other constraints such as nonexistent normative data. As noted in previous chapters, using an idiographic approach for specific clients sometimes provides information that can be used by practitioners and can assist in a better determination of diagnosis and the identification of strengths and weaknesses and treatment goals. In this regard it is critical to recall that in its purest form, and in spite of its inherent weaknesses, the idiographic approach does not include the use of norms but allows the patient to "establish his or her own baseline." This was a proposition in Luria's assessment approach (1966), and the process approach, particularly when the quality of a client's response, not just quantifiable data, is taken into consideration (cf. Kaplan, 1996). The reader may ask under which or what circumstances may such a case emerge? Consider a Hispanic client who recently sustained head trauma and who recently immigrated to the U.S. from a rural town in Guatemala to work in the agricultural industry. He is without formal education, predominantly speaks an indigenous language, with functional (conversational) Spanish but without full literacy in Spanish (this concept used here in the traditional sense), and of course, has very limited exposure to English. It is pivotal to note at this point that no amount of test data, behavioral observations, or other assessment components can supplant clinical judgment, when it is soundly used, and this factor must be given a great deal of consideration when assessing Hispanics, regardless of the quality of instrumentation available to the clinician. In other words, the blind use of instrumentation and dependence on neuropsychological test data should not replace sound interpretation and clinical judgment.[3]

With regard to specific test selection, from an intellectual estimation standpoint for the Latina referral above, it is vital to note that the WAIS-III standardization sample did not stratify individuals who meet some of the demographics described for this client. For example, there are no "Hispanics" in the WAIS-III standardization sample in the 55- to 64-year-old range with ≥ 16 years of education or from the North Central region of the U.S. (covering Chicago, Illinois). Therefore the administration of the WAIS-III, even though the client speaks English, probably does not represent the best evaluative course of action for this client. In contrast, the standardization sample of the WJ-III includes individuals meeting all the aforementioned criteria. Therefore, in this case, an ethical, increasingly valid, and prudent approach to test selection, inference, and application would result in a decision to employ the WJ-III (cognitive abilities) over the WAIS-III. However, had the client been a 54-year-old Hispanic female with the same characteristics from Texas or California with the same educational level as the referred client, the administration of either the WAIS-III or WJ-III would have been appropriate and fundamentally sound, all other factors and assumptions being held equal (e.g., community size, impact of her bilingual nature on tests). (Incidentally, the fact that there are no

---

[3] Although the senior author is fully fluent in Spanish, and is cognizant of the client's background having visited, trained students, and collaborated with colleagues in Guatemala, the chief reason behind this referral to his service, he subsequently referred this client to a colleague with greater competency in assessing clients from such an indigenous background. In some instances, the senior author has assisted individuals and families obtain assistance from their respective embassies so that they can receive financial support to travel to be assessed by a clinician that is versed in the assessment of specific clients from unique backgrounds or other ethnic minority groups (e.g., Middle Eastern).

Hispanics meeting her demographics in the WAIS-III Standardization sample from the Midwest was most likely, and indirectly, affected by patterns of American immigration as noted in Chapter 2.) To underscore the importance of paying attention to demographic factors, the reader is asked to consider a similar decision where the patient is an 85-year-old African-American female with a high school education or, to make the point ridiculously evident, to consider the assessment of memory systems using the WMS-III to rule out memory difficulties in an individual suspected of being afflicted by an amnesic episode when the patient is a 24-year-old "White" person with 8 years of education or less. As mentioned in previous chapters, these examples are not provided to criticize, mock, or ridicule an inanimate object such as a test, nor to belittle the efforts of individuals who have dedicated a lifetime attempting to create objective neuropsychological instruments (the senior author would fall in this category). Rather, it is provided to alert neuropsychologists to the complexity of assessing a Hispanic client, and in fact, any client at all (see footnotes 7, 8, and 9).

The assessment for the Latina client also should include measures capable of assessing memory functions across various modalities if we are to be able to address the referral question appropriately. Therefore, procedures such as measures of visual and verbal memory should be included. However, before getting into details related to test selection, let us assume for a moment that the Hispanic woman was fully fluent in Spanish rather than English, from California (Los Angeles metropolitan area), minimally bilingual (English), or acculturated to American society, and that actual academic, language, and acculturation instruments suggested that to be the case. Such findings indicate that the assessment and test use should be in Spanish rather than in English. Therefore, the WHO-UCLA Auditory Verbal Learning Test (AVLT) (cf. Pontón et al., 1996) or subtests from the SENAS (Mungas et al., 2004) would provide appropriate indices of rote verbal memory functioning in most instances, as they are tests with published norms that provide a better coupling with the patient's demographic characteristics. In this case, we clearly would abstain from administering the WMS-III in English or to translate, most egregiously through the use of a family member or other interpreter, the verbal components of the test into Spanish, and then use the test's extant norms developed for the U.S. population, particularly because the test was only standardized on individuals who were fluent in English. What if the woman had been from Spain? In that case, neither the SENAS, the AVLT, nor the WMS-III would represent appropriate measures, and the reader is left with homework exercise to perform. A similar approach should be taken to address contextual verbal memory, and most important, given the referral question, to address visual memory. Clearly, similar approaches should be taken for language functions (expressive, receptive) and should include word fluency and confrontational naming, as well as verbal abstraction, to detect difficulties in these areas (e.g., dysnomia, dysfluency, problems in verbal abstraction) and other domains, including complex visual constructional tasks, in order to address the specific referral question. Table 6.1 provides a list of procedures, along with information found in Chapter 5, which could be used with the referred patient. For example, the WJ-III and the Batería, along with other tests (e.g., SENAS), provide appropriate subtests to examine such issues, whether the patient speaks English or Spanish. Finally, her level of adaptation and behavioral and emotional functioning should also be examined, not simply to be used for diagnostic purposes or to establish a rule-out, as requested, of AD if possible, but additionally to determine her relative strengths and weaknesses in order to establish appropriate interventions and treatments if required, with specific emphasis on quality of life, safety, social, legal, and career implications, should the assessment results fail to permit a rule-out of AD.

Although the present examples have been brief and limited by space considerations, it is sincerely hoped that the reader begins to develop a sense of the awesome responsibilities faced by the ethical and thoughtful clinician when evaluating Hispanics. A sample report is included in the Appendix to this volume that underscores many of the issues addressed here and in previous chapters.

Summary and Concluding Remarks

This chapter briefly covered theoretical and pragmatic factors associated with the practice of neuropsychology with Hispanics. Factors that influence assessment in this population include acculturation, immigration trends, language, educational levels, socioeconomic status, and examiner knowledge and characteristics of such populations. The pressure to decrease the disparities in special education placement of children, the health status of Americans, judicial outcomes across ethnic groups, in addition to regulations and mandates addressing fairness in psychological assessment, and in particular in neuropsychology, and the economic incentives of test publishers, are likely to shape the future of assessments with Hispanic populations in the U.S. and abroad.

To accommodate the increasing diversity within the context of neuropsychological practice and theory, neuropsychologists should develop theoretical models and instruments that are capable of accounting for the amount of variance in total performance associated with culture. From an applied standpoint, tests that are developed for Hispanics that emphasize fluid reasoning skills and that are normed for such populations, should be of paramount importance to cross-cultural neuropsychology. In addition, a global approach should be taken during the course of assessment of Hispanic populations that emphasize a framework that permits the examination of unique strengths and weaknesses. Some of the aforementioned test batteries, including the Woodcock-Johnson Tests of Cognitive Ability, the SENAS, and others, accomplish some of these goals, but more research and productivity in test development and standardizations are required. In addition further research that examines the utility of these tools is necessary. In addition, cross-cultural neuropsychology, applied to Hispanics, needs to consider within-group differences and the impact of geographical regions and immigration status on assessment outcomes. In fact, within-group differences can be even more pronounced than differences across ethnic groups in some instances. Results from cross-cultural studies also emphasize the importance of conducting longitudinal assessment. It is also critical to note that neuropsychologists gain a greater understanding of brain-behavior relationships through their use of improved assessment tools, and some researchers have advocated revisiting research through the use of single-subject designs that examines aptitude-treatment interventions (Braden and Kratochwill, 1997). Such an assessment posture has the potential to broaden our understanding of Hispanic populations.

When neuropsychologists work with Hispanics, a group that they may not be familiar with, it is important that they routinely consult with other neuropsychologists who may be more familiar with such populations. This recommendation is consistent with the *Ethical Principles of Psychologists* (APA, 2002). Furthermore, issues of acculturation and language proficiency must be taken into account when assessing patients. The tendency to evaluate clients' behaviors and performance within a framework that ignores culture must be discarded.

Chapter 7
Hispanics and Cultural Bias: Test Development and Applications

Peter Smith, Eric Lane, and Antolin M. Llorente

The cultural and ethnic landscapes of the United States (U.S.) are becoming increasingly more diverse, as noted in Chapter 2. Although large-scale migrations historically have exhibited geographical predilection, diversity is no longer manifested only in selected border towns or large metropolitan areas, since small cities and suburbs across the country are reflecting an increasingly diverse population, particularly large-scale increases in the Hispanic population. The effects of multiculturalism are acutely felt in the decision-making processes associated with educational placement, diagnostic formulation, legal proceedings, and treatment planning. Clearly, the important role that neuropsychological evaluations play in the aforementioned decision-making processes will only continue to be effective if the impact of bias in neuropsychological practice, and in particular, test bias, is adequately addressed. For decades neuropsychology has grappled with the effects of such potential biases.

Cultural Bias, Assessment and Instrumentation: Presenting Problem and Historical Antecedents

Cognitive ability testing (CAT) has made an effort to address the effects of multiculturalism and test bias. Helms (1992) wrote that while "many CAT developers have attempted to reduce cultural influences on CATs through construction of culture-fair tests, these devices represent attempts to control the influences of different cultures rather than to measure them" (p. 1091). In fact, the position adopted here suggests that it has been such inadequate attempts to control for culture and its various manifestations that have partially led to bias. In particular, the attempts to define and operationalize culture, race, and ethnicity have proven difficult even within the multicultural literature. As such, "It seems reasonable to ask whether it is possible to control something that one has not conceptualized adequately" (Helms, 1992, p. 1091).

These poor definitions and inappropriate attempts to control or eradicate such factors, including the impact of language and ethnicity, led to the early development of procedures believed to be "culture-fair," yet later proven to be just as biased as existing measures (Sattler, 2001). For example, the notion that the development of the System of Multicultural Pluralistic Assessment (SOMPA; Mercer and Lewis, 1978) was a "culture-free" procedure was later dispelled (cf. Sattler, 2001), partially as a result of lack of established validity for minority populations and poor standardization based on a small sample of children from California. It is our opinion that part of the problem at this early stage in the development of tests for use with ethnic minorities, including Hispanics, was due to a poor understanding of brain-behavior relationships, leading to the development of procedures that allegedly reduced the effects of cultural factors, for example linguistic skills. This was based on the assumption that tests assessing a specific set of skills or a specific skill (e.g., visual reasoning) would not involve or would be partially devoid of the concurrent use of other skills (e.g., language). As noted in the Preface and Chapter 1, brain-behavior relationships are not discrete or culture-free, and therefore the development of a measure on the basis of such an erroneous assumption led to the emergence of procedures that failed to accomplish their intended purpose.

While the impact of cultural variables on neuropsychological measures in relation to standardized administration, psychometric properties, and other factors will be addressed later, empirical evidence has not been presented thus far in this chapter to support an argument buttressing the need to address such variables. However, extant neuropsychological research has investigated a broad range of cultural factors that unequivocally impact brain-behavior relationships. Although space limitations prevent a comprehensive discussion of this research, relatively recent data-based investigations include the relationship between culture and lateralization (Ardila et al., 1989a; Mandal, Ida, Harizuka, Upadhaya, 1999); hemispheric specialization and culture (Best and Avery, 1999; Moss, Davidson, and Saron, 1985); and various investigations showing that differences in cultural context probably affect performance (León-Carrión, 1989). Studies have additionally demonstrated that culture may be related to self-reports of emotional and behavioral functioning (e.g., DuPaul et. al., 2001; Carlson, Uppal, and Prosser, 2000). Although the research did not focus on Hispanics, empirical investigations also have shown the impact of cultural variables on the accuracy of self-perception of neurological impairment post head injury (Prigatano, Ogano, and Amakusa 1997).

Although the relationship of culture to neuropsychology, in particular neuropsychological assessment, cannot be denied, even when empirical evidence is taken into consideration, it is difficult to disentangle the specific mechanisms of how culture, however defined, affects the assessment of people from cultural and racial minorities. In effect, "the absence of clearly articulated, theoretically based models for examining the influence of race-related cultural factors on cognitive ability is reflected in the ambiguous language used to discuss racial factors and CATs" (Helms, 1992, p. 1089). Part of the difficulty has been the use of cultural bias and cultural equivalence without a clear contrast of these terms. As noted in Chapter 1, any measurement on a test ($X_{test\ score}$) is comprised of a true score (X_{true}), representing the actual characteristic or trait under investigation, and error (X_{error}). The error noted in this equation, and assumed to enter the measurement process, is considered to be random in nature, not systematic, and statistical and experimental design methods can control for such random error (Kirk, 1990). However, such methods do not control for systematic error or bias. Bias refers to systematic error that maybe encountered when estimating some value (Anastasi and Urbina, 1997). This systematic error is believed to be constant and greatly diminishes the accuracy of inferences made regarding an individual, sample, or population with regard to a psychological construct, educational performance, or other variable. Therefore, the incorporation and consideration of bias in test construction and interpretation are essential. When discrepancies emerge between different groups on a particular measure, the terms *item bias* or *differential item functioning* (DIF) may appropriately describe the observed discrepancies (American Educational Research Association, 1999), rather than the term *brain-based performance differences*.

Generally speaking, test developers and psychometricians historically have examined cultural test bias via mean differences between dominant and nondominant groups, as well as unequivalent distributions, and have focused on raw and transformed (indexed, scaled, and standardized) scores (Anastasi, 1997). A patent example of such work was conducted between majority and minority children examining intellectual (IQ) scores (e.g., Jensen, 1979). In that study, "a significant age decrement in verbal and non-verbal "IQ" of minority children, but not in the children from the majority culture, was noted. Although this and similar studies were conducted to demonstrate the pernicious impact of a depriving environment on negative cumulative effects on intellectual scores, and the focus of this study was to delineate the effects of "environmental disadvantages" (Jensen, 1979), this investigation, using mean differences between comparisons, was not appropriate. Jensen's inappropriate conclusions were reached based on the erroneous assumption that the tests utilized were measuring the same constructs for separate groups of children.

In general, equivalence in measurement has been "inferred from studies of cultural bias," supposedly to determine if psychological constructs share meaning between or across separate cultural groups. Oftentimes, cultural equivalence has been thought to be established when cultural bias has been minimized through statistical analysis of the factor structure, regression lines, or other procedures. However, "none of these statistical strategies necessarily demonstrates the presence of cultural equivalence in either standardized CATs or the criteria that the tests are used to predict" (Helms, 1992, p. 1089). These procedures do not incorporate the theoretical impact that cultural factors have on the statistical procedures themselves. Could there be separate nonmeasured factors that contribute to cultural equivalent results from statistical procedures? For example, may "a significant correlation between a predictor and criterion across racial groups" reflect the overlap of this other factor?

Reynolds (2000) used the term *cultural test bias hypothesis* (CTBH) to refer to the argument that mean differences of performance across ethnic groups (or between the sexes) are the result of test artifacts and do not represent "true" differences in performance across ethnic groups (or between the sexes). In general, this form of bias renders neuropsychological measures invalid and unreliable for certain populations due to cross-cultural differences and nuances that are not reflected in the measured construct. For example, a Eurocentric view of intelligence, which consists of philosophical dualism, assumption of Eurocentric cognitive strategy superiority, and an emphasis upon logical positivism, may not allow for an adequate evaluation of intellect for people from minority cultures. Since many of the tests are constructed by scientists from majority cultures for use with people from the majority culture, the inherent definition of intelligence and how to measure it may not be valid for people from minority groups (see Helms, 1992).

These facets of a Eurocentric view may be seen in many of the types of questions asked or tasks required on tests of cognitive abilities, including neuropsychological tests. The reliance on right or wrong answers on select subtests reflects an underlying emphasis on a dualistic approach to problem solving. It is the intrinsic assumption that the tests used measure an underlying trait or general ability, such as "g" (Cattell, 1963), in the absence of alternative definitions of intelligence or other construct that reflects the Eurocentric reliance upon the scientific method. As such, it is not surprising to find that there are significant correlations between the test used and the criteria to be measured (cf. Helms, 1992).

Possible sources of test bias include multiple factors that may or may not be within the complete control of a test developer. Although other investigators besides Reynolds (2000) have addressed such issues (cf. Scar and Weinberg, 1978), Reynolds has provided a comprehensive set of potential sources of bias, including inappropriate content, inequitable social consequences, measurement of different constructs, differential predictive validity, inappropriate standardization samples, examiners' and language bias, as well as qualitatively distinct minority and majority aptitude and personality.

Inappropriate content refers to the potential bias inherent in a test whose content is written by members of a majority culture, which does not adequately reflect the unique cultural differences with regard to language and values of a minority culture. Thus, it has been argued that minority test takers are at a distinct disadvantage on certain measures because the content of the test does not reflect the proposed construct as it applies to other cultures. Their experiences, knowledge, and strengths are not reflected in the questions or tasks they are asked to complete, likely resulting in deflated performance when compared to a majority population (Reynolds, 2000). For example, in many instances Hispanic or Latino children from an inner city environment may not have been exposed to the educational or social experiences required to do as well as children from the majority culture from a suburban environment on standardized measures. Bond (1987) notes, as the discrepancy between cultural value systems increase, the discrepancy may be reflected as scoring inconsistencies. This is best exemplified by the inappropriate administration of a test whose content would adversely affect the performance of a child who recently emigrated from Mexico and who has not received formal education in the U.S. (e.g., Who is Hunpty Dumpty? Or Who is Honest Abe?). His lower score on such a test, may actually reflect differential cultural exposure and language discrepancies as a result of inappropriate test content rather than different levels of underlying cognitive abilities as defined by a majority culture. Yet, it is important to note that these factors are external to the testing situation as noted by Reynolds (2000).

Another hypothesized source of cultural test bias stems from inequitable social consequences. This argument points out that minority group members have unjustly suffered from extensive past discrimination, labeling, and inequality of educational opportunities. Therefore, poor test performance is a reflection of a lack of exposure to the content being examined, leading to inappropriate inferences being made from low scores. This process actually continues the cycle of inequitable social consequences. These children are labeled as having cognitive impairments, which then leads to special education services and decreased academic expectations. When children graduate or are discharged from the educational system after being promoted as a result of their chronological age, they are ill prepared to break the cycle of inequitable social consequences by obtaining employment that has lower educational requirements and less opportunity for advancement. Again, the culmination of these factors renders the minority test taker at a distinct disadvantage on these tests (Reynolds, 2000). In summary, the labeling of minority children as intellectually or academically deficient in early elementary school may result in an academic trajectory that is lower than the trajectory of a child from the majority culture. The children from the minority culture are set up, early on, by factors out of their control, to have restricted or limited future academic experiences, likely reducing their performance on future standardized measures.

It is also believed that when a test is extended from the majority culture and given to a minority test taker, attributes such as intelligence, neuropsychological functions, and personality that are allegedly being assessed may not be tapped equivalently in the minority test taker (Reynolds, 2000; Sattler, 2001). Thus a measure of intelligence may measure discrepant constructs of intelligence or other abilities among children of two different cultures. In essence, such constructs are partly culturally defined and tests developed by and for the majority culture likely do not capture the nuances, both subtle and otherwise, of intelligence or other cognitive ability tests as it manifests itself within the minority culture.

Other clinicians and researchers argue that culturally biased measures do not hold the same predictive validity between cultures. Since issues related to the validity of the underlying constructs purported to be measured have been raised, it follows that the predictive value of the purported skills tapped may be lower when applied to minority test takers. Thus, the utilization of various measures to predict behavior does not extend across lines of culture, which raises the question as to what purpose the administration and scoring of the measure with questionable predictive validity serves. This is especially pertinent because neuropsychology is being increasingly used to establish treatment planning, to predict behavior, and to provide consultation with significant economic and social implications. In fact, many Hispanic researchers and educators question the validity of the inferences derived from current standardized measures as they apply to Hispanic populations (Reynolds, 2000).

An additional and significant source of cultural bias likely stems from the underrepresentation of minorities in the measure's standardization sample (cf. Llorente et al., 1999, 2000; Reynolds, 2000). As noted in Chapter 2, when a normative sample is stratified according to the U.S. census, a significantly smaller sample of people from a minority culture is obtained. In fact, many cells in such stratifications, particularly for Hispanics and other ethnic minorities, remain "empty" without individuals stratified into them. This limitation greatly affects clinical judgment by the inappropriate comparison of a minority patient's performance to an inadequate sample, simply because the proportion of minority test takers matches the latest census proportions. Although such a comparison is inappropriate from a psychometric standpoint, from a conceptual standpoint, as noted in Chapter 2, more egregious is the fact that scrutiny of the U.S. Census reveals "that Hispanics, regardless of their actual 'ethnic' background, are classified under the same racial category as "Hispanics," erroneously confusing "ethnicity" with racial background. Such a posture is "problematic for neuropsychology because it is the cultural and ethnic background of the individual that influence the factors that are being assessed by the psychological procedure such as his or her cognitive abilities, not his racial background." Unfortunately, this practice has both historical and practical foundations. One need only look at the standardization samples of many early versions of the neurocognitive tests to see the low sample sizes and reliance upon "White" samples.

Reynolds (2000) additionally notes that the majority of psychologists in the United States are of European ancestry. Thus, lower test scores for minority ethnic groups may be the result of differences in language content and use between the neuropsychologist and patient. This discrepancy may also amplify the already profound power differential between the two parties, thus increasing the chances that decreased performance is not reflective of actual impairment.

Finally, some researchers have hypothesized that different cultures are just that, different, and require separate measures of psychological and neuropsychological constructs (Helms. 1992; Reynolds, 2000). Helms (1992) argued that the intelligence quotient for African Americans is distinct from that of Caucasian Americans, thus requiring the development and implementation of separate measures, and this issue may be applicable to Hispanics as well. In fact, these differences may likely extend beyond aptitude into such constructs as personality. This emphasizes the need for the development of mechanisms to address test bias with different populations across multiple domains. Wong, Strickland, Fletcher-Janzen, Ardila, and Reynolds (2000) offer a number of practical suggestions for mediating the effects of cultural bias on one's clinical practice. The foundation of these suggestions involves recognizing the need for multicultural competence and seeking out training regarding cross-cultural diversity and sensitivity. Additionally, clinicians are advised to consider cultural nuances and the importance of providing a culturally sensitive environment for interviewing and assessment. As always, the importance of a sound and through clinical interview is underscored. Sufficient time and research are essential to a competent clinical interview for a culturally dissimilar patient. The fourth suggestion involves making a concerted effort to find a competent neuropsychologist in the region who speaks the patient's dominant language. Recognize that other cultural factors, especially gender, aside from language barriers, may require one to refer the patient to a more culturally appropriate clinician. Every effort to avoid the utilization of interpreters is advised, as noted in

Chapter 1. Translated tests should be avoided unless score interpretations have been validated for that version of the test and for the individual under consideration. Additionally, the test battery should be the result of a thoughtful process that keeps culturally salient issues at the forefront. Finally, cross-cultural issues should be clearly and effectively communicated in the final report (Wong et. al., 2000).

Although these recommendations provide good guidelines, before specific recommendations are provided in this chapter addressing methods and tactics to reduce bias in test development to be applied with Hispanic populations, it is critical to examine in a detailed fashion a factor that has accounted for a great deal of methodological problems in the development of assessment measures. Such a factor is at the core of problems related to limited validity and reliability.

The U.S. Census, Test Standardization, Sampling Procedures, and Neuropsychology

The U.S. Census has a long and distinguished history. Originally mandated by *Article One* of the *U.S. Constitution* in 1787, the charter census was conducted in 1790 and terminated approximately two years later. The census has been conducted every decade thereafter, with its original goal in mind, governmental applications.

The original Census only consisted of six questions (see Figure 7.1). However, it is critical to examine those questions. Several of those queries have significant historical importance as a result of their demographic content, predominantly addressing race, not ethnicity or culture, which bears significantly on the development of subsequent and modern censuses and, indirectly and most unfortunately, the current standardization of neuropsychological tests. One question in the original census inquired how many "Free White" males of 16 years of age or "upward" lived in the household, men able to participate in the U.S. military or available for work. The original census also queried the number of Free "White" males under the age of 16 years that lived in the household (e.g., collected to estimate the future military potential). Two other items inquired about the number of "White females" and "Slaves" of other members in the household.

Unfortunately, although the U.S. census has since its inception served our nation well, particularly when its *intended* use is taken into consideration (e.g., appropriation of resources, taxation, military potential), the census was not devised for

U.S. Census (1790)
List the number of:

Name of Head of house hold   _____

Free White males of 16 years and upward   _____

Free White males under 16 years of age   _____

Free White females   _____

All other free persons (by sex and color)   _____

Slaves   _____

Figure 7.1 The U.S. Census (1790)

purposes of collecting complex demographic data to be used at a later date by psychologists to develop norms for tests – particularly intricate and complex neuropsychological procedures impacted by ethnicity, not race, and capable of assessing brain-behavior relationships with applications using a nomothetic approach. The U.S. census was originally mandated for purposes of correct apportionment of representation and taxation "according" to the respective number of inhabitants among the States. Its original goals, coupled with its inherent, inappropriate interchange of race for culture or ethnicity (it is inappropriate for neuropsychology but not necessarily for its intended purposes throughout the years), has led to its misapplication, creating problems for neuropsychology (as well as other fields), which will be addressed later.

Although significant changes have been made, close scrutiny of the last two U. S. Censuses reveals the continued difficulties in utilizing such instruments as sources of stratification of normative data for psychological procedures for Hispanics or other ethnic minority populations (We contend that it is even incorrect for "majority" groups; see footnote 9). Perusal of questions addressing race and nationality (not ethnicity) in questions 4 and 7 in the 1990 U.S. Census and questions 5 and 6 in the 2000 Census (see Figures 7.2 and 7.3) reveals that Hispanics, regardless of their actual "ethnic" background, are classified under the same racial category as "Hispanics," albeit with nationality, as a proxy or attempt to get to the issue of ethnicity. In other words, the U.S. Census, not unlike other governmental entities and lay individuals, erroneously confuses "ethnicity" with racial background or nationality, a common mistake, as noted in Chapter 1. Although the 2000 U.S. Census partially attempts to address this issue through the use of more specific questions related to demographic criteria and queries (see Figure 7.3) by providing a better delineation of the "nationality" and racial background of the respondent(s) (e.g., "Non-Hispanic White"), it nevertheless continues to fail to enumerate the ethnicity of individuals but focuses on their race and nationality as a proxy for ethnicity. This is not surprising given the original questions found in the 18th-century U.S. Census. Although this approach to stratification may be appropriate for the intended purpose of the U.S. Census (e.g., allocation of economic resources), it is extremely problematic for neuropsychology on several fronts. It is problematic for psychology because it is the cultural or ethnic background of the individual that influences the factors that are being assessed by neuropsychological and psychological procedures, not his or her *racial* background or *nationality*. This issue is quite evident during the course of evaluation of an individual born in the U.S. (Miami, Florida) from a family whose ancestors came from the Dominican Republic, who originally arrived in that nation from Africa at the turn of the 20th century, who does not speak English but only fluent Spanish, and who (and not until recently as far as the U.S. Census was concerned) is "Black." Despite his Hispanic origin and heritage, this individual may meet a criterion originally intended by the U.S. Census to be based on his race. In this regard his classification may be based on misleading inferences when his race is confounded with his cultural or ethnic identity, particularly if the norms of a neuropsychological procedure are incapable of capturing such ethnic nuance.

Figure 7.2 The U.S. Census (1990)   **U.S. Census (1990)**

4. Race

Fill one circle for the *race that person considers himself/herself to be.*

If **Indian (Amer.),** print the name of the of enrolled or principal tribe → _____

White
Black or Negro
Indian (Amer.)
Eskimo
Aleut

        Asian or Pasific Islander (API)

Chinese	Japanese
Filipino	Asian Indian
Hawiian	Samoan
Korean	Guamanian
Vietnamese	Other API

Other race

7. Is this person of Spanish/Hispanic Origin?

Fill one circle for each person

No (not Spanish/Hispanic)
Yes, Mexican, Mexican, Am., Chicano
Yes, Puerto Rican
Yes, Other Spanish/Hispanic
      (Print one group, for example:
      Argentinian, Colombian, Nicaraguan,
      Salvadorean, Spaniard, and so on)

What is most unfortunate is the fact that Eurocentric and other test publishers have depended for decades on the U.S. Census to stratify samples of the U.S. population, using census data as the standard for identifying individuals of all ethnic backgrounds, and in particular, Hispanics living in the U.S. Clinicians unfortunately have subsequently used those tests, with such poor samplings, to generalize to all Hispanics living in the U.S., and in some instances living abroad, or to those that have recently immigrated to the U.S. What might be wrong with such a process?

There are so many theoretical and methodological problems with such an approach that it is difficult to find a good explanatory starting point. For example, the basic idea behind sampling is that of studying the attributes of a larger group of people (population) on the basis of studying a smaller group of individuals (sample). However, not all individuals in the "population" under investigation are alike, and samples must then choose people from the population that best reflect all the different characteristics and attributes of the larger group or population. Because the first step in sampling is definition of the population, in this case "Hispanics,"

Figure 7.3 U.S. Census (2000) Questions 5 and 6 related to race and nationality

U.S. Census (2000)

5. Is this person Spanish/Hispanic/Latino? *Mark x The "No" box if not Spanish/Hispanic/Latino.*

No, *Not Spanish/Hispanic*

Yes, Mexican, Mexican, Am., Chicano
Yes, Puerto Rican
Yes, Cuban
Yes, Other Spanish/Hispanic/Latino

6. What is this person's race? *Mark x one or More races to indicate what this person considers Himself/herself to be.*

White
Black, African-Am., or Negro
American Indian or Alaska Native — Print name of enrolled or principal tribe

Asian Indian	Native Hawaiian
Chinese	Guamanian or
Filipino	Chamorro
Japanese	Samoan
Korean	Other Pacific
Vietnamese	Islander
Other Asian	Print Race

Some other Race — Print race

(even though Hispanics have been ill-defined because race was interchanged with ethnicity), the first major problem encountered is in the definition of the population itself. Because the population was initially ill defined, the inferences derived from the sample about the population will have poor validity, and therefore generalizations will be of equally poor value.

Clearly, the more a sample represents or reflects attributes of a larger population, the more confidence can be placed on the inferences derived from such a sample about the larger population, and this is a basic tenet of sampling procedures (Yamane, 1967). In order to attain such a level of confidence, several sampling procedures can be used, including random, nonprobability, cluster, and stratified random sampling. Standardization sampling procedures commonly use the last-named procedure to sample the population of the U.S., as noted earlier, to create a standardization sample that is representative of the U.S. population. Unfortunately, although such a procedure is appropriate for age and race, because of the confusion between race and ethnicity whereby the latter has been inappropriately interchanged for the latter, the representation of ethnicity is inaccurate, and a sample based on such a definition

will not be representative of the U.S.'s Hispanic population. Furthermore, let us prepos-
terously assume for a moment that a better definition of "Hispanic" than the one
used by the U.S. Census was available. It is possible that such a definition, as captured by the U.S. Census, may only be applicable to selected groups of Hispanics from
the U.S. but not from other parts of the U.S. or other parts of the world, and in that
sense the sample would still not be representative of the "universe of Hispanics,"
but only of those living in the U.S., who may have varying degrees of acculturation to American society, bilingualism, or other characteristics, as noted in
previous chapters.

Another critical issue is sample size. Most test publishers attempt to standardize
tests using stratified random samples that represent the U.S. population, using the
U.S. Census to mimic the population of the U.S., including Hispanics. The sample
size depends on many factors, including the level of confidence, desired precision
and, most important, as far as Hispanic culture and ethnic identity are concerned,
the variation in the population. Therefore,

$$[(\text{confidence level} \times \text{population variance})/\text{desired precision}]^2 = \text{sample size } (n)$$

Although the data provided by the U.S. Census are appropriate when they are used
for specific demographic variables such as "percentage" of individuals living in the
"West" with "20–34" years of age with "greater than 8 years of education," they are
not appropriate when used to develop psychological or neuropsychological tests
through the use of a stratified variable such as ethnicity. They are not appropriate
because the variation in the population of these two variables is quite distinct.
Therefore, although such a method is appropriate for U.S. government purposes, it
is not appropriate for neuropsychologists or test publishers to establish sample sizes
for Hispanics on the basis of data published by the U.S. Census.

Another major problem is the fact that although standardization samples might
be randomized stratification samples, they still represent the convenience sampling
method associated with data collection specifics such as data collection centers and
other variables that are not captured by the U.S. Census. For example, for many
children's tests, standardization data are collected in school districts that are able
and willing to participate in such studies. Similar situations arise with adults, which
in the final analysis lead to a convenience sample. In fact, standardization testing
sites frequently are not available from specific metropolitan or rural areas, and in
some instances data are not available from every state within the U.S. or representative regions in the U.S. where specific populations with unique ethnicities are
encountered (e.g., Utah, Louisiana). The U.S. Census and, indirectly, standardizations based on such stratification data may thus be biased. Finally, how about the
racial classification of children and data reported to the U.S. Census by their parents or other caretakers?

Other factors could be addressed related to this topic, namely the misuse of the
U.S. Census and its inability to serve as a tool to establish appropriate representative samples that appropriately represent the U.S. population, including complex
variables and interactions between other factors described above, such as levels of

acculturation, bilingualism or language proficiency, the definition(s) of Hispanic in the U.S. Census, and patterns of American immigration as noted in previous chapters. To add to the problem, sampling and data collection difficulties encountered by the U.S. Census Bureau during the process of actual census development and sampling methods, particularly the collection of data from populations with great mobility and large-scale shifts as is the case for Hispanics, exacerbate the difficulties. Lack of space prohibits an expansion of these topics; however, it is sincerely hoped that the reader will begin to obtain a rudimentary idea of the inherent problems of using the U.S. Census to guide stratification of sampling procedures.

In summary, test developers and publishers historically have depended on the U.S. Census to obtain demographic variables to establish normative data for psychological and neuropsychological procedures. Although the use of census data may have reduced economic and time burdens for test developers and publishers, which to a certain extent justifies their use, it is argued here that the use of the census as an index of stratification of demographic characteristics led the field of neuropsychology astray and that such an approach is partially responsible for the current predicaments in this field (see Llorente et al., 1999, 2000). Such a historical and methodological posture, with significant consequences for modern assessment, failed to consider that the census was not intended for such purposes, not to mention that it permitted an important confound, namely race in lieu of culture or ethnicity, to enter the standardization process, leading to norms based on samples that poorly represented their intended populations, particularly for Hispanics, and indirectly to inappropriate assessments and inferences derived from such procedures with catastrophic and pernicious economic, personal, and societal consequences as noted in our nation's record during the last 50 or more years.

Cultural Bias, Hispanics, and Neuropsychology: Extant and Potential Solutions

With regard to test development and utilization, several techniques may lead to decrements in potential biases, including those identified above. These techniques and practices vary in complexity, content, method, scope, and their effects on potential sources of nonrandom error. Such techniques may include alterations in test content, statistical methods including item analysis and oversampling of non-dominant groups, and other methods presented below.

Guiding factors behind the development of tests for Hispanics should be undergirded with respect to cultural differences – not out of necessity, mandate, or economic gain but out of genuine effort to develop instruments that are cross-cultural and fair. Tests and procedures should enhance assessment in cross-cultural contexts in general, as well as neuropsychological procedures and screening batteries designed to assess the effects of conditions affecting neurological functioning, including brain injury, demanding instruments that are as sensitive and as culturally relevant as possible. For example, the use of color or other alterations in test content that may be more universally employed across cultures may reduce bias during the course of test development and utilization. Although the cognitive neuropsychology literature guards against the broad assumption that color perception is a completely culture-free phenomenon (Bornstein, 1973), hues may be used in some circumstances as stimulus because they transcend cultural distinctions. The use of color (e.g., yellow, red) in neuropsychological test procedures has substantially increased during the last three decades. Although unpublished, a manuscript by Llorente and colleagues (Llorente et al., unpublished manuscript) noted that the Wechsler Scales for Children increasingly used color in its content throughout its different subtests and restandardizations. For example, in 1974 (WISC-R; Wechsler, 1974), all of the plates in Picture Completion were in black and white (0% in color). By 1991, or 17 years later (WISC-III, Wechsler, 1991), 23/30, or 76% of all the plates in Picture Completion, were in rich colors. By 2004, or 30 years later (WISC-IV; Wechsler, 2004), 37/38 plates, or 97% of all the plates in Picture Completion were produced in color. Similar, increases in color are evident in other subtests. However, this is not the case for other tests. For example, tests frequently used in neuropsychological assessment continue to use black and white line work, which poorly depicts stimuli. This issue is important to note, because it is not only applicable to Hispanics, but to all examinees: Such poor depiction of stimuli leads to inaccurate test results and poor inferential processes, partially because the test does not represent accurately the stimuli as it appears in the environment ("real world") or the examinee's phenomenological "reality." As a good exemplar, the plate for "Asparagus," in one of the most commonly used tests of confrontational naming in neuropsychology is submitted for the reader's consideration. No wonder large numbers of clients, adults or children, fail such item.

In Chapter 1, we addressed the importance of increased reliability during the course of assessment with Hispanics. Albeit illegal and unethical, neuropsychological tests and procedures are sometimes photocopied (Mitrushina et al., 1999). Such a practice has often resulted in distorted target stimuli, introducing uncontrolled error variance, particularly when used with Hispanic populations – groups of individuals for which studies addressing validity and reliability may not be available. Such problems also significantly impact the comparability of research and clinical findings from studies employing altered procedures. Therefore the creation of tests that use color not reproducible by readily available commercial photocopying equipment eliminates these alterations by using professionally printed color protocols with tints and tones that ensure stable test performance and therefore comparability with normative studies and previous research investigations.

The development of multiple forms of the same test when possible provides for repeated administrations of a test, permitting repeated administration of an equivalent test to the same Hispanic patient, thus permitting the comparison of his or her performance over time with his or her own baseline (cf. Llorente et al., 1999), without dependence on normative samples. Such a method is especially helpful in neuropsychological rehabilitation in which the patient's performance is tracked longitudinally subsequent to insult over short periods of time in the acute setting. Such alternate forms may be developed by using the standard test form as the basis for the development of other forms through mirror imaging or rotation by 180 degrees of the original form, or similar methods, whenever possible (see Llorente et al., 2003). Such methods of developing alternate retest forms of the test assure that stimulus placement and distance traveled between stimuli will remain generally equivalent for all forms of the protocol.

Although space limitations in this volume preclude an expansive description, item analysis is another procedure that may be used to control for cultural bias. Item analysis may constitute either qualitative or quantitative means of addressing cultural test bias. It is an analytical procedure used to evaluate the appropriateness of individual test items to identified traits (cf. Camilli and Shepard, 1994). When applied in a general sense, item analysis can be conceptualized as ensuring that individual items do not differentially discriminate one person's performance or that of a group from other groups. How individuals or groups are organized is of less interest than whether an individual or group performs differently on that individual item. This allows for the development of test items that are appropriate for groups. This procedure can be carried out in a variety of settings from market research surveys, classroom evaluation of the fairness of test questions on a final, to development of unbiased neuropsychological tests for Hispanics. Qualitative item analysis is concerned with content and face validity and item construction. In addition, qualitative item analysis may focus on test content and language use. Experts from different cultures can be utilized to help reduce and eliminate offensive or overtly monoculturally relevant items from tests. A quantitative approach to item analysis is concerned with the statistical properties of the items and the overall test comprised by such items. Individual item characteristics such as item difficulty, item discrimination, guessing, and differential functioning are typically considered within the realm of this approach. As such, Item Response Theory attempts to integrate the first three aspects (difficulty, discrimination, and guessing) into a mathematical formula that can guide test construction (Camilli and Shepard, 1994; Sattler 2001). Item difficulty is framed in terms of the percentage of people who answered a specific item correctly. The range for item difficulty varies between 0.0 (everyone obtains an incorrect answer) to 1.0 (everyone obtains a correct answer). Many tests and procedures currently in use (e.g., Wechsler scales, Stanford-Binet, Differential Abilities Scale, and Woodcock-Johnson) arrange test items in terms of increasing difficulty. As it applies to cross-cultural neuropsychology, item analysis can be used to ensure that any item on a particular test exhibits the same degree of difficulty for all test takers, including Hispanics. A secondary gain associated with this approach to item development and item placement within a test is that it allows for the test taker to have a sense of efficacy as he or she approaches ever increasingly difficult items.

Item discrimination can be understood as "how an item discriminates between examinees who do well on the test as a whole and those who do poorly" (Sattler, 2001, p. 113). Scores range from −1.0 to +1.0. Similar to correlations coefficients, scores at the ends of the spectrum reflect strong relationships while scores in the middle reflect the absence of a relationship between someone's performance on an individual item and the total test. Clearly, an item on a test that is culturally unbiased should exhibit similar levels of discrimination for all individuals regardless of cultural background.

The third aspect used in item response theory is the guessing parameter, which attempts to identify the "probability that a correct response will occur by chance" (Sattler 2001, p. 113). From a cross-cultural neuropsychology standpoint, it should be evident that regardless of cultural background individual test items should reflect similar guessing parameters.

This information is placed into a mathematical formula that can be graphically represented as an item characteristic curve (ICC). It is these curves that can be calculated for groups to determine if the individual items are measuring the same underlying construct. A comparison of the curves can be made, and the items can be assumed to be measuring the same construct(s) if the curves are similar. If the curves are different from each other, they may reflect how group membership according to culture may affect that item.

Another method that can be used to reduce bias associated with cultural background during the course of test development within an item analysis methodology is the Differential Item Functioning (Camilli and Shepard, 1994). This procedure attempts to determine whether groups of "items function differently in different groups". This process assumes that "if different groups of examinees have the same level of proficiency, then they should perform similarly" on test items. Their level of performance should be similar without regard for their group membership. When there are differing probabilities of successfully answering questions, then an item is said to have a differential functioning.

In summary, examining how members of different cultural groups respond to individual items on a test can help to identify those items that are differentially affected by culture. If a significant number of members from at least two different groups respond to an item in a different manner, then an inference may be reached suggesting that cultural factors unduly may have influenced how members responded to that item, even if a content expert(s) has cleared the test item. Item analysis (including IRT and DIF) make it possible to shorten a test, yet enhance its reliability and validity (Anastasi and Urbina, 1997). As discussed earlier, item analysis may be a useful tool for the reduction of cultural test bias, and several potential sources of cultural test bias may be reduced through the use of such procedures (Reynolds, 2000). Item analysis could markedly increase the appropriateness of content within a measure for a particular minority group. It may also allow for the selection of items that better tap into a particular construct for that minority group. For example, items that do not reflect the general educational experience of a minority population may very well be eliminated, thus reducing the chances that these items lend bias to the validity of the results.

Oversampling can be used to address several of the possible sources of cultural test bias noted earlier, particularly some of the problems raised related to the use of the U.S. Census to guide data collection for Hispanics during the course of test standardization. Most appropriately, this practice may help to reduce the bias attributed to poorly constructed standardization samples and aid in collecting large representative samples to allow for effective quantitative item analysis to address differences in subtle content or other factors that might impact the inferential process. It may also be applied to instances in which colloquialism, such as geographically anchored phrasing for everyday items or events, are hypothesized to have the potential to interfere with item construction and administration. Oversampling can be conducted according to specified parameters addressing cultural and ethnic individualities of specific groups of ethnic minorities, not depending on specific census data that use inaccurate pan-ethnic terminology and definitions that were not meant to be used in psychology, and in cross-cultural neuropsychology in particular. For example, it was noted in Chapter 2 that "Mexican" individuals comprise the largest number of "Hispanic" immigrants living in the U.S. In addition, as noted earlier, even if restrictions are placed on the definition of "Mexican" to individuals who were born in Mexico who immigrated to the U.S., such a pan-ethnic term for "Mexican" fails to take into account the complexity of such group of individuals with their rich and significant ethnic and language differences. Therefore, when sampling this population, an oversampling approach could be employed to ensure that enough individuals are included to address such ethnic and language differences. At first glance, this could be perceived as an overwhelming task, yet it is not as difficult as perceived. For example, information can be collected related to their language(s) of origin to determine any specific subgroup, particularly when specific subgroups might be overrepresented in the U.S., and that subgroup then can be oversampled. Doing so may reduce bias during the course of test development related to this specific group of individuals. Most recently, the use of oversampling has been adopted by several test publishers to obtain a selected number of Hispanics and their specific and unique cultural and ethnic characteristics a welcomed approach (cf. McGrew and Woodcock, 2001).

However, oversampling is not applicable to the other sources of cultural test bias, particularly if conducted using the existing pan-ethnic terms derived from the U.S. Census (cf. Reynolds, 2000), unlike the approach described above. These sources of bias are all based on the assumption that minority cultures' experiences, development, and manifestation of such constructs as intelligence and personality are significantly discrepant from the majority culture. Thus, no degree of sampling will be able to rectify these fundamental differences and assist with the provision of more valid results unless the stratification approach is conducted in such a way as to reduce such effects, and doing so can be extremely prohibitive from an economic standpoint.

While item analysis and oversampling are seen as useful tools to reduce cultural test bias, some sources of bias are likely not mitigated by this practice. These untouchable sources may include eliminating the effects of inequitable social consequences, all the effects of language differences, and measurement of different constructs. In addition, these types of strategies do not aid a clinician once the patient has entered the office and is ready to begin a neuropsychological evaluation. Increasing the knowledge of base rates of disorders within certain populations can aid the clinician in understanding discrepant results obtained on standardized measures.

Another issue that requires discourse in this volume is the concept of base rates. Base rates are understood as the frequency of a trait (such as abnormal test finding or presence of symptom) in a population. Since many signs, symptoms, and test score discrepancies are not pathonogmonic to a particular mental health disorder, understanding how often these aforementioned entities are present in a given population aids in determining whether or not there is a pathological state or normal variation within a population, including Hispanics (Lezak et al., 2004; McCaffrey et al., 2003). This is especially important since a large portion of the nosology and nomenclature of clinical syndromes and disorders is actually delineated by a description of the associated cluster of symptoms. Therefore, "the examiner should have an understanding of the base rates of the neurobehavioral symptoms" associated with the patients they are evaluating (Lezak et al., 2004, p. 129).

Understanding how a collection of symptoms is distributed within a certain population therefore aids in the attempt to make a valid diagnosis. This process can have direct relevance in obtaining and conducting culturally sensitive assessments. While many tests use base rates to examine the frequency of discrepancy scores based on nondemographic variables, such as discrepancies in IQ scores or index scores, this process could also be applied to rates of score distributions of nonmajority populations. If conducted correctly, this would allow clinicians to examine a patient's profile and compare his or her performance to a group defined by their shared cultural, ethnic, or socioeconomic status to determine clinically relevant differences from age-determined norms.

In order to understand how the use of base rates may reduce bias during the course of neuropsychological assessment, a brief explanation of how base rates of particular traits or discrepancies affect neuropsychological assessment and clinical decision making is required. The usefulness of a particular trait in clinical decision making is directly related to how frequently that entity occurs in the clinical population being studied. Stated differently, "Because the diagnostic utility of a test is relative to the base rate of the diagnosis in the population of interest, the extensive use of tests in neuropsychological assessment makes knowledge of the use of base rates in this context highly relevant" (McCaffrey, Palav, Bryant, and Labarge, 2003, p. 3).

For these reasons, an examination of the psychometric properties of a test's sensitivity, specificity, positive and negative predictive value as they are applied to different cultural groups instead of clinical groups is required. A brief introduction to the terminology associated with base rates is presented to facilitate this understanding. One aspect of test construction that will be examined first is related to a test's ability to accurately diagnose or differentiate between groups of people with or without a specified disorder based on the presence or absence of a sign. There are six terms related to this ability. The initial four terms include True Positive (TP), False Positive (FP), True Negative (TN), and False Negative (FN) (see Table 7.1). The table attempts to indicate the appropriate location of each term when the presence of a condition is known with a group of people and their result on the test is used to identify that condition.

As can be observed from Table 7.1, a True Positive refers to the ability of an instrument or test to accurately identify or detect an entity when the entity or

Table 7.1 Contingency Table Used to Describe Base Rate, Sensitivity, and Specificity

		Condition	
		Present	Absent
Test (Diagnostic)	Positive Result	True Positive	False Positive
	Negative Result	False Negative	True Negative

condition is actually present. A True Negative refers to the ability of an instrument to accurately identify the absence of an entity or condition when the entity is not present. These terms refer to beneficial detection or identifying aspects of an assessment instrument. A False Positive refers to an instrument's inaccurately identification or detection of an entity or condition when the entity is not actually present and a False Negative refers to the failure of an instrument to identify a condition when the condition or entity is present. These terms refer to errors or lack of benefits in a test (McCaffrey et al., 2003).

By combining these four aspects of population labels into ratios, an instrument's overall ability to accurately identify the presence or absence of a condition reflected by the presence or absence of a trait are referred to as a test's sensitivity or specificity. In particular, sensitivity can be understood as a test's "ability to make true positive identification, or the probability that a sign will be positive when the disorder is present" (McCaffrey et al., 2003, p. 3). Another way to understand sensitivity is as a ratio of the number of true positives to the total of true positives summed with false negatives (or incorrectly identified positives).

For a test to have 80% sensitivity it would have to accurately identify 8 of 10 people who have a condition on the basis of a presence of a trait or sign (see Table 7.2). Specificity can be understood as a test's "ability to make a true negative identification, or the probability that a sign will be negative when the disorder is not present" (McCaffrey et al., 2003, p. 3). Another way to understand specificity is as a ratio of the number of true negatives to the total of true negatives summed with false positives (or incorrectly identified negatives). For a test to have 90% specificity, it would have to accurately identify 81 out of 90 people who do not have a disorder on the basis of the absence of a sign (see Table 7.2).

Sensitivity (S_{Sy}) and specificity (S_{Py}) are inversely related or $S_{Sy} = 1/S_{Py}$

As the sensitivity of an instrument or test increases, the specificity of the instrument or test decreases. Therefore, it becomes necessary to examine the instrument or test and the purpose and repercussions of specific applications to determine the most appropriate level of sensitivity and specificity for a test. In other words, there are applications in which high sensitivity might be required (detection of a dementia) within a context in which a certain degree of specificity (regardless of type of dementia such as vascular, etc.) might be appropriately sacrificed.

This explication effectively highlights the importance of designing tests for Hispanics that are capable of accurately detecting the presence or absence of a

Table 7.2 Contingency Table - Example

N = 100			Condition		
			Present		Absent
Test (Diagnostic)	Positive Result	n = 8	True Positive	N = 9	False Positive
	Negative Result	n = 2	False Negative	N = 81	True Negative
		80%	Sensitivity	90%	Specificity

disorder within a cultural context or presence (and or) absence of other conditions or disorders or signs. It is especially useful when many people identified as "Hispanic" that have different levels of English proficiency as it has direct implications for CATs (cf. Harris and Llorente, 2005). Such is the case because clinicians who perform neuropsychological evaluations need to understand how environmental considerations may adversely affect patients' performance on "demanding, context-reduced" CATs (Harris and Llorente, 2005, p. 394). Their performance on these types of tests has a direct impact on the types of services and/or what types of educational programs they may receive. In effect, the validity of the measures needs to be questioned when the interpretation of the tests is looking for impairments, when they may be more effective at determining the absence of a disorder through the absence of statistically significant and clinically relevant discrepancies in their performance.

The previous information allows test developers to examine how well an instrument can differentiate between the groups of people with or without a particular disorder. However, it does not address how much value the sign has for prediction when the clinical diagnosis is unknown. The predictive value of a sign is reliant upon the integration of a test's sensitivity, specificity, and the base rate of the trait in the specified population. "Positive predictive value (PPV) is the likelihood that an individual from a specific population has a disorder given a positive sign. Conversely, negative predictive value (NPV) is the likelihood that an individual does not have a disorder given a negative sign." (McCaffrey et al., 2003, p. 4) (see Table 7.3).

While many consider PPV and NPV to be synonymous with sensitivity and specificity, there are distinct differences that require explanation. The primary difference between these terms is the use of actuarial data or base rates to determine the probability of the presence or absence of the disorder from a specified sample. PPV and NPV have been characterized as being inversely impacted by changes in the base rates. As the base rate increases, so does the PPV, while NPV decreases, with all other factors being held equal. (McCaffrey et al., 2003)

The effectiveness of using signs to aid in diagnostic accuracy relies upon understanding the prevalence of disorders within certain populations, including Hispanics. For conditions that are common, and for a test to be useful with Hispanic populations, the use of a sign needs to provide a success rate that must exceed the base rate of that disorder. This becomes especially difficult for signs as the base rates decline, which reflects disorders that can be characterized as rare (McCaffre et al., 2003). An example of this can be observed with Table 7.4.

Table 7.3 Contingency Table Used to Explain Base Rate, Negative Predictive Value and Positive Predictive Value

Condition with 10% base rate (TP+FN)/N		Condition		
		Present	Absent	
Test (Diagnostic)	Positive Result	True Positive	False Positive	PPV
	Negative Result	False Negative	True Negative	NPV
		Sensitivity	Specificity	

Table 7.4 Contingency table - Example

Condition with 10% base rate (TP+FN)/N			Condition				
			Present		Absent		
Test (Diagnostic)	Positive Result	n=8	True Positive	n=9	False Positive	47%	PPV
	Negative Result	n=2	False Negative	n=81	True Negative	98%	NPV
		80%	Sensitivity	90%	Specificity	N=100	

Table 7.4 illustrates the necessity to incorporate base rate information into common practice. Even with a test that has adequate sensitivity and specificity, the PPV has dropped substantially when the condition being detected occurs in only 10% of the population. In such a circumstance, the positive result on the test does not adequately determine the presence of the disorder. However, the negative result on the test ends up having greater significance for determining the absence of the identified condition.

Through the use of base rate information, a discrepancy between the performance of a patient from a minority culture and a normed sample, although statistically significant, may not be clinically relevant, as the discrepancy may occur with great frequency, thereby diminishing the impact of the statistical significant difference and, indirectly, the value of the test. Neuropsychologists can demonstrate culturally sensitive case conceptualization and test interpretation when they can explain, through the use of base rates, that a minority patient's performance does deviate from the norm (and classified as abnormal), but occurs so frequently in a given population (minority status) that the result is not clinically relevant.

When it comes to determining the appropriate frequency for determining clinical relevance there is not one accepted standard. According to Sattler (2001), "whether an occurrence is unusual or rare depends on how one defines 'unusual.'" What is the appropriate delineation between unusual or rare? "A difference that occurs in 15% or 20% of the population may be considered unusual by some, whereas others may consider a difference unusual only if it occurs in 5% or 10% of the population." (p. 447). Part of what this dilemma addresses is the confidence that clinicians can have in their interpretation of the data that they are presented with, their knowledge of cultural factors for a specific patient, and so on. The more infrequent the occurrence, the greater confidence a clinician can have in their interpretation that an observed difference is meaningful. Sattler (2001) suggests that "in order to be considered unusual or rare, the difference should occur in 15% or less (in one direction) of the standardization sample" (p. 447). As such, these discrepancies can have a direct impact upon the diagnostic formulations when they are not understood with the use of base rates. For example, if an intelligence test is utilized as part of an educational or neuropsychological assessment with a client from a minority culture, there may be an increased rate of reported borderline intellectual functioning when this test is utilized as a sole marker of cognitive functioning. This increased rate of a diagnostic label within a minority population would be an artifact of blind interpretation of test scores rather than a demonstration of how a different cultural background may affect test performance, which would be minimized if the examiners had an understanding of how to use base rates to influence interpretation, case conceptualization, and diagnostic accuracy. Because many assessment measures are normed using figures based on the U.S. Census to create the normative sample, there is an underlying assumption that the distributions of scores within the two groups are equivalent. In fact, different patterns of performance across ethnic groups or between the sexes may be due to test artifacts and, therefore, may not represent true differences in performance between these groups (cf. Llorente, 1999; Reynolds, 2000). This assumption may lead to erroneous inferences based on an individual patient's performance when he or she is from a nondominant group. By using base rates, the clinical relevance of differing patterns of performance on neuropsychological measures can be addressed in a culturally sensitive manner.

However, what if multiple groups do differ on a particular test and therefore have different distributions of scores? The creation of independent norms per culture may be extravagant, but the use of the base rate of discrepancies between majority and nonmajority cultures may be an appropriate alternative to allow for the appropriate interpretation of a patient's performance. This type of data analysis could be cultivated from the norms that have already been developed for a large number of tests. In this manner, updated norm samples would not have to be ascertained. Instead, an analysis of the distribution of scores obtained via different cultures could be analyzed and discrepancy tables developed as the basis of majority versus nonmajority cultures.

There are additional methods that can be utilized to address the aforementioned concerns related to neuropsychological assessment and cultural sensitivity, including the use of epidemiological research, modified data collection and analysis, and enhanced future test development. Epidemiological research is primarily concerned with the description and study of proximal and distal factors that affect public health. Utilizing primarily descriptive and analytical approaches to the study of factors affecting public health, data can be collected in ways that are broader in perspective than many neuropsychological studies allowing for broader generalizations of societal trends within particular populations. Incorporating this type of research into neuropsychological practice would provide neurophysiologists with information about a multitude of risk factors that may be related to health concerns, such as lower cognitive scores. It may also reveal relationships between different factors, such as those mentioned by Reynolds (2000), that have not been implicated in previous research studies across society. Examples of research can include examining the base rates of different neurological and neuropsychiatric disorders based on identified culture to see if there are different base rates of certain disorders.

As noted above, the use of Eurocentric constructs in test development may be seen in many procedures in the types of questions asked or tasks required on tests of cognitive abilities, including neuropsychological tests that rely on right or wrong answers reflecting an underlying emphasis on a dualistic approach to problem solving. However, this approach has diminished with recent revisions and updates of the many existing tests (e.g., Wechsler Intelligence Tests), whereby a process approach has been incorporated into the test allowing for reduction in the reliance upon a dualistic evaluation of responses, as well as qualitative components of such responses. The increased range and acceptance of alternative responses also reflects the recognition that there may be different cognitive strategies that are utilized during problem solving, partially the result of different cultural backgrounds. This has direct implications for people from minority groups who may utilize alternative strategies that differ in process not content, from the majority culture or vice versa. For example, when a Hispanic male is required to respond in an appropriate form to a social dilemma, his cultural background may dictate that he incorporate culturally appropriate responses that focus on family before personal gain. While the content of his answer may have been regarded as incorrect according to majority culture standards in prior evaluative settings, the increased focus on the presence of different strategies allows for more valid assessment of his underlying ability and cultural factors impacting his response.

In addition, future data collection and research should begin to address the concerns raised in the past related to cultural insensitivity during the course of neuropsychological assessment and test development. Data collection strategies that include a qualitative approach to describe cohorts of subjects and their related or shared experiences could begin to address such questions by providing additional factors that can later be operationalized in studies examining different performances across neuropsychological tests. This would include examining how certain diagnostic signs or symptoms may be affected by culture, leading to the development of classification systems based on neuropsychological and/or neuropsychiatric functions that are influenced by cultural factors.

The present state of affairs in the discipline also argues in favor of comparing an ethnic individual's performance with various normative data sets when possible and available (see Mitrushina et al., 1999), and with the standardization sample most similar in terms of demographic characteristics of the individual undergoing evaluation. Although this issue may seem elementary, it is not unusual in clinical practice to discover that an inappropriate set of norms has been used simply because that individual belongs to the same minority group (e.g., Hispanics). Of course, one major problem is the lack of extant samples, a situation that supports an assessment posture favoring the use of longitudinal examinations for these populations. As noted by Llorente et al. (2000), the present findings "also have implications for private and governmental bodies responsible for the development of policies funding neuropsychological research and norm development." For example, the geographical predilection of certain ethnic minority groups for select metropolitan areas suggest that funded attempts to acquire norms for these groups should be conducted at several centers throughout the U.S., that would allow for proportional stratification according to the U.S. Census Bureau data with full representation of specific ethnic groups and subgroups through the use of over sampling as noted above. In the same vein, racial definitions used by governmental bodies in lieu of ethnicity, including by the U.S. Census Bureau, should be modified to accurately reflect the complexity of ethnic differences found in the U.S. confounding ethnicity with racial characteristics. New categorical definitions should be created by the U.S. Census Bureau and other governmental agencies, and by the Immigration and Naturalization Service, to account for these differences since the development of many psychological procedures used in the U.S. with ethnic minority individuals rely heavily on these data to create stratified normative samples. The need for the development of standardized and published guidelines for the appropriate acquisition of normative data for minority groups also is critical. Future normative studies with Hispanics should be required to describe in more detail their research cohorts while alerting potential users of their possible shortcomings and possible misapplication(s). In addition to information historically critical to normative data sets in neuropsychology (e.g., age, education [parental education in the case of children], gender, lateralization, medical criteria, sample size), norms for ethnic minority populations should minimally report the level of acculturation of the sample, location of data collection, language fluency, and similar demographic factors associated with the sample.

Cultural Bias, Hispanics, and Test Standardization: A Specific Example

The WISC-III (Wechsler, 1991) was for years frequently employed to assess and evaluate intellectual functions in children, including Hispanics in the U.S. It was normed employing youths ages 6 to16 years. The normative sample was comprised of 200 children (100 boys, 100 girls) at each of the aforementioned age levels for a total sample of 2,200 youths. The normative sample for the WISC-III (Wechsler, 1991) was stratified using updated data from the 1980 U.S. Census according to the following characteristics: age (6 years, 0 months to 16 years, 11 months), gender (male, female); Race, *not ethnicity* ("White, Black, Hispanic, and Other"); parental education ("average number of years of school completed by the parents or parents living with the child," or the highest level of education of a single parent, using ≤8, 9–11, 12, 13–15, and ≥16 years of education as stratification cutoffs); and geographical region (North East, North Central, South, West) as well as Community Size (Metropolitan Statistical Area or MSA, greater than 100,000 inhabitants, etc.). Tables 2.2 to 2.6 in the test's manual show these data. Table 2.2 in the manual displays demographic characteristics by "Age, Race/Ethnicity" and mean years of

"Parental Education." Close scrutiny of this table reveals that 200 children at age 6 years comprised the overall 6–0 to 6–11 sample, nominally characterized as 6-year-olds. When the Hispanic group is further examined at this age level, 3.5, 3.0, 3.0, and 1.5% of the 200 children or 7 ([3.5 × 200]/100), 6, 6, and 3 youths (a total of 22 children), respectively, comprise the subsample. Immediately, it becomes critical to note that no Hispanic child with parents with average education equal or greater than 16 years is found at this age level (see Table 2.2.). Further scrutiny of this group, using Table 2.4 (percentages by Age, Gender and Race) indicates that of the 22 6-year-olds, 5.5% are boys and 5.5% are girls of Hispanic origin for a total of 11 ([5.5 × 200]/100) boys and 11 girls. Clearly, of these children, none of them come from parents with 16 or more years of education. Further perusal of Table 2.5 reveals that 0.5% of 6-year-old Hispanic children come from the North Central region of the U.S. (including Chicago) comprising a total of one child ([200 × 0.5]/100)! Is this child 1 of the 11 boys or 1 of the 11 girls? Clearly, it is not a child whose parents averaged 16 or more years of education. Is the child then from the group of parents who averaged 8 or less, 9 to 11, 12, or 13 to 15 years of education? With regard to the application of these norms, are there no 6-year-old Hispanic youths requiring placement in schools or necessitating neuropsychological assessment who come from backgrounds where both parents have a Bachelor's degree residing in Chicago? Most unlikely! What if the child had been a 14-year-old Hispanic from the Northeast, or a 9-year-old with highly educated parents (>16 years of education)? Again, no Hispanic child is represented in such groups. Although it may appear that such weaknesses in the test standardization sample have little relevance, such an assumption would be erroneous. In fact, critical decisions are constantly made about Hispanic patients, including adults, children, and the elderly in the U.S. and abroad, related to school placement and judicial and vocational issues on the bases of these norms, in some instances life-and-death decisions in the case of individuals undergoing criminal proceedings and facing the possibility of capital punishment!

Unfortunately, it is only when tests are examined with this detailed degree of scrutiny that a proper examination of the issues so far discussed can be best elucidated, underscoring the importance of all these factors during the course of neuropsychological assessments with Hispanics. It is also critical to note that these issues are not unique to the Wechsler Scales and that they impact a large number of tests and procedures. It is not surprising, then, yet interesting, because it displays in a clear fashion his acumen, that Professor Wechsler himself argued against the use of normative data for his scales (see Kaufman, 1994; Preface). Again, the issues discussed above should not be perceived as an attack on the test. As test authors ourselves, we understand the painstaking intricacies of developing neuropsychological procedures and acquiring good normative data for tests in the U.S. and abroad. Rather, the example and criticism are provided to underscore the importance and potential consequences of the misuse of such data and tests by poorly trained, biased, or ignorant individuals. It is also provided for readers so they can understand the limitations of such tests and standardization samples as a result of problems in their acquisition, with significant negative repercussions if used inappropriately when using a nomothetic approach with Hispanics.

Cultural Bias, Hispanics, and Test Development: Extant and Future Potential Solutions

In the final section of this chapter, an attempt will be made to describe examples of modern tests that attempted to address the potential cultural biases discussed. Examples of cognitive, behavioral-emotional, and neuropsychological procedures will be presented. Although several issues referenced above related to cultural bias have not been addressed in these measures, they represent some of the best examples available to date of instrumentation that has been developed using a concerted effort to address cultural bias in test development.

Although during the development of the *Wechsler Intelligence Scale for Children - Fourth Edition* (WISC-IV, Wechsler, 2004) an effort was made to address cultural issues by closely following the U.S. Census, including a large stratification of Hispanics with oversampling in some instances, the use of the U.S. Census to stratify a test's standardization sample left much to be desired for obvious reasons, particularly as noted for the *Wechsler Intelligence Scale for Children - Third Edition* (WISC-III; Wechsler, 1991). To complicate matters further, the *WISC IV* was developed in English, and its application, therefore, was limited to individuals who were fluent in English and whose families identified themselves as Hispanic. In addition, the use of the test was limited for a large number of Hispanic children who possess different levels of English proficiency. Therefore, the publisher of the *Wechsler Intelligence Scales* developed the *WISC-IV in Spanish* (Wechsler, 2004). In addition to the stratification described above, additional samples of Hispanic children were collected whose families had originated from Cuba, Central America, the Dominican Republic, Puerto Rico, and South America. In addition, items were designed to minimize the impact of cultural bias as a result of cultural differences between countries, allowing for a statistical examination of item bias using IRT methods of analysis" (Wechsler et al., 2004, p. 21). Supplemental demographic data provided in the test manual allows for a comparison with subgroups of the Hispanic population comprising the standardization sample, enhancing the inferential process. It is clear that such a process of test development is far superior to old translations and simple adaptations of tests, a significant leap forward in the development of tests that attempt to address cultural factors, and worthy of commendation, an ethical approach to test development for Hispanics.

The *Behavior Assessment System for Children - Second Edition* (BASC-II; Reynolds and Kamphaus, 2004) provides another good example. For this test, its developers and publisher created a Spanish version of the BASC-II concurrent with the English version. This process allows for the scales to be used with "Spanish-speaking individuals residing in the United States" (Reynolds and Kamphaus, 2004, p. 247), and the Spanish version includes all of the items in the same order as the English version.

To accomplish such a goal, a professional group was used to translate test items from the original BASC. Bilingual psychologists subsequently were used to express each item in a manner that would be comprehensible "across dialects and would be culturally appropriate for use among with multiple U.S. Spanish-speaking populations" (Reynolds and Kamphaus, 2004, p. 247). The items these individuals reviewed were then distributed to a separate group of psychologists throughout the United States with instructions to compare the English and Spanish versions and to make suggestions "to clarify or improve item wording" while maintaining the "psychological content" and "appropriateness" of the translation (Reynolds and Kamphaus, 2004, p. 247). The suggestions were submitted to the translation service through repeated review rounds until final decisions on the items were reached.

Once the Spanish-language forms were created, they were subjected to a "number of statistical comparisons" to "ensure that both sets of forms could adequately measure their intended constructs" prior to completion of the final Covariance Structure Analysis (CSA), which is also known as a Confirmatory Factor Analysis, and reliability studies (Reynolds and Kamphaus, 2004, p. 247). During the standardization process, parents and children were allowed to complete the appropriate forms in either Spanish or English. Approximately 400 parents and 150 children completed the Spanish versions, allowing for a comparison of the effects of culture and language. The protocols were divided into three groups depending on the identified ethnicity of the child and the language of the form that was used. The groups were non-Hispanic and English form, Hispanic and English form, and Hispanic and Spanish form.

Separate CSAs were conducted for each group resulting in a standardized factor loading for each item on its scale. The magnitude and rank order were compared across groups. Those with an acceptable loading (>.30) in the three groups were retained. If the results were not similar across groups the item was excluded from further analysis. The Spanish language forms were used within the norm sample, as it was "more representative" of the general population (Reynolds and Kamphaus, 2004, p. 248). However, these forms were not included in the internal-consistency and scale correlational studies of the norm sample.

An assumption of similar psychometric properties between the Spanish and English forms was not assumed just because "the Spanish forms consist[ed] of translated versions of items from the English form" (Reynolds and Kamphaus, 2004, p. 248). With regard to the Parent Report Scales (PRS) "the median reliabilities are lower than those obtained in the English-form samples," and they were considered "adequate." (Reynolds and Kamphaus, 2004, p. 247) A similar pattern was obtained with regard to the Self Report Scales in that the median reliability values "are slightly lower than those obtained on the English (SRP) forms" (Reynolds and Kamphaus, 2004, p. 249). This is an admirable example of the development of tests in Spanish that are not separate from the English version, but include and have an appreciation of how culture affects a test's development and its psychometric properties.

Similar advances were used in the development of the Spanish and English Neuropsychological Assessment (SENAS; Mungas, Reed, Haan, and Gonzalez, 2005). They developed an instrument to identify cognitive abilities relevant for the

Table 7.5 SENAS Scales (Mungas et al., 2004)

Ability	Verbal measure	Nonverbal measure
Conceptual thinking	Verbal conceptual thinking	Nonverbal conceptual thinking
Semantic memory	Object naming	Picture association
Attention span	Verbal attention span	Visual attention span
Episodic memory	Word list learning I	Spatial configuration learning
	Word list learning II	
Nonverbal/spatial abilities		Pattern recognition
		Spatial localization
Verbal abilities	Verbal comprehension	
	Verbal expression	

neuropsychological evaluation of older people from different ethnic groups. The authors developed this test using entirely new scales, which are listed in Table 7.5.

Methods based on Item Response Theory (IRT) were used to refine the initial scales. This approach is based on item characteristic curves describing the probability of answering an item in a certain direction. Theoretically, IRT parameters are thought to be stable across samples, provided enough variability is present in the population tested; in other words, the distribution of a given trait (e.g., dementia) in a sample should not impair scale properties of the SENAS. All items were translated by a team of bilingual English/Spanish speakers (mostly Mexican Americans), then back-translated and revised if necessary. Differential item functioning was examined in detail in order to identify differences between English and Spanish versions on verbal scales. For details of the construction process, see Mungas, Reed, Crane, Haan, and Gonzalez (2004).

SENAS first underwent pilot testing using a sample of 208 English-speaking and 200 Spanish-speaking individuals 60+ years of age. Scales were then revised based on IRT and covariance structure analysis (CSA).

The revised scales were then administered to a variety of samples for different scales. Object Naming, Picture Association, Verbal Attention Span, Verbal Conceptual Reasoning, and Pattern Recognition were administered to 547 English- and 582 Spanish-speaking participants. Word List Learning I was administered to 995 English- and 1,094 Spanish speakers. The remaining scales were administered to 385 English and 327 Spanish speakers. Reliabilities of all subscales averaged .85 for the English, .86 for the English-speaking Hispanics, and .88 for the Spanish scales, ranging from .79 to .92 (Mungas et al., 2004). This is comparable to reliabilities of the WAIS-III and the WMS. As Mungas and colleagues noted, "the extent of psychometric matching between the English and Spanish versions is exceptional" (Mungas et al., 2004, p. 357). In terms of construct validity, dimensional structure was found to be similar in both the English and the Spanish version of the SENAS, with some group differences in factor loading, most notably for the conceptual thinking factor (Mungas et al., 2004).

In order to evaluate concurrent validity, a sample of 367 Hispanics and 160 non-Hispanic Whites were administered the SENAS and two measures of cognitive status (3MS and IQCODE). All SENAS parameters were associated with cognitive status independent of demographic variables. Overall, there were no significant differences in concurrent validity between Hispanics and non-Hispanic Whites (Mungas et al., 2005).

The study (Mungas et al., 2005) demonstrated robust effects of education and language use on SENAS variables, whereas gender and age effects were weak to modest. Spanish language use was associated with lower test scores. Acculturation effects were limited after controlling for education and language use. Likewise, ethnicity effects were eliminated by controlling for education and language use. Mungas and colleagues provide a sound instrument for assessing cognitive functioning in older adults of Hispanic (and non-Hispanic) origin. The authors caution that education and language exert measurable effects on test scores, but note that assessment of these confounds seems relatively manageable and should provide clinicians with enough data to interpret results appropriately.

In conclusion, although the aforementioned tests are not perfect by any means, they represent meritorious attempts to include cultural factors in test development. This is a critical issue because clinicians who use neuropsychological assessment measures assume a large amount of responsibility for providing accurate and valid information about a Hispanic patient's current functional abilities, in some instances with significant economic, personal, and societal dispositions. Modern tools developed to be used with Hispanics should reflect comprehensive cultural factors and specific characteristics, yet appropriate and sound psychometric properties. The use of base rates and other information, sometimes available, should allow clinicians to examine a multitude of factors beyond discrepancy scores and differences in performance among minority groups, including Hispanics.

Chapter 8
Rehabilitation

Julie K. Ries, Brian Potter, and Antolin M. Llorente

It should be patently clear that the historical record provided in most rehabilitation textbooks is Eurocentric in its perspective. For example, although Eurocentric history tends to note the emergence of trephination in Egypt, it fails to note that in the "New World," the advanced Chinchoros culture of Northern Chile, precursors to the complex, eminent, and sophisticated Inca State, perfected artificial mummification as a means to protect the body and soul in the afterlife. However, unbeknownst to large number of students in the field of neuropsychology, psychology, and rehabilitation, is the fact that the Chinchoros perfected this process in the third millennium BC, most likely before or temporally concurrent with the Egyptians (Mosely, 1993). This example is provided because it underscores the importance of attending to our cultural biases, even when addressing a discipline's history, an issue that should be taken into consideration when rehabilitating individuals from ethnic minority backgrounds, including Hispanics.

It is also important to examine the precursory roots and historical foundations of neuropsychological rehabilitation in detail to foster greater appreciation of the current state of the field and its future, providing a better context for cross-cultural perspectives and their specific applications to Hispanics. Such a rich history actually spans across cultures, particularly views and positions addressing rehabilitation.

As note by León-Carrión (1997), some of the oldest discoveries of treatment and interventions for brain damage can be dated as early as the Mesolithic Age. Skulls were discovered with holes on their left side that appear to be a form of surgical intervention, trephination. Physicians practicing during the Hippocratic period noted brain-behavior connections such as the brain's intellectual capacities, regulating a majority of body functions, allowing it to make judgments. In keeping with tradition, Hippocratic physicians used trephinations for the treatment of selected mild brain injuries.

According to León-Carreón (1997), quoted in Ries, Potter, and Llorente (2007), "The first hospitals and convalescence homes for the treatment of physical lesions were founded in 499 to 429 BC Greece, which indicates an important shift in the treatment of illness in Western societies. Previously, children born with deformities were displayed in public places for a period of time or were thrown off of Mount Taigeto. In Imperial Rome, it was acceptable to take the life of children who were born with any type of physical lesion, abandon them, or release them into the Tiber River in flower baskets."

"In the Second Century B.C., Galen was among the first to require a detailed clinical examination of all patients, noting all symptoms in order to provide information for diagnosis and treatment. Through anatomical dissection of monkeys, he provided detailed findings regarding the anatomy of the nervous system and of brain trauma" (Ries et al., 2007).

The 18th century marked a period of intellectual and scientific advances that led to new theories and hypotheses about functional anatomy, specifically neuroanatomy. The French Revolution (1789) prompted the emergence of equal treatment for the ill, whereas advances in science and medicine prompted the use of electricity for rehabilitation of hemiplegias (León-Carrión, 1997), as well as a greater understanding of the nervous system. The 19th century was marked by a scientific continuation of the discovery of localization of functions as well as systems within the brain. According to many neuroscientists, most influential were the discoveries by Paul Broca and Carl Wernicke regarding the language system subsequent to neuropathological investigations and, as noted in Chapter 1, the proposition by the Spanish histologist Ramón y Cajal (1889) describing the neuron system and the discovery of chemical neuronal transmission (cf. León-Carrión, 1997). Advances also were possible as a result of the contributions made by the English neurologist Hughlings Jackson, which addressed the hierarchical nature of the central nervous system, an often forgotten contribution in the neurosciences.

In the 20th century, the Russian scholar Vygotsky provided a framework noting the importance of cultural factors in human development (cf. LeFrancois, 1995), which had significant applications, particularly from a theoretical perspective for neuropsychology. One of Vygotsky's colleagues, Alexander Luria, would use this framework to make significant theoretical and applied contributions to the field of rehabilitation. Luria also reportedly had direct impact on the field through the establishment of rehabilitative centers in the Soviet Union after World War II.

Despite concurrence with previous writings that brain injury was well recognized and and its rehabilitation perhaps attempted by ancient civilizations as noted above (cf. Courville, 1967), it is an accepted fact by most serious students in the field of rehabilitation that the modern, evidence-based "history of modern neurorehabilitation had its humble yet most influential beginnings in association with the emergence of the Industrial Revolution and World War I, as well as with advances in technology and Western medicine" (cf. Ries et al., 2007). This evolution and renaissance were partially the result of pragmatic factors impacting rehabilitative medicine, including low survival rates of victims who had sustained central nervous system (CNS) trauma before that time and, indirectly, the investigation of rehabilitative methods and their impact on recovery after injury (cf. Gurdjian, 1973). As noted by Ries et al. (2007), "Technological advances in the treatment of infections additionally led to increased survival, and advances in technology itself played a major role (e.g., angiography) leading to the study of previously untreatable injuries or poorly understood CNS diseases" and their treatments (e.g., strokes) (DeJong, 1982).

"Although several programs of rehabilitation for wounded war veterans or industrial accident victims were established in the earlier part of the Twentieth Century (Harris, 1919), particularly in England and France, modern neurorehabilitation owns a great deal of debt to early programs established in Germany (Camus, 1917/1918; Harris, 1919)." Although most programs established during the early part of the last century focused on physical and occupational rehabilitation (cf. Camus, 1917/1918), partially due to significant advances in orthopedic medicine as a result of the development of the x-ray and limited knowledge in the neurosciences, the charter programs begun in Germany were original interventions that included the rehabilitation of brain injuries in a comprehensive fashion, including the social reintegration of brain-injured individuals and an effort to understand the effects of brain injury on vocational and occupational outcomes (cf. Poser, Kohler, and Schönle, 1996). Kurt Goldstein (1919; 1942), who was responsible for such programs in collaboration with his student Frieda Fromm-Reichmann and colleagues (Goldstein and Reichmann, 1920), was in charge of the development and documentation of rehabilitative programs that included the comprehensive assessment of and intervention for patients. Those assessments were comprehensive in scope and included the assessment of several domains of functioning (e.g., attention, perception, memory), similar to extant neuropsychological examinations. According to Ries et al., 2007, "Rehabilitative programs also were quite advanced and included the use of techniques employing relatively preserved cognitive strengths to address relative weaknesses, specific rehabilitative interventions including treatments for aphasias and other disorders, and an examination of specific outcomes of rehabilitation and social reintegration, including return-to-work, that employed the results of neuropsychological assessments as well as behavioral observations in the work setting" (cf. Goldstein and Reichmann, 1920). Figure 8.1 shows data from one of their investigations reporting the percentage of individuals returning to work according to their premorbid occupational allegiance grouping (Prozentzahl innerhalb der Berufsarten) (WWI German veterans). These data suggested to Goldstein and Reichmann that patients who had been employed in the farming industry (*Landwirte*) enjoyed the best vocational outcomes often traumatic brain injury, whereas, patients who had been employed in the mining industry (*Bergleute*) exhibited the poorest vocational outcomes. Returning brain injured veterans in the farming industry had the best overall outcomes as measured by the percentage of patients who were able to return to their previous occupations (*in alten Beruf*). In comparison, patients employed in the mining industry were more likely to change to new occupations (*im neuen Beruf*) or remain unemployed (*beschäftigungslos*) post injury. Interestingly, neither of these two groups had the smallest number of unemployed, and this poor outcome was mostly associated with postal service (Post-u. Bahnunterbeamte) and other occupations (*Sonstige Berufe*). These programs were the progenitors of modern rehabilitation programs throughout the world and led to eventual and modern collaborations by the European Union and eventually to the formation of the European Brain Injury Society in 1986 and to modern standards in clinical practice on the European continent.

The information presented above underscores the multicultural aspects of the history and genesis of modern neurorehabilitation. However, prior to engaging in

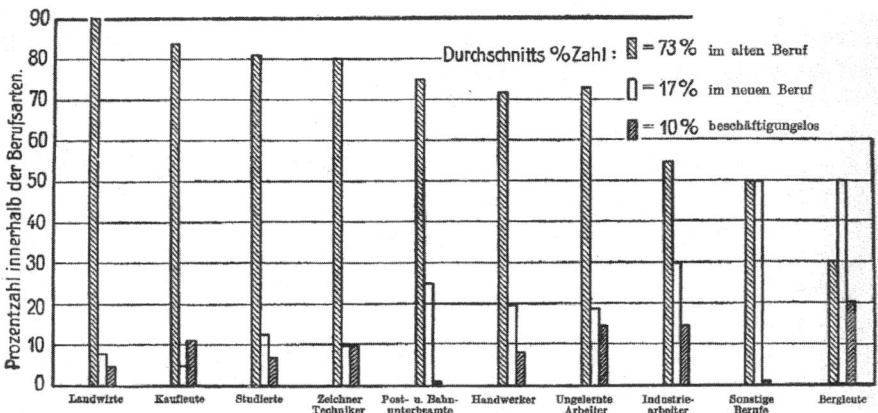

Figure 8.1 Premorbid Occupation and rehabilitation outcomes after brain injury. Study showing percentages of "return-to-work" WWI German veterans (brain-injured patients) as a function of premorbid occupational allegiance (see text for explanation). From Goldstein and Reichmann (1920), with permission from the publisher

an examination of the literature investigating the importance of multicultural aspects of neuropsychological rehabilitation in the U.S., it is critical to examine why such a need emerges. An examination of culture, ethnicity, and inherent factors associated with such constructs, including the epidemiology of injuries and its relation to ethnicity and patterns of American immigration, as noted in Chapter 2, and their impact on neuropsychology, are proper places to begin.

Epidemiology of Brain Trauma or Acquired Brain Diseases

Is the epidemiology of traumatic brain injury (TBI), or acquired brain injury, impacted by ethnicity or cultural factors? Although a close examination of epidemiological factors is clearly beyond the scope of this chapter and this volume, a brief glance at the epidemiology of brain trauma or acquired brain diseases buttresses the need to attend to cultural factors. Although unfortunately confounding ethnicity with race, a nevertheless comprehensive investigation, conducted by the Centers for Disease Control and Prevention (CDC), revealed that deaths in the U.S. attributed to traumatic brain insults as a result of vehicular accidents, including automobile accidents, was equivalent in Caucasian and African-American populations. In contrast, the same investigation indicated that African-Americans had a higher rate of TBI than Caucasians subsequent to firearm injuries (CDC, 1999). Clearly, in selected areas of the U.S., higher rates of such types of injuries also are applicable to Hispanic populations, including those in metropolitan counties such as Los Angeles County, California, and Hudson County, New Jersey, partly the result of patterns of American immigration as noted in Chapter 2 in this volume – particularly the geographical affinity of selected groups of immigrants. Similarly, a previous report published by the CDC (CDC, 1998) noted that "cerebrovascular disease is twice as high among African-American men (53.1 per 100,000) as among white men (26.3 per 100,000) and twice as high among African American women (40.6 per 100,000) as among white women (22.6 per 100,000)." Similar health disparities are applicable to Hispanics. In addition, although the contrasts between ethnic minority groups, including Hispanics, and the dominant cultural group have revealed meaningful epidemiological differences, modern investigations also have shown the emergence of interethnic differences in the epidemiology of TBI. For example, in an elucidating study, Kraus et al. (1986) found differential epidemiology rates of TBI in "Hispanics" compared to "African-Americans" and "Asians/Native Americans" related to median income in these groups.

Although many other examples could be provided for other injuries and disorders, it should be sufficient to note that racial, and more important and critical, ethnic differences, in conjunction with other variables such as socio-economic status, health care access, and other variables, have historically led to differential rates of incidence and prevalence of brain injuries or acquired diseases of the brain requiring rehabilitation. Therefore, the close relationship between the epidemiology of acquired brain injury and ethnic minority status, namely Hispanic, buttresses the importance of attending to such factors' capability to impact neuropsychological interventions and rehabilitation in the U.S.

The Nature of Culture in the United States

Although culture and ethnicity were discussed in detail in previous chapters, they are briefly addressed here, in some instances from different perspectives, to note their impact on the rehabilitation process. The term culture has been described by the American Psychological Association (APA, 2003) as "the embodiment of a worldview through learned and transmitted beliefs, values, and practices, including religious and spiritual traditions. It also encompasses a way of living informed by the historical, economic, ecological, and political forces on a group" (p. 380). As noted by Ries et al. (in press), "culture embodies and influences all facets of the individual including cognition and emotions." "Differences in cultural background include not just language differences, but also differences in group identity, beliefs, and values" (Dana, 1993), all of which influence the use of services including rehabilitation, the presentation of neuropsychological symptoms, the assessment and interventional techniques employed by the field, and all or most aspects of treatment including neuropsychological rehabilitation.

Although as noted by Ardila (2003), culture is in the brain, and as noted in Chapter 1, there may be an intricate interaction between culture and brains mediated by genetic mechanisms. In addition, race unfortunately has been used interchangeably with the term *ethnicity*. As noted by Llorente et al. (2000) and Harris and Llorente (2005), such a definitional interchange unfortunately has been a source of significant confusion. This is partially the result of the fact that race and ethnicity are distinct constructs. In this regard, Jalali (1988) defined ethnicity as "the culture of [a] people [that] is thus critical for values, attitudes, perceptions, needs, and modes of expression, behavior, and identity" (p. 10). Therefore, one's culture and ethnicity are similar as they are learned and passed down from generations, whereas race typically refers to cultural groups with permanent attributes that are not learned nor can be changed because they are biologically-based (cf. Carter and Qureshi, 1995). The subtle but significant definitional differences noted above are important.

For example as it relates to Hispanics, the term has been used to describe a heterogeneous group of individuals, and as stated by Llorente et al. (2000), has been misused because it has been used as a racial category rather than an ethnic label. Harris and Llorente also note that this "panethnic label" fails to "capture the unique attributes" of an individual including, oddly enough, his or her racial background in some instances. Even when referring to a specific Hispanic group, such as Mexican or Puerto Rican, there are several unique attributes to consider. For example, whether they are Mexican-American of Mexican descent born and raised in the U.S. or Mexican immigrants born and raised in Mexico from dozens of possible ancestral backgrounds, including one or more of 50 aboriginal origins, should be included when considering ethnicity. Similarly, level of acculturation to American society and dominant language should be included (cf. Harris and Llorente, 2005). These distinctions are critical if we are to understand specific triggers that lead to variations in rates of interethnic outcomes during TBI after rehabilitation. Such distinctions are required because it is possible that specific demographics (e.g., level of education, literacy, specific occupational predilections or opportunities), interacting with specific ethnic subgroup, may be associated, or may modulate or moderate, interethnic and intraethnic TBI rates. Most important, as noted by Ries et al. (2007), culture can have significant impact on brain injury rehabilitation and prospective outcomes whether addressing pediatric or adult populations (cf. Yeats et al., 2002; Uomoto and Wong, 2000).

Ries and her colleagues (in press) also note that "general treatment adherence" in multicultural clients "[is] more likely to end treatment prematurely, due to frustration, misunderstanding, and role ambiguities of treatment," and the role of such factors in the rehabilitation process of ethnic minority individuals has found support in the literature (cf. Sue and Zane, 1987). Sohlberg and Mateer (2001) indicate that identity and self-concept are influenced and impacted by culturally mediated norms about assertiveness, aggression, emotional expression, and individual goal attainment versus sacrificing for the greater good. In fact, as noted in previous chapters, cultural identity and ethnicity also may underlie beliefs about illness and disability by the patient and clinician, as well as its meaning and interpretation. "Whereas personal independence is highly valued in Western culture, it is not necessarily a goal in other cultures, which have different beliefs about (1) person's degree of responsibility and control over health and (2) the role of family in dealing with illness, according to Ries et al. (in press; cf. Watanabe et al., 2001; Uomoto and Wong, 2000).

Finally, it is critical to note that population predictions indicate marked increases in all minority groups; most notably, the Hispanic population grows

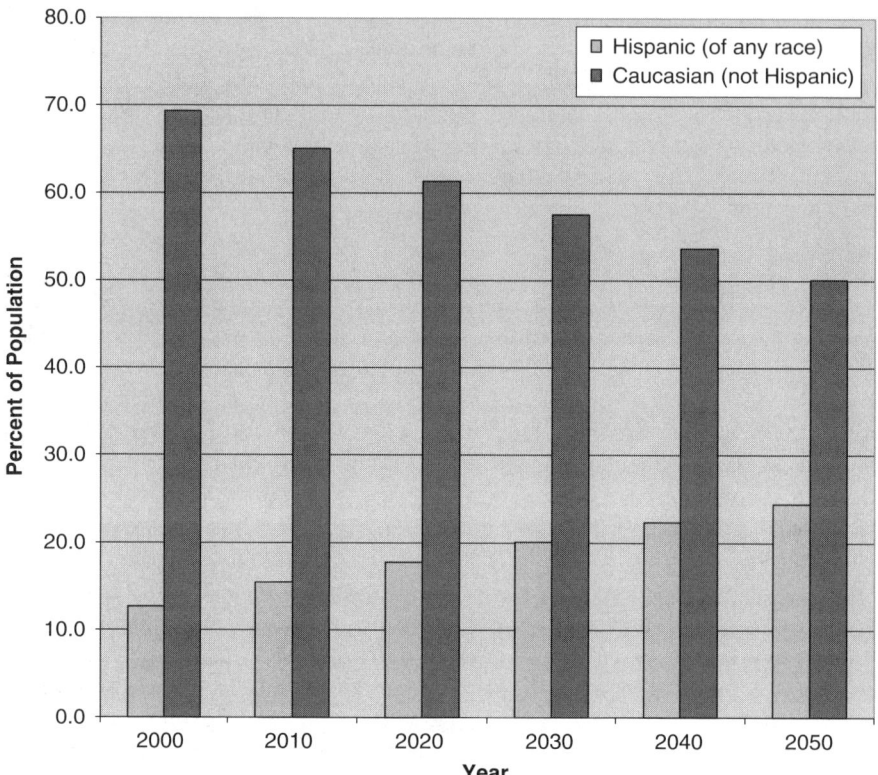

Figure 8.2 Expected percent of Hispanic relative to non-Hispanic White population across decades (U.S. Census, 2004)

at significantly faster rates, nearly doubling their percentage in their share of the total U.S. population. This trend is predicted to continue and by the end of the 21st century, the number of inhabitants of Hispanic origin is predicted to be nearly half the number of inhabitants of Caucasian origin living in the U.S. (see Figure 8.2) (U.S. Census, 2004).

More important, as it relates to neuropsychological intervention, patterns of American immigration, moderating demographic variables of large numbers of individuals, including Hispanics, are not the result of mechanisms driven by chance processes as noted in Chapter 2 with significant repercussions for neuropsychology and neuropsychological assessment and rehabilitation.

In summary, the predicted changes in the cultural and ethnic diversity in the U.S. population buttress the increasing importance of understanding the interplay between such factors and neuropsychological rehabilitation. Finally, it is critical to recognize that culture may interact with other variables, such as SES, access to medical care, nutritional variables, beliefs, rituals, and other cultural factors to create specific brain injury epidemiology.

Multicultural Assessment and Intervention

Neuropsychological assessment continues to be a significant component of empirically based neurorehabilitation, as was the case for Goldstein and his colleagues during the early part of the last century in Germany. However, neuropsychologists depend on normative data during the course of assessment to inform their research or clinical practice, including the application of specific treatments, unless an idiographic approach is used. Normative data provide a context or empirical frame of reference for which test scores can be understood (Mitrushina, Boone, D'Elia, and D'Elia, 1999), and normative data are considered the "gold standard" by many practitioners as a way of comparing individual performance (Mitrushina et al.,1999). In fact, the combination of sound clinical judgment and the use of appropriate normative comparison groups allow neuropsychologists to better understand individuals (Lezak, 1995). Ideally, the normative reference groups should be as narrow as possible (representative of the individual being compared), as long as the norms on which they are based are stable and do not fluctuate significantly (Rorer and Dawes, 1982).

Unfortunately, the ideal process of comparison sometimes does not take place and while a normative reference group may reflect overall population statistics, the norms may not reflect the specific demographic of an individual from a given ethnic group (Harris and Llorente, 2005), particularly the individual undergoing rehabilitation. Such issues merit significant attention because they can lead to inaccurate inferences and interpretations of the data with ethnic minorities, particularly Hispanics, unless measures are taken to reduce such potential biases. For example, modern versions of tests (e.g., WISC-IV-Spanish Edition) oversample ethnic minority populations in order to represent a specific minority group more adequately (Harris and Llorente, 2005; Prifitera, Saklofske and Weiss, 2005). Such overrepresentation also permits additional and supplemental statistical analyses capable of informing test publishers of potential limitations of their procedures (see Chapter 7).

Multicultural Aspects of Neuropsychological Intervention

The Rehabilitation of the Hispanic Client and Multi-Cultural Models

Blonder (1991) examines the concept of culture within the context of neuropsychological theories and research. Blonder noted that the effects of cultural variations on linguistics impact the cerebral organization of language and reveal both organizing principles as well as the impact of neuroplasticity on the brain and language functions. In spite of variation in syntactic markers in languages, aphasic speakers show similar patterns of problems following lesions to Broca's area. The grammatical endings are lost or used incorrectly, and words are produced in their uninflected form as stems or infinitives. Blonder proposes that language is a brain-mediated cognitive system proceeding from a limit set of structural features that underlie the world languages, and at this juncture the reader is challenged to examine the sign language and brain injury literature.

Condeluci (1997) has extensively studied the transition from rehabilitation to one's community for people with chronic or acquired disabilities. Initially, the goal is saving a person's life or stabilizing their vital functions. Then the rehabilitation focus shifts to returning the individual to their community. Condeluci challenges the deficit-based medical model of rehabilitation in which the physician is empowered to fix deficits, or if the deficits are unable to be alleviated or mitigated, they must be accepted. Patients and families following this model may end up in placement in settings that are less than optimal for the individual, particularly settings in which the patient may be labeled or stereotyped, lack privacy or control, become dependent on this system, and subsequently lower standards and expectations. In contrast, Condeluci proposes a community-based, interdependent model that identifies the individual's capacities and supports, and encourages empowerment of the person with the disability through choice and participation in decision making (as age appropriate), in which the individual and/or family is in charge of the outcome. The interdependence model focuses on the culture and community as the more effective change agents than the individual. In this context, culture is defined as "common rituals, rules, boundaries, and jargon" (p. 491). A cultural group is unified by their common belief system and has either formal or informal leaders. Membership is based on "proving" oneself before the individual is invited to join this group. Several types of cultures may be relevant in rehabilitation, according to Condeluci, including family, spiritual, work, age, neighborhood, ethnic, gender or sexual orientation, and common interests. As the supportive systems of the person with a brain injury understand the diverse cultures and their influences, it will be easier for the patient to then experience "culturation," an informal process by which the patient is appreciated and understood by the group. This process is critical for the successful reentry of the patient into his or her environment. As Condeluci notes:

> Life is a tight ecological web with links up and down the scale. Our micro worlds – our abilities, personality, and character – are uniquely related to our macro world – family, friends, community, and greater society. One cannot be considered without the other. (p. 494)

Based on Condeluci's interdependent model, integration of the patient within the culture and the community and empowerment of individuals to make decisions regarding their future course is paramount to successful recovery.

The American Psychological Association (APA, 2003) guidelines are focused on psychotherapeutic intervention: "Cross-culturally sensitive practitioners are encouraged to develop skills and practices that are attuned to the unique worldviews and cultural backgrounds of clients by striving to incorporate understanding of a client's ethnic, linguistic, racial, and cultural background into therapy" (p. 391). Therefore, the neuropsychologist must extrapolate how to interpret these guidelines for specific interventions. Empirically validated, culturally sensitive neuropsychological interventions are rare, and there is a need for increased research in this area, as noted in the following statement by Christophersen and Mortweet (2001):

> Although numerous discussion articles have highlighted the importance of the issues of cultural diversity, there are virtually no published research studies that have compared the outcomes of two or more ethnic groups that were exposed to identical treatments. When clients in different countries have presented with the same problems, similar treatments have reportedly produced comparable results. For example, when children with encopresis, enuresis, or habit disorders have been treated using empirically supported or probably efficacious procedures, the outcomes have been essentially similar. The lack of empirical data on cultural diversity makes it impossible to estimate when and where cultural differences are important. (p.7)

Multiculturally sensitive neuropsychological intervention poses unique challenges to practitioners, given the limitations in our assessment tools that guide this intervention, the need for developing a greater understanding of the impact of culture on one's practice, developing empirically validated culture specific interventions, and interpreting the results of our findings within a culturally sensitive context (cf. Gannotti and Handwerker, 2002). Groce and Zola (1993) propose that this cultural sensitivity begins with self-reflection:

> Everyone has a cultural heritage that influences his or her health beliefs and practices. It is thus not practical to learn in detail the infinite details of specific cultures, but rather to assume that such variations occur and learn how they might affect one's health practices. Rather than teaching every health practitioner to be a mini-medical anthropologist, it is more important for practitioners to be sensitive to the patient's heritage, to their own heritage, and to what happens when different heritages and belief systems come together. (p. 1054)

These are questions that should guide a practitioner's interactions with patients from different cultures.

Fadiman (1997) exemplifies what can occur if there is a lack of understanding of different cultures in the medical setting, including the rehabilitation milieu. This book examines the potential cultural conflict between Western beliefs and an individual culture when a seizure disorder is perceived as a gift within a specific culture, but as a disorder in Western medicine. The author provides some questions to ask to promote greater understanding of a patient's culture such as "What do you call the problem? What do you think has caused the problem? How severe is the sickness? What are the most important results you hope to receive from this treatment?" Additional studies have supported the use of similar questions in understanding a patient's perspective of illness, disease, and disability within their culture (García Coll and Magnuson, 2002; Reeve, Groce, Persing, and Magge, 2004).

Li (2003) proposes a unique model that incorporates the dynamic interplay of culture and biology across the lifespan. This framework highlights "how interactive processes and developmental plasticity at different levels are closely connected to each other and unfold across different time scales. Consequently, together they channel reciprocal cultural experiential influences on behavioral, cognitive, and brain development throughout the life span" (p. 173). Li describes the reciprocal and dynamic process by which genetics and neuronal mechanisms interface with environment and culture to determine development.

Empirically Validated Rehabilitation Models[1]

Attempts have been made to incorporate culture into specific models of rehabilitation as a moderating variable rather than as an independent variable. Such a modeling posture has assisted investigators to better understand the role of culture in rehabilitation. For example, ethnicity has been hypothesized to be intricately related to SES, accounting for a portion of the findings that implicate ethnicity in TBI. In this regard, culture interacts, as a moderator variable, with SES to create a pattern of performance that is unique to a specific individual. Although related to race, not ethnicity, this is depicted in individuals who come from specific African-American populations in which the rates of TBI as a result of violence are greater than those for European-Americans, most likely as a result of lower levels of SES combined with other factors. In this case, TBI severity related to violence, for example, could be associated with SES yet moderated by a specific ethnic background within a race construct (e.g., African-American, Hispanic), or other variable(s). Such methods of examining culture and other factors, as moderator variables, have been postulated by various investigators (e.g., Baron and Kenney, 1986; Holmbeck, 1997) and have received limited yet sound empirical validation. In the case of children, for example, an investigation has shown that African-Americans compared to Whites (race), independent of SES, were able to moderate differences in injured groups (TBI v. Orthopedic) in parental and family outcomes (Yeats et al., 2002). In contrast, Handwerker (2002) proposes methods of analyses of transposed matrices to take advantage of the unique point of view that ethnography offers – its focus on similarities and differences among informants rather than among variables. According to Handwerker:

> Without explicit construct validation of the cultures, one cannot know which groups to compare. If one divides one's data by identity (ethnicity, class, gender, age, etc), counts the responses for each, and compared the results, one imposes cultural differences by assumption, not evidence. (p. 2095)

Although limited, in light of the dramatic increase in use of unconventional medical therapies and complementary treatments over the past 20 years, research has focused on the development of empirical models. One such model, for example, incorporates Eastern medicine into traditionally Western medicine delivery systems. Wu (2004) developed a model for the use of complementary and alternative health care options to determine factors contributing to health care use among a cohort of Chinese-American families. The full and partial research models reveal that the factors contributing the most to their medical preferences were their acculturation level and health beliefs. Additionally, this culturally specific model showed that adding acculturation and health beliefs as enabling factors in the model, rather than predisposing factors, resulted in increased predictive power over predisposing factors for Chinese-American attitudes toward Western medical practices. Golomb,

---

[1] Portions of this chapter one from Ries et al. (2007)

Hune, MacGregor and deVeber (2003) found that the combination of Eastern and Western medicine occur frequently without knowledge. They studied the prevalence of use of Eastern medicine practices in first-generation Chinese-Canadian children with stroke and cerebrovascular disease. They found that over 53% of the children received some sort of alternative (Eastern) medicine (e.g. acupuncture, herbal medications) in addition to the Western medicine they received. Interestingly, Western doctors were unaware of most of the alternative medicine use until a Cantonese-speaking nurse practitioner interviewed them. This stresses the importance of the impact of culture and the role language has in the treatment of pediatric and adult populations. In contrast, integration of Western and Chinese traditional medicine has been proposed as the treatment for primary nephrotic syndrome in China (Zhimin, 2003).

Although strides have been made in this area, a great deal of work remains. For example, in the Yeats et al. (2002) and other studies (cf. CDC, 1998), it is unclear who constituted the group labeled as African-American. Is it possible that specific subgroups of African-American families, from specific backgrounds (e.g., where violence is explicitly accepted or exhibited) or other demographic variables, are mostly responsible for such effects? In fact, to date, although we are aware that "African-Americans" have a higher rate of TBI as a result of violence, for example, a limited understanding of the specific variables that moderate this relationship is known. Clearly, factors such as acculturation-assimilation, education, geographical areas, climate, and substance abuse may play a role on how violence is exhibited, and such moderators must be examined within the African-American context, and other cultures, including Hisporics in such investigations and future studies to determine whether more precise intraethnic factors can lead to specific prediction. It is also critical to mention that such distinctions are important because they may reduce stereotypes that paint all "African-American" families (or other ethnic groups) with the same brush. It is also critical to note that sometimes such investigations cannot be conducted as a result of the small number of participants from different backgrounds within a specific ethnic group, and this issue plagues many studies, including our own investigations. Nevertheless, it is an issue that merits significant attention and resources. Acknowledgement of the importance of more specifically defining the conceptual frameworks results in the call to provide accurate and thorough information about study sample characteristics by various journals and federal funding agencies (García Coll and Magnuson, 2002).

Culturally Sensitive Interventions and Rehabilitation Outcomes

Pontón, Gonzalez, and Mares (1997) describe a culturally based intervention used in the rehabilitation of a Hispanic population who experienced brain damage. Four well-grounded therapeutic techniques are utilized as intervention: *symptom validation, journaling, structuring, and reframing*. Symptom validation is defined as, "to verbalize concretely the subjective experience of vague and diffuse symptoms and to make the patient feel understood" (p. 515). This technique involves active listening and informing the patient about the symptoms commonly experienced in brain injury rehabilitation. Journaling involves recording symptoms and subjective experience ("How does the symptom make you feel?") with reasonable frequency in order to define the symptoms, provide a baseline of symptoms, foster coping style, and to provide a concrete measure of progress. Structuring involves establishing or returning an individual to a routine to increase his or her productivity and adjustment. It is defined as, "a predictable, purposeful set of activities that allows patients to channel their energy productively. It gives them a sense of control over their immediate environment, provides them with positive feedback on their progress, and helps them achieve short-term realistic goals" (p. 522).

Finally, the purpose of reframing is defined as, "shifting the perspective of the process – from tragedy to challenge, from future to present, from unmanageable issues to manageable issues" (p. 524). This technique involves paradoxical/cognitive-behavioral interventions (e.g., guided imagery), as well as reframing of spiritual issues ("spiritualizing"). Pontón, Gonzalez, and Mares describe three case studies in which these techniques were used and found to be effective. They also discuss the limitations to these specific techniques, and readers should aware of the study's limitations as a result of its small sample size.

Unfortunately, the majority of the empirically validated treatments has been based on White Americans and does not reflect the cultural diversity of the United States. Christophersen and Mortweet (2001) note that the lack of empirical data (e.g., base rates, treatment efficacy) on cultural diversity makes it difficult to estimate when and where cultural differences are important. Guidelines to improve cultural awareness and understanding were created by the American Psychological Association (2003) due to:

> the continuing evolution of the study of psychology, changes in society at large, and emerging data about the different needs of particularly individuals and groups historically marginalized or disenfranchised within and by psychology based on their ethnic/racial heritage and social group identity or membership. (p. 377)

These guidelines recognize the importance of influences of the larger environment (e.g., social, political, historical, and economic) on one's behaviors: (1) Psychologists are encouraged to recognize that, as cultural beings, they may hold attitudes and beliefs that can detrimentally influence their perceptions of and interactions with individuals who are ethnically and racially different from themselves; (2) psychologists are encouraged to recognize the importance of multicultural sensitivity/responsiveness to, knowledge of, and understanding about ethnically and racially different individuals; (3) as educators, psychologists are encouraged to employ the constructs of multiculturalism and diversity in psychological education; (4) culturally sensitive psychological researchers are encouraged to be cognizant of the importance of conducting culture-centered and ethical psychological research among persons from ethnic, linguistic, and racial minority backgrounds, (5) psychologists are encouraged to apply culturally appropriate skills in clinical and other applied psychological practices, (6) sychologists are encouraged to use organizational change processes to support culturally informed organizational development and practices.

With regard to interventional outcomes, the literature supports the fact that racial-ethnic differences exist in outcomes. For example, in a recent study published by Hanks et al. (2003), data supported the fact previously reported that ethnic and racial minorities showed greater frequency of TBI associated with violence than Whites. In fact, they showed rates of violent TBI to be approximately twice as high in ethnic minorities (74%) compared to Whites (46%). Most important, these results suggested the presence of poorer outcomes in minorities as a result of violent TBI. It should be noted that this disparity is similar, for example, to that for strokes in African-Americans populations and other diseases and conditions impacting Hispanics as well. One of the most comprehensive studies assessing TBI outcome to date was sponsored by the National Institute for Disability and Rehabilitation Research (NIDRR), Traumatic Brain Injury Model Systems (cf. Harrison et al., 1996), established in "1987 to demonstrate the benefits of a coordinated system of neurotrauma and rehabilitation care and conduct innovative research on all aspects of care for those who sustain traumatic brain injuries" and establish a national TBI database. In this study, a comparison was made again between the ethnic "minority" group (e.g., African-American, Asian/Pacific Islander) and Whites. This investigation revealed the presence of poorer outcome as measured by the Community Integration Questionnaire assessing role performance in the community, with the "minority" group scoring lower than Whites after significant analyses were made to covariate for various potential demographic and injury confounders, including age, gender, and trauma cause and severity. While there may be many moderating variables implicated in outcome studies, recognition of health and mental health care needs and access to them may negatively impact minority populations. In this regard, a study by Slomine et al. (2006) examined "White" and "non-White" children and adolescents with moderate to severe TBI from four trauma centers. Approximately 12 months post injury, non-White youth were significantly more likely to have unrecognized needs and lack of appropriate service utilization despite need when compared to the White youth, and according to the authors these findings may provide an explanation related to poorer outcome in youth from poorer family functioning. The most common unmet need in their study was appropriate treatment and targeting of cognitive dysfunction impacting performance in the classroom and neurobehavioral sequelae.

In another study recently published using existing Veterans Administrations records (Stansbury et al., 2004), they note the importance of appropriately documenting ethnicity, as it has high significance in adult stroke rehabilitation. More important, they note the pitfalls associated with methodological issues when using race (ethnicity) as a predictor with dichotomous response variables. Similar findings have been obtained for other outcome measures in other studies for various types of brain injury and its rehabilitation, but their detailed examinations are beyond the scope of this chapter (cf. Burnett et al. 2003). Finally, a U.S. volunteer surgical team performed approximately 100 craniofacial surgeries to repair cleft lip/palate in the Middle Amazon region of Brazil, which is composed of mixed Amerindian, European, and African ancestry. The team inquired, through a Portuguese translator, about the patients' and their families' expectations after surgery, traditional beliefs, attitudes toward surgical intervention, and outreach efforts. The study found that growing international clinical exchange programs to provide services to underserved populations in less developed countries can potentially make significant contributions; however, authors caution, they must understand the patients' sociocultural matrix in which the meaning of the condition they are treating and the future they face are determined by a host of factors over and above the specific procedures they are performing (Reeve, Groce, Pering, Magge, 2004).

Additional support for culturally sensitive approaches to intervention was examined by Zhimin (2003). This study examined the interplay between Western and Chinese traditional medicine and education to promote increased adherence through self-care practices in Chinese school-age children with primary nephrotic syndrome. Results of the study indicated high levels of self-care (90%) for children ranging in age from 6 to 12 years of age, the older children were most adherent to their self-care regimen.

Summary and Concluding Comments

In summary, despite the great advances attained by Goldstein and his colleagues during the early part of the last century, particularly related to the outcome of specific vocational groups subsequent to habilitation, neuropsychological rehabilitation remains in a state of immature development as it relates to the understanding of the impact of culture on treatment outcomes, particularly ethnic minority populations including Hispanics living in the U.S. Nevertheless, it is critical for clinicians to be cognizant of epidemiological and demographic issues that impact their daily duties with Hispanic clients, which in the U.S. encompass a large number of individuals. It is also important for multicultural models to guide empirically validated rehabilitative methods, and Groce and Zola (1993) offer useful advice to overcome the challenge of providing culturally sensitive neuropsychological evaluations: They note that "No one individual can anticipate all the problems that might arise in an attempt to understand chronic illness and disability in a multicultural society, but we can all have enough sensitivity to realize that there might be significant difference, and enough respect for others to ask questions and listen carefully to the replies (p. 1055). This level of sensitivity, or the aspirations of the work underscored in this chapter relative to cultural sensitivity, should not be exclusively applicable to clinical settings but should permeate research studies examining TBI, an issue that has not received due attention despite governmental efforts to include Hispanics in national research protocols. It is also important for the reader to recognize that many of the issues raised here are applicable when providing feedback to Hispanic families.

The information presented above clearly underscores the importance of considering cultural factors as an intricate component, not a corollary, of intervention during the course of neuropsychological rehabilitation with Hispanic populations, because as noted by Vygotsky: humans "create cultures, and cultures have a vitality, a life of their own. They grow and change and exert a very powerful influence on their members." In other words, as noted by Ries et al. (in press), "individuals are forged within their cultural context" with significant repercussions for a rehabilitative discipline and clinical outcomes squarely impacted by such interventions.

Summary and Concluding Remarks

Antolin M. Llorente

Neuropsychology faces daunting tasks and exciting challenges and opportunities in the 21st century if it is to remain a viable science and applied discipline. Although different demands are currently being placed on the field from various sources and directions, including economic, ethical and practical, the specific challenge referred to in this volume arises out of its need to be able to develop comprehensive theoretical models and applied methods that are capable of incorporating culture into integrated explanations of complex brain-behavior relationships. Intricacies associated with the neuropsychological assessment of Hispanic populations is an area that also demands greater attention, as individuals of Hispanic descent are the fastest growing minority members in the United States (U.S. Census, 2004). The cultural, ethnic, and linguistic heterogeneity of Hispanic populations also poses unique challenges and opportunities for neuropsychology and its applications as it strives to develop such comprehensive explanatory frameworks not to mention the development of assessment procedures capable of accounting for such heterogeneity. It is also paramount to understand that the changes occurring in this field related to multiculturalism are not result of a simple addition to knowledge, but may represent a paradigmatic shift as noted by Thomas Kuhn (1970, 1996), and as it occurs in the natural sciences. It is also important to recognize, that the inclusion of culture in models within neuropsychology, and more general, in cognitive mechanisms, is not the result of recent discoveries or scholarly thought, but rather, that they had their earlier and nascent formulations within psychology in the theoretical foundations and propositions of the environmentalists including the Russians Lev Vygotsky and Alexander Luria, and neopragmatics such as the American John Dewey, and outside psychology in the works of the German-American Franz Boas among many other giants. Given our recent advances in genetics, it would appear as if brain and culture are interwoven by biological mechanisms, and humans may actually posses "culture" genes that mediate such an interaction between biology and the environment, providing an interactive mechanism capable of permitting humans to assimilate complex cultural variables into its biological makeup, particularly the central nervous system.

As indicated in this volume, it is not easy to simply label "Hispanics" using pan-ethnic definitions and comprehend the variability and heterogeneity observed within such populations. In the United States, they are usually defined as people with Spanish as primary language or individuals from Hispanic backgrounds. According to this definition, "Hispanics" would include people with origins from Spain, Mexico, Central and South America, Puerto Rico, Cuba, and others regions of the world, yet as noted in previous chapters, individuals may identify themselves as Hispanic even though they do not meet such criteria, and may include individuals from Brazil or Portugal or other regions. Obviously, their beliefs, cultural values, practices, rituals, and other factors at the core of their self-identity fundamentally vary substantially. Furthermore, the distribution of the Hispanic population in the United States is not uniform, and there are regional idiosyncrasies as well as significant geographical affinity for specific groups of Hispanics. Large variability also can be found in the acculturation levels of U.S.-born versus foreign-born Hispanics, and among these subgroups, including their linguistic skills. For these reasons, it is not sufficient, for example, simply to conduct an assessment in Spanish, to use norms based on a "Hispanic" sample, or to assume certain cultural similarities, in order to work competently with heterogenic Hispanic populations. In addition, race is often confused with culture and ethnicity, as are the latter two. Race reflects common descent and physical characteristics, while culture reflects a set of social beliefs and behaviors (Ardila, Rosselli, and Puente, 1994). Although culture and ethnicity can be considered to be similar because they may be learned and flexible (Smedley, 1993), culture, as noted above, can be perceived as a complex manifestation or expression or symbolic elements that define a group of individuals or society from which an individual may adopt specific characteristics which over time are learned and lead to their own, unique ethnic identity (cf. Smedley, 1993). Whereas an individual adopt several characteristics capable of leading to his unique ethnic identity, there can be many ethnicities in a culture.

This book therefore made an attempt to discuss multiple factors that should be considered in understanding neuropsychological functions within a cultural context, and providing assessment and consultation to this unique population. In addition, it is hoped that a message was conveyed indicative of the large numbers of risk factors often encountered in these individuals, as a result of specific demographic characteristics, including low educational attainment, literacy broadly defined, high risk occupations, and other factors such as SES, etc. Education, in particular, is a variable that has been found to have significant impact on neuropsychological performance, in all ethnic groups, including Hispanics (Ardila, Rosselli, and Rosas, 1989). Low levels of formal education (i.e., fewer than eight years) has been found commonly among immigrants (Wong et al., 2000), and the levels of educational achievement are often lower for Hispanics than for other ethnic groups in the United States (Shorris, 1992). The reasons for such educational differences may be socioeconomic and sociopolitical, yet present in the population. According to relatively recent U.S. Census Bureau survey (1999), Hispanics tend to drop out of school at a rate greater, almost three times more, than Anglo- or European Americans and African Americans. Hispanics also are starting school later than average relative to other groups (Shorris, 1992). As noted by Harris and Llorente (2005), "As many neuropsychological test scores are correlated with education level," it is important to be cognizant of differences in educational opportunities, quality of education, educational experiences, and attitude toward education among Hispanics. Moreover, in the process of establishing normative data for neuropsychological instruments, people with ten to twelve years of education and below are usually combined into a homogeneous educational group. However, reliable differences due to years of educational attainment have been found in the neuropsychological performance among people who attained less than 10 years of education, while little differences have found in the upper end (Ardila et al., 1989b). These factors lead to increased chance of errors in the inferences derived from neuropsychological assessment with Hispanics with low educational levels. Neuropsychological profiles of Hispanics with limited education, for example, could mimic educated, brain-damaged persons (Ardila et al.).

Without question, a great portion of group differences observed in neuropsychological performances can be attributed to cultural differences (e.g., Shepherd and Leathem, 1999), yet another proportion to other variables such as socioeconomic status differences, particularly interacting with culture. Variables that play important roles in neuropsychological evaluation may include poverty, poor nutrition, health care as well as other characteristics. Each or various combinations of these factors could act as causes, mediators, and/or moderators affecting individuals' performances on neuropsychological assessment, and also influence attitude toward, access to, and quality of health care received (Center for Disease Control and Prevention [CDC]; McKenzie and Crowcroft, 1994). Although an argument is not being made here that all Hispanics fit categories associated with lower SES, many of them do, and in many instances it is such individuals who end up across the clinician's assessment desk, or rehabilitation centers, partly the results of such risk factors.

Aside from the aforementioned factors, many Hispanic cultures, or specific Hispanics from a unique ethnic background within a specific cultre, hold strong religious and other beliefs and thereby have different understandings for the causes of illness, influencing their perceptions about neuropsychological evaluations (Puente and Ardila, 2000). Such factors also impact their decision to assimilate and adopt American values and customs and whether or not to learn English or assimilate other aspects of American society and culture. To many, their concept and use of time are different from mainstream individuals, which could put them at a disadvantage when administered timed tests. The culture also emphasizes the importance of harmonious human relationships than academic or other competitions, which might influence their motivations during evaluations (Puente and Ardila, 2000). There may be additional cross-cultural differences in the expression of symptoms of diseases (cf. Clark et al., 2005; Llorente et al., 2000, 2001). In addition, different cultures, including Hispanics, have different degrees of role, status differentiations between males and females. Therefore, the effects of gender on neuropsychological performance might be moderated by culture as well, and this issue should be given due weight.

Another critical issue is strongly related to the application of tests. Because most neuropsychological tests have been normed using prevailing, majority populations, the use of such norms is not appropriate when examining selected individuals with a Hispanic background. Furthermore, it cannot be assumed that norms ascertained with Hispanics in one geographical region of the U.S., or in a foreign country, would be applicable to Hispanic individuals from other (or all) geographical areas in the U.S., solely because the patient undergoing assessment belongs to the same ethnic group as the standardization sample or because he or she speaks Spanish (Llorente et al., 2000). Further, the level of acculturation must be taken into consideration (Dana, 1993).

Individual differences in linguistic skills acquisition, fluency and mastery as well as the differences in the nature of English and Spanish as languages also create significant challenges. Although a value judgment is not being made, many Hispanics in the U.S. use both Spanish and English in varied degrees of proficiency and frequency, and oftentimes combine these two languages to create what many have termed Spanglish (cf. Cruz and Teck, 1998), in some instances with positive and/or negative consequences due their inability to truly master either language. Significant differences also exist in the structure of these two languages further complicating the assessment process. Oral and written proficiencies, language preferences, and the patterns of use depend on multiple factors, such as the age, language learning sequence, reasons behind learning these two or more languages, method of acquisition, early versus late exposure to the languages, degree of cultural identification, and individual differences in verbal abilities (cf. Ardila, 1998). Some patients may only speak Spanish, while children may have more exposure to English through school, friends, media and leisure activities with greater frequency than adults. Some are more concerned about maintaining their cultural heritage (therefore speaking primarily Spanish), while others are more concerned about adapting the mainstream culture (therefore speaking primarily English). These and other factors influence individuals' performance not only on tasks measuring language development and functions and abilities, but also on tasks that are intended to measure other abilities (e.g., attention, memory, processing speed, etc.) but often requiring verbal mediation and processing. It is clear that language may present a barrier for neuropsychological test administration. How could neuropsychologists accurately assess the brain-behavior relationship of bilingual patients? As discussed above, there are considerable limitations to conducting neuropsychological evaluations with non-English speakers. For example, there is a misunderstanding that only a translation of the text is needed (Echmendia, Harris, Congett, Diaz, and Puente, 1997). Translating individual test items during evaluation procedures is not adequate, as it deviates from standardized procedure, and the accuracy and appropriateness of the translations would likely to vary significantly among examiners. Translations must be conducted in a standardized fashion, and appropriate norms must be established. Brislin (1983) emphasized the use of back translation to ensure the comparability of the translated instrument. The changes in the nature and cognitive equivalency of the translated-tests must be considered because of the differences in language and culture. For example, an object that is easy to name in one language may require significantly more sophisticated proficiency in another language, or a word may contain a greater number of syllables in one language than the other. The International Test Commission has also provided guidelines for the adaptation of tests (Muniz and Hambleton, 1996). The guidelines not only address issues associated with translations, but also discuss the selection of appropriate tests, consideration of potential biases, appropriate scoring methods, appropriate communication of findings, revision of tests, etc. Even when using validated translated instruments, the test results should be interpreted with caution, and within an appropriate cultural context. Individuals assessing these patients should be competent to conduct such evaluations. It is also important to be aware of the unique needs of Spanish-English bilinguals living in the United States. For many, using either Spanish or English testing materials and norms can underestimate their cognitive abilities (Puente and Ardila, 2000). To reduce bilingualism effects in testing, it would be ideal to have special norms for Spanish-English bilinguals (until test are developed that are not biased), and a bilingual examiner who can provide instructions and understand answers in either language or any mixture of both languages. If this is not feasible, their results could perhaps be interpreted using both norms (English and Spanish versions).

As noted in Chapter 7, modern neuropsychological procedures have used more complex methods of tests development using operating-receiver curves or item analytic procedures creating standards for test development far more advanced and sophisticated that a simple adaptation, or worst, a translation of a test. If a patient's primary language is unfamiliar, it is best to refer the patient to a neuropsychologist who can competently perform an evaluation in that language. Only as a last resort and if necessary, an interpreter should be used for clinical interviews and consultations. In such cases, clinicians must select interpreters carefully, and rapport should be established between a neuropsychologist and an interpreter prior to meetings with patients. It is important that interpreters are familiar with neuropsychological principles and terms as well as different Hispanic cultures and regional languages. Still, it is crucial that clinicians are aware of the increased possibility of miscommunications and misunderstandings. Having an interpreter in a room may change the comfort level and dynamics during meetings, and the subtleties in communications, such as nonverbal cues and complex language responses can be lost easily through interpretations. It is also pivotal to note the use of interpreters during the course of neuropsychological assessment was not advocated or recommended in this volume, and such a practice should be avoided at all costs, particularly in forensic proceedings, and the use of family members as interpreters completely discarded.

In conclusion, significant attention towards ethical considerations should be given to scientific models and applied methods in neuropsychology addressing cross-cultural issues related to Hispanics, using irreproachable standards of practice in clinical, educative, and research endeavors.

References

Adams, R.L., Boake, C., and Crain, C. (1982). Bias in neuropsychological test classification related to education, age and ethnicity. *Journal of Consulting and Clinical Psychology, 50,* 143–145.

Adrenal, A. (2002). Spanish-English bilingualism in the United States of America. In F. Fibber (ed.) *Advances in the neurolinguistics of bilingualism. Essays in honor of Michael Paradis.* (pp. 49–67). Udine (Italy).

Ahmad, A., Mohamed, T., and Ameen, N.M. (1997). A 26-month follow-up of posttraumatic stress symptoms in children after the mass-escape tragedy in Iraqi Kurdistan. *Nordic Journal of Psychiatry, 52,* 357–366.

Ajdukovic, M. (1995). Mothers' perception of their relationship with their children during displacement: A six month follow up. *Child Abuse Review, 5,* 34–39.

Ajdukovic, M., and Ajdukovic, D. (1993). Psychological well being of refugee children. *Child Abuse and Neglect, 17,* 843–854.

Ajdukovic, M., and Ajdukovic, D. (1998). Impact of displacement on the psychological well being of refugee children. *International Review of Psychiatry,* 10, 186–195.

Alden, K., Poole, C., Chantavanich, S., Ohmar, K., Aung, N.N., and Mollica, R.F. (1996). Burmese political dissidents in Thailand: Trauma and survival among young adults in exile. *American Journal of Public Health, 86,* 1561–1569.

Alegria, M., Vila, D., Woo, M., Canino, G., Takeuchi, D., Vera, M., Febo, V., Guarnaccia, P., Aguilar-Gaxiola, S., and Shrout, P. (2004). Cultural relevance and equivalence in the NLAAS instrument: Integrating etic and emic measures in the development of cross-cultural measures for a psychiatric epidemiology and services study of Latinos. *International Journal of Methods in Psychiatric Research, 13,* 270–288.

Almqvist, K., and Brandell-Forsberg, M. (1997). Refugee children in Sweden: Post-traumatic stress disorder in Iranian preschool children exposed to organized violence. *Child Abuse and Neglect, 21,* 351–366.

Almqvist, K., and Broberg, A.G. (1999). Mental health and social adjustment in young refugee children 3 1/2 years after their arrival in Sweden. *Journal of the American Academy of Child and Adolescent Psychiatry, 38,* 723–730.

American Educational Research Association. (1999). *Standards for educational and psychological Testing.* Washington, DC: AERA Publications.

American Educational Research Association, American Psychological Association, and National Council on Measurement in Education. (1999). *The standards for educational and psychological testing.* Washington, DC: American Psychological Association.

American Psychiatric Association. (1987). *Diagnostic and statistical manual of mental disorders* (3rd ed.) revised. Washington, DC: Author.

American Psychiatric Association. (1994). *Diagnostic and statistical manual of mental disorders* (4th ed.). Washington, DC: Author.

American Psychiatric Association. (2000). *Diagnostic and statistical manual of mental disorders* (4th ed.) text revision. Washington, DC: Author.

American Psychological Association. (1991). *Guidelines for providers of services to ethnic, linguistic, and culturally diverse populations*. Washington, DC: American Psychological Association.

American Psychological Association. (1992). Ethical principles of psychologists and code of conduct. *American Psychologist, 47*, 1597–1611.

American Psychological Association. (2002). *Ethical principles of psychologists and code of conduct*. Retrieved Jan. 5, 2006, from http://www.apa.org/ethics/code2002.html.

American Psychological Association. (2001). *Guidelines on multicultural education, training, research, practice, and organizational change for psychologists*. Retrieved Nov. 3, 2005, from http://www.apa.org/divisions/div45/resources.html.

American Psychological Association. (2003). Guidelines on multicultural education, training, research, practice, and organizational change for psychologists. *American Psychologist, 58*, 377–402.

American Psychological Association. (1985, 1999). *The Standards for educational and psychological testing*. Washington, DC: Author.

American Speech-Language-Hearing Association. (1982). Committee on language, speech and hearing services in the schools. Definitions: Communicative disorders and variations. *American Speech-Language-Hearing Association, 24*, 949–950.

Anastasi, A., and Urbina, S. (1997). *Psychological testing* (7th ed.). Upper Saddle River, NJ: Prentice Hall.

Angel, B., Hjern, A., and Ingleby, D. (2001). Effects of war and organized violence on children: A study of Bosnian refugees in Sweden. *American Journal of Orthopsychiatry, 71*, 4–15.

Anger, W.K., Cassitto, M.G., Liang, Y.X. et al. (1993). Comparison of performance from three continents on the WHO-recommended Neurobehavior Core Test Battery. *Environmental Research, 62*, 125–147.

Applebaum, H. (1987). *Perspectives in cultural anthropology*. Albany, NY: State University of New York Press.

Ardila, A. (1993). Future directions in the research and practice of cross-cultural neuropsychology. *Journal of Clinical and Experimental Neuropsychology, 15*, 19 (abstract).

Ardila, A. (1998). A note of caution: Normative neuropsychological test performance: Effects of age, education, gender and ethnicity: A comment on Saykin et al. (1995). *Applied Neuropsychology, 5*, 51–53.

Ardila, A. (2003). Culture in Our Brains: Cross-Cultural Differences in the Brain-Behavior Relationships. In A. Toomela (ed.), *Cultural Guidance in the Development of the Human Mind*. London: Greenwood Publishing.

Ardila, A. (2005). Cultural values underlying psychometric cognitive testing. *Neuropsychological Review, 15*, 185–195.

Ardila, A., and Moreno., S. (2001). Neuropsychological test performance in Aruaco Indians: An exploratory study. *Journal of the International Neuropsychological Society, 7*, 510–515.

Ardila. A., Ardila. O., Bryden M.P., Ostrosky F, Rosselli. M., and Steenhuis. R. (1989a). Effects of cultural background and education on handedness. *Neuropsychologia, 27*, 893–897.

Ardila, A., Rosselli, M., and Rosas, P. (1989b). Neuropsychological assessment of illiterates: Visuo-spatial and memory abilities. *Brain and Cognition, 11*, 147–166.

Ardila, A., Rosselli, M., and Puente, A. (1994). *Neuropsychological assessment of the Spanish speaker*. New York: Plenum Press.

Arroyo, W., and Eth, S. (1996). Post-traumatic stress disorder and other stress reactions. In R.J. Apfel and S. Bennett (eds.), *Minefields in their hearts: The mental health of children in war and communal violence* (pp. 52–74). New Haven, CT: Yale University Press.

Artioli i Fortuny, L., and Mullaney, H.A. (1998). Assessing patients whose language you do not know: Can the absurd be ethical? *The Clinical Neuropsychologist, 12*, 113–126.

Artioli i Fortuny, L., Garolera, M., Hermosillo, R.D., Feldman, E., Fernandez Barillas, H., Keefe, R., et al. (2005). Research with Spanish-speaking populations in the United States: lost in the translation. A commentary and a plea. *Journal of Clinical and Experimental Neuropsychology, 27*, 555–564.

Athey, J.L., and Ahearn, F.L. (1991). The mental health of refugee children: An overview. In F.L. Ahearn and J.L. Athey (eds.), Refugee children: Theory, research, and services. *The Johns Hopkins series in contemporary medicine and public health* (pp. 3–19). Baltimore, MD: The Johns Hopkins University Press.

Auffrey, J., and Robertson, M. (1972). Case history information and examiner experience as determinants of scoring validity on the Wechsler intelligence tests. *Proceedings of the 80th Annual Convention of the American Psychological Association, 7*, 553–554.

Axelrod, B.N. (2002). Validity of the Wechsler Abbreviated Scale of Intelligence and other very short forms of estimating intellectual functioning. *Assessment, 9*, 17–23.

Badcock, K.A., and Ross, M.W. (1982). Neuropsychological testing with Australian aborigines. *Australian Psychologist, 17*, 297–299.

Baker, D., Stevens, C., Brook, R. et al. (1996). Determinants of emergency department use: Are race and ethnicity important? *Annals of Emergency Medicine, 28*, 677–682.

Ballard, W.S., Tighe, P.L., and Dalton, E.F. (1989). *IDEA Oral Language Proficiency Test Pre- IPT – Spanish*. Brea, CA: Ballard and Tighe Publishers.

Ballard, W.S., Tighe, P.L., and Dalton, E.F. (1996a). *IDEA Oral Language Proficiency Test IPT 1 – Spanish*. Brea, CA: Ballard and Tighe Publishers.

Ballard, W.S., Tighe, P.L., and Dalton, E.F. (1996b). *IDEA Oral Language Proficiency Test IPT II – Spanish*. Brea, CA: Ballard and Tighe Publishers.

Baron, I.S. (2004). *Neuropsychological evaluation of the child*. Oxford: University Press.

Baron, R.M., and Kenny, D.A. (1986). The moderator-mediator variable distinction in socialpsychological research: Conceptual, strategic and statistical considerations. *Journal of Personality and Social Psychology, 51,* 1173–1182.

Bates, E., Dale, P.S., and Thal, D. (1995). Individual differences and their implications for theories of language development. In P. Fletcher and B. MacWhinney (eds.), *Handbook of child language*. Oxford: Basil Blackwell.

Bates, E., Thal, D., and Janowsky, J. (1992). Early language development and its neural correlates. In S. Segalowitz and I. Rapin (eds.), *Handbook of Neuropsychology: Vol. 7. Child Neuropsychology* (pp. 69–110). Amsterdam: Elsevier.

Bates, E., Thal, D., Finlay, B., and Clancy, B. (2003). Early language development and its neural correlates. In I. Rapin and S. Segalowitz (eds.), *Handbook of neuropsychology: Child neuropsychology* (Vol. 8, 2nd ed.). Amsterdam: Elsevier.

Bayley, N. (1993). *Bayley Scales of Infant Development* (2nd ed.). San Antonio, TX: Psych Corp.

Becker, D.F., Weine, S.M., Vojvoda, D., and McGlashan, T.H. (1999). Case series: PTSD symptoms in adolescent survivors of "ethnic cleansing." Results from a 1-year follow up study. *Journal of the American Academy of Child and Adolescent Psychiatry, 38*, 775–781.

Bedore, L.M. (1999). The acquisition of Spanish. In O.L. Taylor and L.B. Leonard (eds.), *Language acquisition across North America: Cross-cultural and cross-linguistic perspectives* (pp. 157–207). San Diego, CA: Singular Publishing Group, Inc.

Beery, K.E., and Taheri, C.M. (1992). *Beery Picture Vocabulary Test*. Odessa, FL: Psychological Assessment Resources, Inc.

Beiser, M., Dion, R., Gotowiec, A., Hyman, I., and Vu, N. (1995). Immigrant and refugee children in Canada. *Canadian Journal of Psychiatry, 40*, 67–72.

Belyaev, D.K. (1979). Destabalizing selection as a factor in domestication. *Journal of Hereditz, 70*, 301–308.

Bemak, F., and Timm, J. (1994). Case study of an adolescent Cambodian refugee: A clinical, developmental and cultural perspective. *International Journal for the Advancement of Counselling, 17*, 47–58.

Benson, D.F. (1993). Aphasia. In K.M. Heilman and E. Valenstein (eds.), *Clinical neuropsychology* (3rd ed., pp. 17–36). New York: Oxford University Press.

Benton, A.L., Hamsher, K. de S., Rey, G.J., and Sivian, A.B. (1994). *Multilingual Aphasia Examination* (3rd ed.). Iowa City, IA: AJA Associates.

Berman, H. (2001). Children and war: Current understandings and future directions. *Public Health Nursing, 18,* 243–252.

Berry, J.W. (1997). Immigration, acculturation and adaptation. *Applied Psychology, 46,* 5–68.

Berry, J.W. (2001). Contextual studies of cognitive adaptation. In J.M. Collis and S. Messick (eds.), *Intelligence and personality: Bridging the gap in theory and measurement* (pp. 319–333). Mahwah, NJ: Lawrence Earlbaum.

Berry, J. W. (1999). Emics and etics: a symbiotic conception. *Culture and Psychology, 5,* 165–171.

Berthold, S.M. (1999). The effects of exposure to community violence on Khmer refugee adolescents. *Journal of Traumatic Stress, 12,* 455–471.

Best, C.T., and Avery, R.A. (1999). Left-hemisphere advantage for click consonants is determined by linguistic significance and experience. *Psychological Science, 10,* 65–70.

Bird, H.R. (1996). Epidemiology of childhood disorders in a cross-cultural context. *Journal of Child Psychology and Psychiatry and Allied Disciplines, 37,* 35–49.

Bland, J.M., and Altman, D.G. (1986). Statistical methods for assessing agreement between two methods of clinical measurement. *Lancet, i,* 307–310.

Blau, T. (1998). *The psychologist as expert witness* (2nd ed.). New York: Wiley.

Blonder, L.X. (1991). Human neuropsychology and the concept of culture. *Human Nature, 2,* 83–116.

Bond, L. (1987). The golden rule settlement: A minority perspective. *Educational Measurment: Issues and Practice, 6,* 23–25.

Bornstein, M.H. (1973). Color vision and color naming: A psychological hypothesis of cultural difference. *Psychological Bulletin, 80,* 257–285.

Bos, C.S., and VanReusen, A. K. (1991). Academic interventions with learning disabled students: A cognitive/metacognitive approach. In J.E. Obrzut and G.W. Hynd (eds.), *Neuropsychological foundations of learning disabilities* (pp. 659–684). San Diego, CA: Academic Press.

Botwinick, J. (1967). *Cognitive Processes in Maturity and Old Age.* New York: Springer.

Boydston, J.A. (ed.). (1981). *Dewey, J. The Later Works, 1925–1953.* Carbondale: Southern Illinois University Press.

Braden, J.P., and Kratochwill, T.R. (*1997). Treatment utility of assessment: Myths and realities.* School Psychology Review, 26, 475–485.

Brandt, J. (February, 2005). *Neuropsychological Crimes and Misdemeanors,* Presidential Address, 33rd Annual Meeting of the International Neuropsychological Society, St. Louis, Missouri.

Brislin, R.W. (1983). Translation and content analysis of oral and written material. In H.C. Tridndis and J.W. Berry (Eds.), *Handbook of Cross-Cultural Methodology.* Boston: Allyn & Bacon.

Broca, P. (1861). Perte de la parole, ramollissement chronique et destruction partielle du lob anterieur gauche de cerveau. *Bulletins de la Societe d'Anthropologie, 62,* pp. 235–238.

Brownell, R. (2001). *Expressive One-Word Picture Vocabulary Test – Spanish Bilingual Edition.* Novato, CA: Academic Therapy Publications.

Bruininks, R.H., Woodcock, R.W., Weatherman, R.F., and Hill, B.K. (1996). *Scale of Independent Behavior* (rev. ed.). Itasca, IL: Riverside Publishing Company.

Burnett, D.M., Kolakowsky-Hayner, S.A., Slater, D., Stringer, A., Bushnik, T., Zafonte, R., and Cifu, D.X. (2003). Ethnographic analysis of traumatic brain injury patients in the National Model Systems database. *Archives of Physical Medicine and Rehabilitation, 84,*263–267.

Byrd, D.A., Sanchez, D., & Manly, J.J. (2005). Neuropsychological test performance among Caribbean-born and U.S.-born African-American elderly: The role of age, education, and reading level. *Journal of Clinical and Experimental Neuropsychology, 27,* 1056–1069.

Camilli, G., & Shepord, L.A. (1994). *Methods for identifying biased test items.* Thousand Oaks, CA. Sage.

Campbell, T., Dollaghan, C., Needleman, H., and Janosky, J. (1997). Reducing bias in language assessment: Processing dependent measures. *Journal of Speech and Hearing Research, 40,* 519–525.

Camus, J. (1917/1918). *Physical and occupational re-education of the maimed.* London: Bailliere, Tindal and Cox.

Canadian Psychological Association. (1991). *Canadian Code of Ethics for Psychologists*. Ottawa, Ontario: Canadian Psychological Association.

Carlson, C.I., Uppal, S., and Prosser, E. (2000). Ethnic differences in processes contributing to the self-esteem of early adolescent girls. *Journal of Early Adolescence, 20*, 44–67.

Carroll, J.B. (2005). The three-stratum theory of cognitive abilities. In D.P. Flanagan and P.L. Harrison (eds.), *Contemporary intellectual assessment: Theories, tests, and issues*. New York: Guilford Press.

Carroll, J.B., Davies, P., and Richman, B. (1971). *The American heritage word frequency book*. Boston: Houghton Mifflin.

Carter, R.T., and Qureshi, A. (1995). A typology of philosophical assumptions in multicultural counseling and training. In J.G. Ponterotto, J.M. Casas, L.A. Suzuki, and C.M. Alexander (eds.), *Handbook of Multicultural Counseling* (pp. 239–262). Thousand Oaks, CA: SAGE Publications, Inc.

Cascallar, E.C., and Arnold, J. (2001). Second language acquisition. In M.O. Pontón and J. León-Carrión (eds.), *Neuropsychology and the Hispanic patient: A clinical handbook* (pp. 59–74). Mahwah, NJ: Lawrence Erlbaum Associates.

Cattell, R.B. (1963). Theory of fluid and crystallized intelligence; A critical experiment. *Journal of Educational Psychology, 54*, 1–22.

Ceci, S.J. (1996). *On intelligence (expanded ed.)*. Cambridge, MA: Harvard University Press.

Centeno, J.G., and Obler, L.K. (2001). Principles of bilingualism. In M.O. Pontón and J. León-Carrión (eds.), *Neuropsychology and the Hispanic patient: A clinical handbook* (pp. 75–86). Mahwah, NJ: Lawrence Erlbaum Associates.

Centers for Disease Control and Prevention. (1998). *Tobacco use among U.S. racial/ethnic minority groups - African Americans, American Indians and Alaska Natives, Asian Americans and Pacific Islanders, and Hispanics: A report of the Surgeon General*. Atlanta: Author.

Centers for Disease Control and Prevention. (1999). *Traumatic brain injury in the United States: A report to congress*. Atlanta: Author.

Cervantes, R.C., and Acosta, F.X. (1992). Psychological testing for Hispanic-Americans. *Applied and Preventive Psychology, 1*, 209–219.

Choi, S. (1999). Acquisition of Korean. In O.L. Taylor and L.B. Leonard (eds.), *Language acquisition across North America: Cross-cultural and cross-linguistic perspectives* (pp. 281–334). San Diego, CA: Singular Publishing Group, Inc.

Chomsky, N. (1991). Linguistics and cognitive science: Problems and mysteries. In A. Kasher (ed.), *The Chomskyan turn*. Cambridge, MA: Blackwell.

Christensen, A.L. (1975). *Luria's neuropsychological investigation*. New York: Spectrum.

Christensen, A.L., and Castano, C. (1996). Alexander Romanovitch Luria (1902–1977): Contributions to neuropsychological rehabilitation. *Neuropsychological Rehabilitation, 6*, 279–303.

Christophersen, E.R., and Mortweet, S.L. (2001). *Treatments that work with children: Empirically supported strategies for managing childhood problems* (pp. 3–10). Washington DC: American Psychological Association.

Clark, C.M., DeCarli, C., Mungas, D., Chui, H.I., Higdon, R., Nunez, J., et al. (2005). Earlier onset of Alzheimer disease symptoms in Latino individuals compared with Anglo individuals. *Archives of Neurology, 62,* 774–778.

Clarke, G.N., Sack, W.H., and Goff, B. (1993). Three forms of stress in Cambodian adolescent refugees. *Journal of Abnormal Child Psychology, 21*, 65–77.

Cole, E. (1998). Immigrant and refugee children: Challenges and opportunities for education. *Canadian Journal of School Psychology, 14*, 36–50.

Collier, V.P. (1992). A synthesis of studies examining long-term language minority student data on academic achievement. *Bilingual Education Research Journal, 16,* 187–221.

Collier, V.P. (1995). Acquiring a second language for school. *Directions in Language and Education, 1*, 1–10.

Committee on Minority Representation in Special Education (2002). Representation of minority students in special and gifted education. In M.S. Donovan and C.T. Cross (eds.), *Minority students in special and gifted education*. (pp. 35–90).

Comrie, B. (2000). From potential to realization: An episode in the origin of language. *Linguistics, 38*, 989–1004.

Condeluci, A. (1997). Community inclusion: The ultimate goal of rehabilitation. In J. León-Carrión (ed.), *Neuropsychological rehabilitation: Fundamentals, innovations, and directions* (pp. 483–495). Delray Beach, FL: GR/St. Lucie Press.

Connelly, J., and Schweiger, M. (2000). The health risks of the UK's new asylum act. *British Medical Journal, 321*, 5–6.

Courville, C.B. (1967). *Injuries of the skull and brain as described in the myths, legends and folk-tales of the various peoples of the world.* New York: Vantage Press.

Coutinho, M.J., and Oswald, D.P (2000). Disproportionate representation in special education: A synthesis and recommendations. *Journal of Child and Family Studies, 9*, 13–156.

Crago, M.B., and Allen, S.E.M. (1999). Acquiring Inuktitut. In O.L. Taylor and L.B. Leonard (eds.), *Language acquisition across North America: Cross-cultural and cross-linguistic perspectives* (pp. 245–278). San Diego, CA: Singular Publishing Group, Inc.

Crowley, M. (1992). Behavioural difficulties and their relationship to language impairment. In J. Law (ed.), *The early identification of language impairment in children: Therapy in practice* (pp. 63–83). London: Chapman and Hall.

Cruz, B., Teck, B. (1998). The official spanglish dictionary: Un user's guide to more than 300 words and phrases that aren't exactly Espanol or Ingles. New York: Fireside Books.

Crystal, D. (1987). *Cambridge encyclopedia of language.* Cambridge: Cambridge University Press.

Cummins, J. (1979). Linguistic interdependence and the educational development of bilingual children. *Review of Educational Research, 49*, 222–251.

Cummins, J. (1981). The role of primary language development in promoting educational success for language minority students (pp. 3–49). In *Schooling and language minority students.* Sacramento, CA: California Department of Education.

Cummins, J. (1984). *Bilingualism and special education: Issues in assessment and pedagogy.* San Diego, CA: College-Hill Press.

Cummins, J. (1989). *Empowering language minority students.* Sacramento, CA: California Association for Bilingual Education.

Cummins, J., and Gulutsan, M. (1975). Set, objectification and second language learning. *International Journal of Psychology, 10*, 91–100.

Cunningham, M., and Cunningham, J.D. (1997). Patterns of symptomatology and patterns of torture and trauma experiences in resettled refugees. *Australian and New Zealand Journal of Psychiatry, 31*, 555–565.

Damasio, A.R., and Damasio, H. (2000). Aphasia and the neural basis of language. In M.M. Mesulam (Ed.), *Principles of behavioral and cognitive neurology* (2nd ed., pp. 294–315). Oxford: Oxford University Press.

Damico, J.S. (1985). Clinical Discourse Analysis: A functional language assessment technique. In C.S. Simon (ed.), *Communication skills and classroom success: Assessment of language-learning disabled students* (pp. 165–204). Austin, TX: Pro-Ed.

Damico, J.S. (1991). Descriptive assessment of communicative ability in limited English proficient students. In E.V. Hayaman and J.S. Damico (eds.), *Limiting bias in the assessment of bilingual students* (pp. 157–217). Austin, TX: Pro-Ed.

Dana, R. (1993). *Multicultural assessment perspectives for professional psychology.* Needham Heights, MA: Allyn and Bacon.

Darwin, C. (1967). *On the origin of species. A facsimile of the first edition.* New York, Atheneum.

Das, J.P, Naglieri, J., and Kirby, J.R. (1994). *Assessment of cognitive processes: The PASS theory of intelligence.* Needham Heights, MA: Allyn and Bacon.

Davies, M., and Webb, E. (2000). Promoting the psychological well-being of refugee children. *Clinical Child Psychology and Psychiatry, 5*, 541–554.

DeBlesser, R. (1988). Localisation of aphasia: Science or fiction? In G. Denes, C. Semenza, and P. Bisiacchi (eds.), *Perspectives on cognitive neuropsychology.* East Sussex, U K: Lawrence Earlbaum Associates.

Dejong, R. (1982). *History of American neurology*. New York: Raven Press.

De Jongh, E.M. (1991). Foreign language interpreters in the courtroom: The case for linguistic and cultural proficiency. *Modern Language Journal, 75*, 285–295.

DeLong, G.R. (1993). Effects of nutrition on brain development in humans. *American Journal of clinical Nutrition, 57*, 286–290 (Supplement).

Delis, O.C., Kaplan, E., & Kramer, J.H. (2001). *The Delis-Kaplan Executive Function System (DKEFS)*. San Antonio, TX: The Psychological Corporation.

Delis, D.C., Kiefner, M.G., and Fridlund, A.J. (1988). Visuospatial dysfunction following unilateral brain damage: Dissociations in hierarchical and hemispatial analysis. *Journal of Clinical Neuropsychology, 10*, 421–431.

Dennett, D.C. (1978). *Brainstorms: Philosophical essays on mind and psychology*. Montgomery, VT: Bradford Books.

Dewey, J. (1938). *Experience and education*. New York: Macmillan Press.

Dodd, W. (1983). Do interpreters affect consultation? *Family Practice, 1*, 42–47.

Donahue, D., and Sattler, J.M. (1971). Personality variables affecting WAIS scores. *Journal of Consulting and Clinical Psychology, 36*, 441.

Drame, E.R. (2002). Sociocultural context effects on teachers' readiness to refer for learning disabilities. *Exceptional Children, 69*, 41–53.

Dreman, S., and Cohen, E. (1990). Children of victims of terrorism revisited: Integrating individual and family treatment approaches. *American Journal of Orthopsychiatry, 60*, 204–209.

Dronkers, N.F., Pinker, S., and Damasio, A. (2000). Language and the aphasias. In E.R. Kandel, J.H., Schwartz, and T.M. Jessell (eds.), *Principles of neural science* (4th ed., pp. 1169–1187). New York: McGraw-Hill.

Dunn, L.M., and Dunn, L.M. (1981). *Peabody Picture Vocabulary Test – Revised*. Cicle Pines, MN: American Guidance Service.

Dunn, L.M., Padilla, E.R., Lugo, D.E., Dunn, L.M. (1986). Test de Vocabulario en Imagines Peabody: Adaptación Hispanoamericana [Peabody Picture Vocabulary Test: Hispanic American Adaptation]. Circle Pines, MN: American Guidance Service.

Dunn, L.M., and Dunn, L.M. (1997). *Peabody Picture Vocabulary Test* (3rd ed.). Circle Pines, MN: American Guidance Service.

DuPaul. G.J., Schaughency, E.A., Weyandt, L.L., Tripp, G., Kiesner, J., Ota, K., and Stanish, H. (2001). Self-report of ADHD symptoms in university students: Cross-gender and cross-national prevalence. *Journal of Learning Disabilities, 34*, 370–379.

Dussell, E. (Ed). (1992). *The Church in Latin America, 1492–1992*. Maryknoll, NY: Orbis.

Dybdahl, R. (2001). Children and mothers in war: An outcome study of a psychosocial intervention program. *Child Development, 72*, 1214–1230.

Echemendía, R., Harris, J.G., Congett, S., Diaz, and Puente, A. (1997). Neuropsychological training and practices with Hispanics: A national survey. *The Clinical Neuropsychologist, 11*, 29–243.

Echemendia, R.J., and Harris, J.G. (2004). Neuropsychological test use with Hispanic/Latino populations in the United States: part II of a national survey. *Applied Neuropsychology, 11*, 4–11.

Echevarria, J., and McDonough, R. (1996). An alternative reading approach: Instructional conversations in a bilingual special education setting. *Learning Disabilities Research and Practice, 10*, 108–119.

Eckberg, D., and Hill, L. (1979). The paradigm concept and sociology. *American Sociological Review, 44*, 925–937.

Efron, R. (1990). *The decline and fall of hemispheric specialization*. Hillsdale, N.J.: Erlbaum.

Egeland, B. (1967). Influence of examiner and examinee anxiety on WISC performance. *Psychological Reports, 21*, 409–414.

Eisenson, J. (1984). *Aphasia and related disorders in children* (2nd ed.). New York: Harper and Row Publishers.

El Habir, E., Marriage, K., Littlefield, L., and Pratt, K. (1994). Teachers' perceptions of maladaptive behaviour in Lebanese refugee children. *Australian and New Zealand Journal of Psychiatry, 28*, 100–105.

Elbedour, S., ten-Bensel., and Bastien, D.T. (1993). Ecological integrated model of children in war: Individual and social psychology. *Child Abuse and Neglect, 17*, 805–819.

Elbert, T., Pantev, C., Wienbruch, C., Rockstroh, P., and Taub, E. (1995). Increased cortical representation of fingers of the left hand in string players. *Science, 270*, 305–307.

Elliot, C.D. (1990). *Differential Ability Scales*. San Antonio, TX: The Psychological Corporation.

Elliott, S.N. (1990). The nature and structure of the DAS: Questioning the test's organizing model and use. *Journal of Psychoeducational Assessment, 8*, 406–411.

Espino, C.M. (1991). Trauma and adaptation: The case of Central American children. In F.L. Ahearn and J.L. Athey (eds.), *Refugee children: Theory, research and services. The Johns Hopkins series in contemporary medicine and public health* (pp. 106–124). Baltimore, MD, US: The Johns Hopkins Press.

Espinosa, G., Elizondo, V., and Miranda, J. (eds.). (2005). *Latino religions and civic activism in the United States*. New York: Oxford University Press.

Evans, J.L. (2001). An emergent account of language impairments in children with SLI: Implications for assessment and intervention. *Journal of Communication Disorders, 34*, 39–54.

Ezkenazi, B., and Maizlish, N.A. (1988). Effects of occupational exposure to chemicals on neurobehavioral functioning. In R.E. Tarter, D.H. van Thiel, and K.L. Edwards (eds.), *Medical neuropsychology: The impact of disease on behavior* (pp. 223–264). New York: Plenum.

Fadiman, A. (1997). *The spirit catches you and you fall down: A Hmong child, her American doctors, and a collision of two cultures*. New York: Farrar, Straus, and Giroux.

Fantino, A.M., Colak, A. (2001). Refugee children in Canada: Searching for identity. *Child Welfare, 80*, 587–596.

Farris, R.E.L., and Dunham, H.W. (1939). *Mental Disorders in Urban Areas*. Chicago: University of Chicago Press.

Felsman, J.K., Leong, F.T., Johnson, M.C., and Felsman, I.C. (1990). Estimates of psychological distress among Vietnamese refugees: Adolescents, unaccompanied minors and young adults. *Social Science and Medicine, 31*, 1251–1256.

Fennell, E.B., and Bauer, R.M. (1989). Models of inference in evaluating brain-behavior relationships in children. In C. Reynolds and E. Fletcher-Janzen (eds.), *Handbook of Clinical Neuropsychology* (2nd ed., pp. 204–215). New York: Plenum Press.

Fenson, L., Dale, P.S., Reznick, S., Bates, E., Thal, D., and Pethick, S. (1994). Variability in early communicative development. *Monographs of the Society for Research in Child Development, 59* (Serial No. 242).

Figueroa, R.A., Sandoval, J., and Merino, B. (1984). School psychology and limited-English proficient (LEP) children: New competencies. *Journal of School Psychology, 22*, 131–143.

Flynn, J.R. (1984). The mean IQ of Americans: Massive gains 1932–1978. *Psychological Bulletin, 95*, 29–51.

Folstein, M.F., Folstein, S.E., and McHugh, P.R. (1975). Mini-mental state: a practical method for grading the cognitive status of patients for the clinician. *Journal of Psychiatric Research, 12*, 189–198.

Fortin, J., and Crago, M.B. (1999). French language acquisition in North America. In O.L. Taylor and L.B. Leonard (eds.), *Language acquisition across North America: Cross-cultural and cross-linguistic perspectives* (pp. 209–242). San Diego, CA: Singular Publishing Group, Inc.

Fox, P.G., Cowell, J.M., and Montgomery, A.C. (1994). The effects of violence on health and adjustment of Southeast Asian refugee children: An integrative review. *Public Health Nursing, 11*, 195–201.

Franco, J.N. (1983). An acculturation scale for Mexican-American children. *Journal of General Psychology, 108*, 175–181.

Fromm, E. (1956). *The Art of Loving*. New York: Harper & Raw.

Fuld, P.A. (1981). *The Fuld Object Memory Evaluation*. Wood Dale, IL: Stoelting Instrument Company.

Galton, F. (1869/1892/1962). *Hereditary genius: An Inquiry into its laws and consequences*. London: Macmillan/Fontana.

Gannotti, M.E., and Handwerker, W.P. (2002). Puerto Rican understandings of child disability: Methods for the cultural validation of standardized measures of child health. *Social Science and Medicine, 55*, 2093–2105.

Garbarino, J., and Kostelny, K. (1996). The effects of political violence on Palestinian children's behavior problems: A risk accumulation model. *Child Development, 67*, 33–45.

Garbarino, J., and Kostelny, K. (1996). What do we need to know to understand children in war and community violence? In R.J. Apfel and S. Bennett (eds.), *Minefields in their hearts: The mental health of children in war and communal violence* (pp. 33–51). New Haven, CT: Yale University Press.

Garbarino, J., Kostelny, K., and Dubrow, N. (1991). What children can tell us about living in danger? *American Psychologist, 46*, 376–383.

García Coll, C., and Magnuson, K. (2002). Cultural differences as sources of developmental vulnerabilities and resources. In J.P. Shonkoff and S.J. Meisels (eds.) *Handbook of early childhood intervention* (2nd ed.) (pp. 94–114). New York: Cambridge University Press.

Garcia, M. (1981). *Desert Immigrants: The Mexicans of El Paso, 1880–1920*. New Haven, CT: Yale University Press.

Gardner, M.F. (1990a). *Expressive One-Word Picture Vocabulary Test – Revised*. Novato, CA: Academic Therapy Publications.

Gardner, M.F. (1990b). *Expressive One-Word Picture Vocabulary Test – Revised, Spanish Edition*. Novato, CA: Academic Therapy Publications.

Gardner, M.F. (2000). *Receptive One-Word Picture Vocabulary Test* (2000 ed.). Novato, CA: Academic Therapy Publications.

Garmezy, N., and Rutter, M. (eds.) (1983). *Stress, Coping, and Development in Children*. Baltimore, MD: The Johns Hopkins University Press.

Geltman, P.L., Augustyn, M., Barnett, E.D., Klass, P.E., and McAlister Groves, B. (2000). War trauma experience and behavioral screening of Bosnian refugee children resettled in Massachusetts. *Journal of Developmental and Behavioral Pediatrics, 21*, 255–261.

Georgas, J. (2003). Cross-cultural psychology, intelligence, and cognitive processes. In Georgas, J., Weiss, L.G., Van de Vijver, F.J.R., and Saklofske, D.H. (eds.). *Culture and Children's Intelligence: Cross-cultural analysis of the WISC-III*. (pp. 23–37). San Diego CA: Academic Press.

Georgas, J., Weiss, L.G., Van de Vijver, F.J.R., and Saklofske, D.H. (2003a). A cross-cultural analysis of the WISC-III. In Georgas, J., Weiss, L.G., Van de Vijver, F.J.R., and Saklofske, D.H. (eds.). *Culture and Children's Intelligence: cross-cultural analysis of the WISC-III*. (pp. 277 –313). San Diego CA: Academic Press.

Georgas, J., Weiss, L.G., Van de Vijver, F.J.R., and Saklofske, D.H. (eds.). (2003b). *Culture and Children's Intelligence: cross-cultural analysis of the WISC-III*. San Diego CA: Academic Press.

German, D.J. (1986). *Test of Word Finding*. Allen, TX: DLM Teaching Resources.

Golden, C.J. (1981). The Luria-Nebraska Children's Battery: Theory and formulation. In G.W. Hynd and J. E. Obrzut (eds.), *Neuropsychological assessment and the school-aged child: Issues and procedures* (pp. 277–302). Orlando, FL: Grune and Stratton.

Golden, C.J. (1986). *Manual for the Luria-Nebraska Neuropsychological Battery: Children's revision*. Los Angeles: Western Psychological Services.

Goldstein, K. (1919). *Die behandlund, fürsorge und begutachtung der hirnverletzen. Zugleich ein beitrag zur verwendung psychologischer methoden in der klinik*. Leipzig: F.C.W. Vogel.

Goldstein, K. (1942). *After effects of brain injuries in war: Their evaluation and treatment; the application of psychologic methods in the clinic*. New York: Grune and Straton.

Goldstein, K., and Reichmann, F. (1920). Über praktische und theoretische ergebnisse aus den erfahrungen an hirnschu verletzten. *Ergebnisse der inneren Medizin und Kinderheilkunde, 18*, 405–305.

Golomb, M. R., Hune, S., MacGregor, D.L., and deVeber, G. (2003). Alternative therapy use by Chinese-Canadian children with stroke and cerebrovascular disease. *Journal of Child Neurology, 18*, 714–717.

Gomez-Tortosa, E., Martin, E., Gaviria, M., Charbel, F., and Ausman, J. (1995). Selective deficit of one language in a bilingual patient following surgery in the left perysylvian area. *Brain and Language, 48*, 320–325.

Gonzalez, J.J. (2001). Pediatric assessment. In: Pontón, M.O., and León-Carrión, J. (eds.) *Neuropsychology and the Hispanic patient* (pp. 105–136). Mahwah, NJ: Lawrence Erlbaum.

Goodglass, H., and Kaplan, E. (1983a). *Boston Diagnostic Aphasia Examination*. Philadelphia: Lea & Febiger.

Goodglass, H., and Kaplan, E. (1983b). *The assessment of aphasia and related disorders* (2ⁿᵈ ed.). Baltimore, MD: Williams & Wilkins.

Green, B., Korol, M., Grace, M., Vary, M., Leonard, A., Gleser, G., and Smitson-Cohen, S. (1991). Children and disaster: Age, gender and parental effects on PTSD symptoms. *Journal of the American Academy of Child and Adolescent Psychiatry*, 30, 945–951.

Greenbaum, C.W., Erlich, C., and Toubiana, Y.H. (1993). Settler children and the Gulf War. In L.A. Leavitt and N.A. Fox (eds.), *The psychological effects of war and violence on children* (pp. 109–130). Hillsdale, NJ: Lawrence Erlbaum Associates.

Groce, N.E., and Zola, I.K. (1993). Multiculturalism, Chronic Illness, and Disability. *Pediatrics, 91*, 1048–1055.

Grossman, F.D. (1978). The effect of an examinee's reported academic achievement and/or physical condition on examiner's scoring and of the WISC-R Verbal IQ. *Dissertation Abstracts International, 38*, 4091A. (University Microfilms No. 77–28,462).

Guarnaccia, P.J., and Lopez, S. (1998). The mental health adjustment of immigrant and refugee children. *The Child Psychiatrist in the Community, 7*, 537–553.

Guarnaccia, P.J., and Rogler, L. H. (1999). Research on culture-bound syndromes: New directions. *American Journal of Psychiatry, 156*, 1322–1327.

Guarnaccia, P.J., Lewis-Fernandez, R., and Marano, M.R. (2003). Toward a Puerto Rican popular nosology: Nervios and Ataque de Nervios. *Culture, Medicine and Psychiatry, 27*, 339–366.

Guilford, J.P. (1967). *The nature of human intelligence*. New York: McGraw-Hill.

Gurdjian, E.S. (1973). *Head injuries from antiquities to the present with special reference to penetrating head wounds*. Springfield, IL: Charles C Thomas Publisher.

Hakuta, K., Ferdman, B.M., and Diaz, R.M. (1987). Bilingualism and cognitive development: Three perspectives. In S. Rosenberg (ed.), *Advances in applied psycholinguistics: Vol. 2. Reading, writing, and language learning* (pp. 284–319). New York: Cambridge University Press.

Hale, J. B., and Fiorello, C. (2002). *Beyond the academic rhetoric of g: Intelligence testing guidelines for practitioners, part I*. National Association of School Psychologists. Retrieved March 25, 2003, from http://www.nasponline.org/ publications/cq312beyondg.html.

Hale, J.B., Fiorello, C.A., Kavanaugh, J.A., Hoeppner, J.B., and Gaither, R.A. (2001). WISC-III predictors of academic achievement for children with learning disabilities: Are global and factor scores comparable? *School Psychology Quarterly, 16*, 31–55.

Haley, S., Coster, W., Ludlow, L., Haltiwanger, J. and Andrellos, P. (1992). *Pediatric evaluation of disability inventory (PEDI)*. Boston: New England Medical Center Hospital and PEDI Research Group.

Hall, C.C.I. (1997). Cultural malpractice: The growing obsolescence of psychology with the changing U.S. population. *American Psychologist, 52*, 642–651.

Halstead, W.C., and Wepman, J.M. (1959). The Halstead-Wepman Aphasia Screening Test. *Journal of Speech and Hearing Disorders, 14*, 9–15.

Hamayan, E.V., and Damico, J.S. (1991). Developing and using a second language. In E.V. Hamayan and J.S. Damico (eds.), *Limiting bias in the assessment of bilingual students* (pp. 39–75). Austin, TX: Pro-Ed.

Hamers, J.F., and Blanc M.H.A. (1989). *Bilinguality and Bilingualism*. Cambridge, England: Cambridge University Press.

Hamilton, N., and Chinchilla, N. (1991). Central American migration: A framework for analysis. *Latin American Research Review, 26*, 75–110.

Handwerker, W.P. (2002). The construct validity of cultures: Cultural diversity, culture theory, and a method for ethnography. *American Anthropologist, 104*, 106–122.

Hanks, R., Wood, D., Millis, S., Harrison-Felix, C., Pierce, C., Rosenthal, M., Bushnik, T., High Jr., W., and Kreutzer, J.S. (2003). Violent traumatic brain injury: Occurrence, patient characteristics, and risk factors from the traumatic brain injury model systems project. *Archives of Physical Medicine and Rehabilitation, 84*, 249–254.

Hannay, H.J., Bieliauskas, L.A., Crosson, B.A., Hammake, T.A., Hamsher, K. deS, and Koffler, S.P. (1998). Proceedings of the Houston Conference on Specialty Training in Clinical Neuropsychology: Policy Statement. *Archives of Clinical Neuropsychology, 13*, 160–166.

Harris, G. (1919). *The redemption of the disabled: A study of the programmes of rehabilitation for the disabled of war and of industry*. London: D. Appleton Publisher.

Harris, J.G., and Llorente, A.M. (2005). Cultural considerations in the use of the Wechsler Intelligence Scale for Children - Fourth Edition (WISC-IV). In A. Prifitera, D.H. Saklofske, and L.G. Weiss (eds.), *WISC-IV Clinical Use and Interpretation Scientist-Practioner Perspectives* (pp. 382–413). Burlington, MA: Elsevier Academic Press.

Harris, J.G., Echemendía, R., Ardila, A., and Rosselli, M. (2001). Cross-cultural cognitive and neuropsychological assessment. In J.W. Andrews, H. Janzen, and D. Saklofske (eds.), *Ability, achievement, and behavioral assessment*. San Diego, CA: Academic Press.

Harris, J.G., Tulsky D.S., and Schultheis, M.T. (2003). Assessment of the non-native English speaker: assimilating history and research findings to guide clinical practice. In D.S. Tusky, D.H. Saklofske, G.J. Chelune, R.J. Heaton, R.J. Ivnik, R. Bornstein et al. (eds.), *Clinical Interpretation of the WAIS-III and WMS-III*. (pp. 343–390). San Diego, CA: Academic Press.

Harrison, C., Newton, C.N., Hall, K., & Kreutzer, J.S. (1996). Deseriptive findings from the Traumatic Injury Model Systems National Data Base. *Journal of Head Trauma Rehabilitation, 11*, 1–14.

Harrison, P.L., and Oakland, T. (2003). *Adaptive Behavior Assessment System* (2nd ed.). San Antonio, TX: Psychological Corporation.

Hart, A.C. (ed.), and Hopkins, C.A. (2002). *International Classification of Diseases – Ninth Revision Clinical Modification* (9th ed.). Reston, VA: St. Anthony Publishing.

Heaton, R.K., Grant, I., and Matthews, C. (1986). Differences in neuropsychological test performance associated with age, education, and sex. In I. Grant and K.M. Adams (eds.), *Neuropsychological assessment of neuropsychiatric disorders* (pp.100–120). New York: Oxford University Press.

Hebb, D.O. (1949). *Organization of behavior*. New York: John Wiley and Sons, Inc.

Hehir, T. (2002). Eliminating ableism in education. *Harvard Educational Review, 72*, 1–31. Boston: Harvard Education Publishing Group.

Helms, J.E. (1992). Why is there no study of cultural equivalence in standardized cognitive ability testing? *American Psychologist, 47*, 1083–1101.

Heptinstall, E., Sethna, V., and Taylor, E. (2004). PTSD and depression in refugee children: Association with pre-immigration trauma and post-migration stress. *European Child and Adolescent Psychiatry, 13*, 373–380.

Hernandez, A.E., Dapretto, M., Mazziotta, J., and Bookheimer, S. (2001). Language switching and language representation in Spanish-English bilinguals: An fMRI study. *Neuroimage, 14*, 510–520.

Herrnstein, R.J., and Murray, C. (1996). *The bell curve: Intelligence and class structure in American life*. Simon & Schuster Adult Publishing Group.

Hicks, R., Lalonde, R.N., and Pepler, D. (1993). Psychosocial considerations in the mental health of immigrant and refugee children. *Canadian Journal of Community Mental Health, 12*, 71–87.

Higgs, T.V. (1985). Language acquisition and language learning: A plea for syncretism. *Modern Language Journal, 69*, 8–14.

Hines, T.M. (1996). Failure to demonstrate selective deficit in the native language following surgery in the left perisylvian area. *Brain and Language, 54*, 168–169.

Hjern, A., Angel, B., and Hoejer, B. (1991). Persecution and behavior: A report of refugee children from Chile. *Child Abuse and Neglect, 15*, 239–248.

Hjern, A., Angel, B., and Jeppson, O. (1998). Political violence, family stress and mental health of refugee children in exile. *Scandinavian Journal of Social Medicine, 26,* 18–25.

Hodes, M. (1998). Refugee children may need a lot of help (Editorial). *British Medical Journal,* 316, 793–725.

Hodes, M. (2000). Psychologically distressed refugee children in the United Kingdom. *Child Psychology and Psychiatry Review, 5,* 57–68.

Holden, C. (1996). Small refugees suffer the effects of early neglect. *Science,* 274, 1076–1077.

Hollingshead, A.B. (1957). *Two factor index of social position.* Unpublished manuscript, Department of Sociology, Yale University. New Haven, CT.

Hollingshead, A.B., and Redlich, F.C. (1958). *Social class and mental illness: A community study.* New York: John Wiley and Sons, Inc.

Holm, A., Dodd, B., Stow, C., and Pert, S. (1999). Identification and differential diagnosis of phonological disorder in bilingual children. *Language Testing, 16,* 271–292.

Holmbeck, G.N. (1997). Toward terminological, conceptual, and statistical clarity in the study of mediators and moderators: Examples from the child-clinical and pediatric psychology literatures. *Journal of Consulting and Clinical Psychology, 65,* 599–610.

Horn, J.L. (1967). Intelligence – Why it grows, why it declines. *Trans-action, 5,* 23–31.

Horn, J.L. (1979). Trends in the measurement of intelligence. *Intelligence, 3,* 229–239.

Horn, J.L. (1989). Cognitive diversity: A framework of learning. In P.L. Ackerman, R.J. Sternberg, and R. Glaser (eds.), *Learning and individual differences* (pp. 61–116). New York: Cambridge University Press.

Howard, M., and Hodes, M. (2000). Psychopathology, adversity and service utilization of young refugees. *Journal of the American Academy of Child and Adolescent Psychiatry, 39,* 368–377.

Hubbard, J. Realmuto, G.M., Northwood, A.K., and Masten, A.S. (1995). Comorbidity of psychiatric diagnoses with posttraumatic stress disorder in survivors of childhood trauma. *Journal of the American Academy of Child and Adolescent Psychiatry, 34,* 1167–1173.

Human Rights and Equal Opportunity Commission. (2001). *Face the facts: Some questions and answers about immigration, refugees and indigenous affairs.* Sydney: Human Rights and Equal Opportunity Commission, Australia.

Hyman, I., Vu, N., and Beiser, M. (2000). Post-migration stresses among Southeast Asian refugees youth in Canada: A research note. *Journal of Comparative Family Studies, 31,* 281–293.

International Dyslexia Association (IDA). (May 2000). Dyslexia basics. *Fact Sheet #962.*

Irvine, S.H., and Berry, J.W. (eds.) (1988). *Human Abilities in Cultural Context.* New York: Cambridge University Press.

Jalali, B. (1988). Ethnicity, cultural adjustment, and behavior: Implications for family therapy. In L. Comas-Diaz and E.E.H. Griffith (eds.), *Clinical guidelines in crosscultural mental health* (pp. 9–32). New York: John Wiley and Sons, Inc.

Jarvis, E. (1866). Influence of distance from and nearness to an insane hospital on its use by the people. *American Journal of Insanity, 22,* 361–406.

Jensen, A. (1980). *Bias in mental testing.* New York: Free Press.

Jensen, A.R., (1979). Cumulative deficit in IQ of blacks in the rural south. In L. Willerman, and R.G. Turner (Eds.), *Readings about individual and group differences* (pp. 83–91). San Francisco; W.H. Freeman and Company.

Johnston, J.R. (1982). Narratives: A new look at communication problems in older language disordered children. *Language, Speech, and Hearing Services in Schools, 13,* 144–155.

Johnstone, B., Holland, D., and Larimore, C. (2000). Language and academic abilities. In G. Groth-Marnat (Ed.), *Neuropsychological assessment in clinical practice: A guide to test interpretation and integration* (pp. 335–354). New York: John Wiley and Sons, Inc.

Jones, R.L. (1996) (ed.). *Handbook of Tests and Measurements for Black Populations.* Hampton, VA: Cobb and Henry.

Joseph, R. (1996). *Neuropsychiatry, neuropsychology, and clinical neuroscience: Emotion, evolution, cognition, language, memory, brain damage, and abnormal behavior* (2nd ed.). Baltimore, MD: Williams & Wilkins.

Joshhi, M.R., Dahlgren, M., and Boulware-Gooden, R. (2002). Teaching reading in an inner city school through a multisensory teaching approach. *Annals of Dyslexia, 55*, 229–242.

Junque, C., Vendrell, P., and Vendrell, J. (1995). Differential impairments and specific phenomena in 50 Catalan-Spanish bilingual aphasic patients. In M. Paradis (ed.), *Aspects of Bilingual Aphasia*. Oxford: Pergamon Pres.

Jupp, J.J., and Luckey, J. (1990). Educational experiences in Australia of Indo-Chinese adolescent refugees. *International Journal of Mental Health*, 18(4), 78–91.

Kalat, J.W. (1998). *Biological psychology* (6th ed.). Pacific Grove, CA: Brooks/Cole Publishing Company.

Kamphaus, R.W. (1993). *Clinical assessment of children's intelligence: A handbook for professional practice*. Boston: Allyn and Bacon.

Kamphaus, R.W., Petoskey, M.D., and Rowe, E.W. (2000). Current trends in psychological testing of children. *Professional Psychology: Research and Practice, 31*, 155–164.

Kaplan, E. (1996). A process approach to neuropsychological assessment. In M. Dennis, E. Kaplan, M. Posner, D. Stein, and R. Thompson (eds.), *Clinical Neuropsychology and Brain Function: Research, Measurement, and Practice*. Washington, DC: American Psychological Association.

Kaplan, E., Fein, D., Kramer, J., Delis, D., and Morris, R. (1999). *Wechsler Intelligence Scale for Children – Third Edition, PI*. San Antonio, TX: The Psychological Corporation.

Kaplan, E., Goodglass, H., and Weintraub, S. (1983). *Boston Naming Test* (Revised 60-item version). Philadelphia: Lea & Febiger.

Kaplan, R.M., and Saccuzzo, D.P. (1997). *Psychological testing: Principles, application, and issues*. Pacific Grove, CA: Brooks/Cole Publishing Company.

Kaufman, A.S., and Flanagan, D.P. (2004). *Essentials of WISC IV assessment*. New York: Wiley.

Kaufman, A.S., and Kaufman, N.L. (1990). *Kaufman Brief Intelligence Test (K-BIT)*. Circle Pines, MN: American Guidance Service.

Kaufman, A.S., and Kaufman, N.L. (1993). *Kaufman Adolescent and Adult Intelligence Test (KAIT)*. Circle Pines, MN: American Guidance Service.

Kaufman, A.S. (1994). *Intelligent testing with the WISC-III*. New York: John Wiley and Sons.

Kaufman, D.M. (2001). *Clinical neurology for psychiatrists* (5th ed.).Philadelphia: W.B. Saunders Company.

Kay, J., and Ellis, A. (1987). A cognitive neuropsychological case study of anomia. *Brain, 110*, 613–629.

Kayser, H. (1993). Hispanic cultures. In D. Battle (ed.), *Communication disorders in multicultural populations* (pp. 114–157). Boston: Andover Medical Publishers.

Keith, T.Z., Quirk, K.J., Schartzer, C., and Elliott, C.D. (1999). Construct bias in the Differential Ability Scales? Confirmatory and hierarchical factor structure across three ethnic groups. *Journal of Psychoeducational Assessment, 17,* 249–268.

Kemeny, M.E., and Gruenewald, T.L. (2000). Affect, cognition, the immune system and health. In E.A. Mayer and C. Saper, (eds.), *The Biological Basis for Mind Body Interactions. Progress in Brain Research Series* (pp. 291–308). Amsterdam: Elsevier Science B.V.

Kennepohl, S. (1999). Toward a cultural neuropsychology: An alternative view and a preliminary model. *Brain and Cognition, 41*, 365–380.

Kessler, R.C., and Cleary, P.D. (1980). Social class and psychological distress. *American Sociological Review, 45*, 463–478.

Kinzie, J.D. (1988). The psychiatric effects of massive trauma on Cambodian refugees. In: Wilson J.P., Harel Z., Kahana B., eds. *Human adaptation of extreme stress: From the Holocaust to Vietnam* (pp. 305–317). New York: Plenum Press.

Kinzie, J.D., and Sack, W. (1991). Severely traumatized Cambodian children: Research findings and clinical implications. In F.L. Ahearn and J.L. Athey (eds.), Refugee children: Theory, research and services. *The Johns Hopkins series in contemporary medicine and public health* (pp. 92–105). Baltimore, MD: The Johns Hopkins University Press.

Kinzie, J.D., Boehnlein, J.K., Leung, P.K., and Moore, L.J., Riley, C., and Smith, D. (1990). The prevalence of posttraumatic stress disorder and its clinical significance among Southeast Asian refugees. *American Journal of Psychiatry, 147,* 913–917.

Kinzie, J.D., Sack, W., Angell, R., and Clarke, G. (1989). A three-year follow-up of Cambodian young people traumatized as children. *Journal of the American Academy of Child and Adolescent Psychiatry, 28,* 501–504.

Kinzie, J.D., Sack, W.H., Angell, R.H., Manson, S.M and Ben, R. (1986). The psychiatric effects of massive trauma on Cambodian children: I. The children. *Journal of the American Academy of Child* Psychiatry, 25, 370–376.

Kirk, R.E. (1990). *Experimental design: Procedures for the Behavioral Sciences* (2nd ed.). Belmont, CA: Brooks/Cole Publishing.

Kleim, J.A., Swain, R.A., Czerlanis, C.M., Kelly, J.L., Pipitone, M.A., and Greenough, W.T. (1997). Learning-dependent dendritic hypertrophy of cerebellarstellate neurons: Plasticity of local circuit neurons. *Neurobiology of Learning and Memory, 67,* 29–33.

Klingman, A. (1994). Children's response to the Gulf War: Assessment via ordinal and nominal quantification of compositions. *School Psychology* International, 15, 235–246.

Kocijan-Hercigonja, D., Rijavec, M., and Hercigonja, V. (1998). Mental health condition and adjustment of refugee and displaced children in a war area. *Psychiatria Danubina, 10,* 23–29.

Kocijan-Hercigonja, D., Rijavec, M., Marusic, A., and Hercigonja, V. (1997). Coping strategies of refugee, displaced, and non displaced children in a war area. *Nordic Journal of Psychiatry, 52,* 45–50.

Kohler, E., Keysers, C., Umilta, M.A., Fogassi, L., Gallese, V., Rizzolatti, G. (2002). Hearing sounds, understanding actions: Action representation in auditory mirror neurons. *Science, 297,* 846–848.

Kohn, M.L. (1973). Social class and schizophrenia: A critical review and reformulation. *Schizophrenia Bulletin, 7,* 60–79.

Kolb, B., and Fantie, B. (1997). Development of the child's brain and behavior. In C.R. Reynolds and E. Fletcher-Janzen (eds.), *Handbook of clinical child neuropsychology* (pp. 17–41). New York: Plenum Press.

Korkman, M., Kirk, U., and Kemp, S. (1998). *NEPSY: A Developmental Neuropsychological Assessment.* San Antonio, TX: The Psychological Corporation.

Krashen, S. (1982). *Principles and practice in second language acquisition.* New York: Prentice Hall.

Kraus, J.F., Fife, D., Ramstein, K., Conroy, C., and Cox, P. (1986). The relationship of family income to the incidence, external causes, and outcomes of serious brain injury, San Diego County, California. *American Journal of Public Health, 76,* 1345–1347.

Kress, G. (2003). *Literacy in the new media age.* London: Routledge.

Krupinski, J., and Burrows, G. (eds.). (1986). *The Price of Freedom: Young Indochinese Refugees in Australia.* Sydney: Pergamon Press.

Kuhn, T.S. (1962). *The structure of scientific revolutions* (1st ed.). Chicago: University of Chicago Press.

Kuhn, T.S. (1970). *The structure of scientific revolutions* (2nd. ed.). Chicago: University of Chicago Press.

Kuhn, T.S. (1996). *The structure of scientific revolutions* (3rd ed.). Chicago: The University of Chicago Press.

Kuper, A. (1999). *Culture: The anthropologists' account.* Harvard University Press.

Kwak, K. (2003). South Korea. In J. Georgas, L. Weiss, F.J.R van de Vijver and D.H. Saklofske (eds.), *Culture and children's intelligence: Cross cultural analysis of the WISC-III* (pp. 227–240). London: Academic Press.

LaCalle, J. (1987). Forensic psychological evaluations through an interpreter: Legal and ethical issues. *American Journal of Forensic Psychology, 5,* 29–43.

Lacelle-Peterson, M.W., and Rivera, C. (1994). Is it for all kids? A framework for equitable assessment policies for English language learners. *Harvard Educational Review, 64,* 55–75.

Lai, C.S.L. et al. (2001). A forkhead-domain gene is mutated in a severe speech and language disorder. *Nature, 413,* 519–523.

Lambert, N., Nihira, K., and Leland, H. (1993). *AAMR Adaptive Behavior Scale – School* (2nd ed.). Austin, TX: Pro-Ed.

Lankshear, C., and Knobel, M. (2003). *New literacies: Changing knowledge and classroom learning*. Buckingham: Open University Press.

Laor, N., Wolmer, L., Mayes, L.C., and Gershon, A. (1997). Israeli preschool children under scuds: A 30-month follow-up. *Journal of the American Academy of Child and Adolescent Psychiatry, 36*, 349–356.

Laor, N., Wolmer, L., Mayes, L.C., and Golomb, A., Silverberg, D.S., Weizman, R., and Cohen, D.J. (1996). Israeli preschoolers under Scud missile attacks: A developmental perspective on risk-modifying factors. *Archives of General Psychiatry, 53*, 416–423.

Laosa, L.M. (1984). Ethnic, socioeconomic and home language influences upon early performance on measures of abilities. *Journal of Educational Psychology, 76*, 1178–1198.

Laosa, L.M. (1996). Intelligence testing and social policy. *Journal of Applied Developmental Psychology, 17*, 155–173.

LaRue, A., Romano, L.J., Ortiz, I.E., Liang, H.C., and Lindeman, R.D. (1999). Neuropsychological performance of Hispanic and non-Hispanic older adults: An epidemiologic survey. *Clinical Neuropsychologist, 13*, 474–486.

Lashley, K.S. (1938). Factors limiting recovery after central nervous system lesions. *Journal of Nervous and Mental Disease, 88*, 733–755.

Laurel, F., and Zimmerman, M. (2001). Posttraumatic stress disorder and major depressive disorder: Investigating the role of overlapping symptoms in diagnostic comorbidity. *Journal of Nervous and Mental Diseases, 189*, 548–551.

Law, J. (1992). Factors associated with language impairment. In J. Law (ed.), *The early identification of language impairment in children: Therapy in practice* (pp. 41–62). London: Chapman and Hall.

LeFrançois, G.R. (1995). *Of children: An introduction to child development* (8th ed.). Belmont, CA: Wadsworth Publishing Company.

Leonard, L.B. (1999). The study of language acquisition across languages. In O.L. Taylor and L.B. Leonard (eds.), *Language acquisition across North America: Cross-cultural and cross-linguistic perspectives* (pp. 3–18). San Diego, CA: Singular Publishing Group, Inc.

León-Carrión, J. (1989). Trail Making Test scores for normal children: Normative data from Spain. *Perceptual and Motor Skills, 68*, 627–630.

León-Carrión, J. (1997). A historical view of neuropsychological rehabilitation: The search for human dignity. In J. León-Carrión (ed.), *Neuropsychological rehabilitation: Fundamentals, innovations, and directions* (pp. 3–39). Delray Beach, FL: GR/St. Lucie Press.

Lezak, M.D. (1995). *Neuropsychological assessment* (3rd ed.). New York: Oxford University Press.

Lezak, M.D., Howieson, D.B., and Loring, D.W. (2004). *Neuorpsychological Assessment* (4th Ed.). New York: Oxford University Press.

Li, S. (2003). Biolcultural orchestration of developmental plasticity across levels: The interplay of biology and culture shaping the mind and behavior across the life span. *Psychology Bulletin, 129* (2), 171–194.

Llorente, A.M. (August, 1997). *Neuropsychologic assessment of Hispanic populations: The influence of immigration on assessment*. Paper presented at the 105th Annual Convention of the American Psychological Association, Chicago, IL.

Llorente, A.M. (2000). Evaluation of developmental neurocognitive and neurobehavioral changes associated with pesticide exposure: Recommendations for the U.S. Environmental Protection Agency on the assessment of health effects of pesticide exposure in infants and young children. In D. Otto, R. Calderon, P. Mendola, and E. Hilborn (eds.), *Assessment of Health Effects of Pesticide Exposure in Young Children* (pp. 22–32). Research Triangle Park, NC: Environmental Protection Agency (EPA/600/R-99/086).

Llorente, A.M. (June, 2004). *Psychological issues affecting unaccompanied immigrant children*. Invited presentation at the 11th National Conference on children and and the law. Washington, DC.

Llorente, A.M., Cassatta, A., Perez, L., Sines, M. (unpublished manuscript). "Not the same old thing:" Alterations in test stimuli across five decades on the Wechsler Intelligence Scale for Children and its probable impact on performance with Hispanic children in three case studies.

Llorente, A.M., LoPresti, C.M., Guzzard. C., Satz, P., and Evans, G. (2000a). HIV-1 infection spectrum disease: Neuropsychological manifestations and cross-cultural considerations in adulthood, adolescence, and childhood. In E. Fletcher-Janzen, T. Strickland, and C.R. Reynolds (eds.), *Handbook of Cross-Cultural Neuropsychology* (pp. 215–246). New York: Kluwer Academic/Plenum Publishers.

Llorente, A.M., Amado, A., Voigt, R.G., Berretta, M.C., Fraley, K.A., Jensen, C.L., & Heird, W.L. (2001a). Internal consistency, temporal stability, and reproductivity of individual index scores of the Test of Variables of Attention (T.O.V.A) in children with attention-deficit, hyperactivity disorder (AD/HD). *Archives of Clinical Neuropsychology, 16,* 535–546.

Llorente, A.M., LoPresti, C.E., Levy, J.K., and Fernandez, F. (2001). Neuropsychological and neurobehavioral correlates associated with HIV infection: Assessment considerations with Hispanic populations. In M. Pontón and J. León-Carrión (eds.), *Neuropsychology and the Hispanic Patient* (pp. 209–242). Mahwah, NJ: Lawrence Erlbaum and Associates.

Llorente, A.M., Pontón, M.O., Taussig, I.M., and Satz, P. (1999). Patterns of American immigration and their influence on the acquisition of neuropsychological norms for Hispanics. *Archives of Clinical Neuropsychology, 14,* 603–614.

Llorente, A.M., Taussig, I.M., Perez, L., and Satz, P. (2000). Trends in American immigration: Influences on neuropsychological assessment and inferences with ethnic-minority populations. In E. Fletcher-Janzen, T. Strickland, and C.R. Reynolds (eds.), *Handbook of Cross-Cultural Neuropsychology* (pp. 345–359). New York: Kluwer Academic/Plenum Publishers.

Llorente, A.M., Williams, J., D'Elia, L., Satz, P. (2003). *Children's Color Trails Test 1 and 2 Manual.* Odessa, FL: Psychological Assessment Resources, Inc (PAR).

Lopez Cardozo, B., Vergara, A., Agani, F., and Gotway, C.A. (2000). Mental health, social functioning and attitudes of Kosovar Albanians following the war in Kosovo. *Journal of the American Medical Association, 284,* 569.

Lopez, S.R., and Taussig, I.M. (1991). Cognitive-intellectual functioning of Spanish-speaking impaired and nonimpaired Elderly: Implications for culturally sensitive assessment. *Psychological Assessment, 3,* 448–454.

Losen, D.J., and Orfield, G. (2002). Introduction: Racial inequity in special education. In D. Losen and G. Orfield (Eds.), *Racial inequity in special education* (p. 1–24). Boston: Harvard Education Publishing.

Loughry, M., and Flouri, E. (2001). The behavioral and emotional problems of former unaccompanied refugee children 3–4 years after their return to Vietnam. *Child Abuse and Neglect,* 25, 249–263.

Lu, F.G., Lim, R.F., and Mezzich, J.E. (1995). Issues in the assessment and diagnosis of culturally diverse individuals. In J. Oldham and M. Riba (eds.), *Review of Psychiatry, 14,* 477–510. Washington, DC: American Psychiatric Press.

Lukman, B., and Bach-Mortensen, N. (1995). Symptoms in children of torture victims: Post traumatic stress disorders? *World Pediatrics and Child Care,* 5, 32–42.

Luria, A.R. (1976). *Cultural Development: Its Cultural and Social Foundations* Cambridge, MA: Harvard University Press.

Luria, A.R. (1979). *The making of mind: A personal account of Soviet Psychology.* In M. Cole and S. Cole (eds.). Cambridge, MA: Harvard University Press.

Luria, A.R. (1966). *Higher Cortical Functions in Man.* London: Tavistock.

Macksoud, M.S., and Aber, J.L. (1996). The war experiences and psychosocial development of children in Lebanon. *Child Development, 67,* 70–88.

MacMillan, D.L., and Speece, D.L. (1999). Utility of current diagnostic categories for research and practice. In R. Galllimore, L.P. Bernheimer, D.L. MacMillan, D.L. Speece, and S. Vaughn (eds.), *Developmental perspectives on children with high incidence disabilities* (pp. 111–133). Mahwah, NJ: Lawrence Erlbaum and Associates.

Malgady, R.G., Rogler, L.H., and Tryon, W.W. (1992). Issues of validity in the Diagnostic Interview Schedule. *Journal of Psychiatric Research, 26*, 59–67.

Malzberg, B., and Lee, E.S. (1956). *Migration and mental disease: A study of first admissions to hospitals for mental disease, New York, 1939–1941*. New York: Social Science Research Council.

Mandal, M.K, Ida, Y., Harizuka, S., and Upadhaya, N. (1999). Cultural difference in hand preference: Evidence from India and Japan. *International Journal of Psychology, 34*, 59–66.

Marin G., and Marin, B.V. (1991). *Research with Hispanic populations*. Newbury Park, CA: Sage.

Marin, G., Sabogal, F., Marin, B., and Otero-Sabogal, R. (1984). Development of a short acculturation scale for Hispanics. *Hispanic Journal of Behavioral Sciences, 9*, 183–205.

Markowitz, F. (1996). Living in limbo: Bosnian Muslim refugees in Israel. *Human Organization, 55*, 127–132.

Marlowe, W.B. (2000). Multicultural perspectives on the neuropsychological assessment of children and adolescents. In E. Fletcher-Janzen, T.L. Strickland, and C.R. Reynolds (eds.), *Handbook of cross-cultural neuropsychology* (pp. 145–165). New York: Kluwer Academic/ Plenum Publishers.

Masser, D.S. (1992). Psychosocial functioning of Central American refugee children. *Child Welfare*, 71(5), 439–456.

Masterman, M. (1974). The nature of a paradigm. In I. Lakatos and A. Musgrave (eds.), *Criticism and the growth of knowledge* (pp. 58–89). New York: Cambridge University Press.

Mather, N., and Woodcock, R.W. (2001). Application of the Woodcock-Johnson Tests of Cognitive Ability-Revised to the diagnosis of learning disabilities. In A.S. Kaufman and N.L. Kaufman (eds.), *Specific learning disabilities and difficulties in children and Adolescents* (pp. 55–96). New York: Cambridge University Press.

Matthey, S., Silove, D., Barnett, B., Fitzgerald, M.H., and Mitchell, P. (1999). Correlates of depression and PTSD in Cambodian women with young children: A pilot study. *Stress Medicine*, 15, 103–107.

McCaffrey, R.J., Palav, A.A., O'Bryant, S.E., and Labarge, A.S. (2003). A brief overview of base rates. In A.E. Puente and C.R. Reynolds (eds.), *Critical issues in neuropsychology* (pp. 1–9). New York: Kluwer Academic/Plenum Publishers.

McCallin, M. (1992). *Living in detention: A review of the Psychological wellbeing of Vietnamese children in the Hong Kong detention centers*. Geneva: International Catholic Child Bureau.

McCloskey, L.A., and Southwick, K. (1996). Psychosocial problems in refugee children exposed to war. *Pediatrics, 97*, 394–39.

McCloskey, L.A., Southwick, K., Fernandez-Esquer, M.E., and Locke, C. (1996). The psychological effects of political and domestic violence on Central American and Mexican immigrant mothers and children. *Journal of Community Psychology*, 23, 95–116.

McGrew, K.S., and Woodcock, R.W. (2001). *Technical Manual. Woodcock-Johnson III*. Itasca, IL: Riverside Publishing.

McNamara, K.M., and Hollinger, C.L. (1997). Intervention-based assessment: Rates of evaluation and eligibility for specific learning disability classification. *Psychological Reports, 81*, 620–622.

McKelvey, R.S., and Webb, J.A. (1997). A prospective study of psychological stress related to refugee camp experience. *Australian and New Zealand Journal of Psychiatry, 31*, 549–554.

McKenzie, K.J., and Crowcroft, N.S. (1994). Race, ethnicity, culture, and science. *British Medical Journal, 39*, 286–287.

Mejia, S., Gutierrez, L.M., Villa, A.R., and Ostrosky-Solis (2004). Cognition, functional status, education, and the diagnosis of dementia and mild cognitive impairment in Spanish-speaking elderly. *Applied Neuropsychology, 11*, 194–201.

Melendez, F. (2001). Forensic assessment of Hispanics. In M.O. Pontón & J. León-Carrión (Eds.), *Neuropsychology and the Hispanic Patient: A Clinical Handbook* (pp. 321–340). Mahwah, NJ: Lawrence Erlbaum and Associates.

Melville, M.B., and Lykes, M.B. (1992). Guatemalan Indian children and the sociocultural effects of government-sponsored terrorism. *Social Science and Medicine, 34*, 533–548.

Mercer, J., and Lewis, J. F. (1978). *System of Multi-Pluralistic Assessment* (SOMPA). San Antonio, TX: Psychological Corporation.

Mezzich, J. E., and Lewis-Fernandez, R. (1997). Cultural considerations in psychopathology. In A. Tasman, J. Kay, and J.A. Lieberman (eds.), *Psychiatry* (pp. 563–571). Philadelphia: W.B. Saunders.

Mghir, R., Freed, W., Raskin, A., and Katon, W. (1995). Depression and posttraumatic stress disorder among a community sample of adolescent and young adult Afghan refugees. *Journal of Nervous and Mental Disease, 183*, 24–30.

Miller, K.E. (1996). The effects of state terrorism and exile on indigenous Guatemalan refugee children: A mental health assessment and an analysis of children's narratives. *Child Development, 67*, 89–106.

Minicucci, C., and Olsen, L. (Spring, 1992). *Programs for secondary limited English proficient students: A California study.* (Occasinal Papers in Bilingual Education, No. 5). Washington, DC: National Clearinghouse for Bilingual Education.

Mitrushina, M.N., Boone, K.B., D'Elia, K.F., and D'Elia, L. (1999). *Handbook of normative data for neuropsychological assessment.* New York: Oxford University Press.

Mollica, R.F., Poole, C., Son, L., Murray, C.C., and Tor, S. (1997). Effects of war trauma on Cambodian refugee adolescents' functional health and mental health status. *Journal of the American Academy of Child and Adolescent-Psychiatry, 36*, 1098–1106.

Montgomery, E. (1998). Refugee children from the Middle East. *Scandinavian Journal of Social Medicine*, Supplement 4.

Montgomery, G.T., and Orozlo, S. (1984). Validation of a measure of acculturation for Mexican Americans. *Hispanic Journal of Behavioral Sciences, 6*, 53–63.

Morrow, R.D. (1994). Immigration, refugee and generation status as related to behavioral disorders. In R.L Peterson and S. Ishii-Jordan (eds.), *Multicultural issues in the education of students with behavioral disorders* (pp. 196–207). Cambridge, MA, US: Brookline Books.

Mosely, M.E. (1993). *The Incas and their ancestors: The archeology of Peru.* New York: Thames and Hudson.

Moss, E., Davidson, R.J. and Saron, C. (1985). Cross-cultural differences in hemisphericity: EEG asymmetry discriminates between Japanese and Westerners. *Neuropsychologia, 23*, 131–135.

Mullen, E.M. (1995). *Mullen Scales of Early Learning.* Circle Pines, MN: American Guidance Service.

Mungas, D. (1996). The process of development of valid and reliable neuropsychological assessment measures for English –and Spanish-speaking elderly persons. I.G. Yeo and D. Gallagher-Thompson (eds.), *Ethnicity and the dementias* (pp. 33–46). Washington, DC: Taylor and Francis.

Mungas, D., Reed, B.R., Crane, P.K., Haan, M.N., and Gonzalez, H. (2004). Spanish and English neuropsychological assessment scales (SENAS): Further development and psychometric characteristics. *Psychological Assessment, 16*, 347–359.

Mungas, D., Reed, B.R., Haan, M.N., and Gonzalez, H. (2005) Spanish and English Neuropsychological Assessment Scales: Relationship to demographics, language, cognition, and independent functioning. *Neuropsychology, 19*, 466–475.

Muñiz, J., and Hambleton, R.K. (1996). Directrices para la tradición y adapción de los tests. *Papeles del Psicologo, 66*, 63–70.

Muñoz-Sandoval, A.F., Cummins, J., Alvarado, C.G., and Ruef, M.L. (1998). *Bilingual Verbal Abilities Test.* Itasca, IL: Riverside Publishing.

Muñoz-Sandoval, A., Woodcock, R.W., McGrew, K.S., and Mather, N. (2005) *Bateria III Woodcock-Munoz.* Itasca, IL: Riverside.

Mushi, S.L.P. (2002). Simultaneous and successive second language learning: Integral ingredients of the human development process. *Early Child Development and Care, 172*, 349–358.

Nagel, J. (1994). Constructing ethnicity: Creating and recreating ethnic identity and culture. *Social Problems, 41*, 152–176.

Naglieri, J.A. (1997). *Naglieri Nonverbal Ability Test.* San Antonio, TX: Psychological Corporation.

Naglieri, J.A., and Ronning, M.E. (2000). Comparison of White, African American, Hispanic, and Asian children on the Naglieri Nonverbal Ability Test. *Journal of Psychoeducational Assessment, 18,* 230–239.

Naglieri, J.A., Booth, A.L., and Winsler, A. (2004). Comparison of Hispanic children with and without limited English proficiency on the Naglieri nonverbal ability test. *Psychological Assessment, 16,* 81–84.

National Center for Education Statistics (February 2000). *Racial and ethnic distribution of elementary and secondary students* [on-line]. Available: http://www.nces.ed.gov/edstats/

Neisser, U., Boodoo, G., Bouchard, T.J., Boykin, A.W., Brody, N., Ceci, S.J., Halpern, D.F., Loehlin, J.C., Perloff, R., Sternberg, R.J., and Urbina, S. (1996). Intelligence: Knowns and unknowns. *American Psychologist, 55,* 77–101.

Nell, V. (2000). *Cross-cultural neuropsychological assessment: Theory and Practice.* Mahwah, NJ: Lawrence Erlbaum Associates.

Oakes, J. (1990). *Multiplying inequalities: The effects of race social class, and tracking on opportunities to learn mathematics and science.* Santa Monica, CA: RAND.

Obradovic, B., Kanazir, V., Zalisevskij, G., Popadic, K., and Simic, I. (1993). A threat to mental health of children and young people in exile. *Psihijat dan, 25,* 91–98.

Ochoa, S.H., Rivera, B., and Ford, L. (1997). An investigation of school psychology training pertaining to bilingual psych-educational assessment of primarily Hispanic students: Twenty-five years after Diana v. California. *Journal of School Psychology, 35,* 329–349.

Ødegaard, Ø. (1932). Emigration and insanity: A study of mental disease among the Norwegian-born population of Minnesota. *Acta Psychiatrica et Neurologica, 4,* 1–206, Supplement.

Office of Special Education Programs (2001). *Twenty-third annual report to congress on the implementation of the Individuals with Disabilities Education Act. Section II, Sudent Characteristics* (pp. 22–30).

Olazaran, J., Jacobs, D.M., and Stern, Y. (1996). Comparative study of visual and verbal short-term memory in English and Spanish speakers: testing a linguistic hypothesis. *Journal of the International Neuropsychological Society, 2,* 105–110.

Oller, D.K. (1986). Metaphonology and infant vocalizations. In B. Lindblom and R. Zetterstrom, (eds.), *Precursors of early speech* (pp. 21–35). New York: Stockton Press.

Oller, K., Eilers, R., Steffens, M., Lynch, M., and Urbano, R. (1994). Speechlike vocalizations in infancy: An evaluation of potential risk factors. *Journal of Child Language, 21,* 33–58.

Orton, S.T. (1937). *Reading, writing, and speech problems in children.* New York: W.W. Norton.

Ostrosky-Solis, F., Ramirez, M., Lozano, A., Velez, A. (2004). Culture or education? Neuropsychological test performance of a Maya indigenous population. *International Journal of Psychology, 39,* 36–46

Otero, M. (2006). Bateria III Woodcock-Munoz (Bateria III). *School Psychologist, 60,* 86–89.

Paardekooper, B., de Jong, J.T.V.M., and Hermanns, J.M.A. (1999). The psychological impact of war and the refugee situation on South Sudanese children in refugee camps in Northern Uganda: An exploratory study. *Journal of Child Psychology, Psychiatry and Allied Disciplines, 40,* 529–536.

Padilla, E.R., Roll, S., Gomez Palacio, M. (1982). The performance of Mexican children and adolescents on the WISC-R. *Interamerican Journal of Psychology, 16,* 122–128.

Palacio, M., G., Padilla, E.R., and Roll, S. (1984). *Escala de Inteligencia Revisada para el Nivel Escolar (WISC-RM).* Mexico, D.F.: Editorial Manual Moderno.

Papageorgiou, V., Frangou-Garunovic, A., Iordanidou, R., Yule, W., Smith, P., and Vostanis, P. (2000). War trauma and psychopathology in Bosnian refugee children. *European Journal of Adolescent Psychiatry, 9,* 84–90.

Paradis, M. (ed.). (1978). *Aspects of bilingualism.* Columbia, SC: Hornbeam Press.

Paradis, M. (1977). Bilingualism and aphasia. In H. Whitaker and H.A. Whitaker (eds.), *Studies in Neurolinguistics, Volume 3* (pp. 65–121). New York: Academic Press.

Paradis, Michel (ed.). (1995). *Aspects of Bilingual Aphasia.* London: Pergamon Press.

Passel, J.S., Capps, R., and Fix, M. (2004). Undocumented immigrants: Facts and figures, http://www.urban.org/uploadedpdf/1000587_undoc_immigrants_facts.pdf

Paul, P.V. (1996). First- and second-language English literacy. *Volta Review, 98*, 5–16.

Peal, E., and Lambert, W.E. (1962). The relation of bilingualism to intelligence. *Psychological Monographs, 76*, 23.

Pedersen, P., and Marsella, A.J. (1982). Ethical crisis for cross cultural counseling and therapy. *Professional Psychology, 13*, 492–496.

Perez-Foster, R.M. (2001). When immigration is trauma: Guidelines for the individual and family clinician. *American Journal of Orthopsychiatry, 71*, 153–170.

Petitto, L.A., and Holowka, S. (2002). Evaluating attributions of delay and confusion in young bilinguals: Special insights from infants acquiring a signed and a spoken language. *Sign Language Studies, 3*, 4–33.

Pigatano, G.P., Ogano, M., and Amakusa B. (1997). A cross-cultural study on impaired self-awareness in Japanese patients with brain dysfunction. *Neuropsychiatry, Neuropsychology, Neuropsychiatry and Behavioral Neurology, 10*, 135–143.

Piper, T. (1993). And *then there were two: Children and second language learning*. Ontario: Pippin Publishing Ltd.

Plank, G.A. (2001). Application of the cross battery approach in the assessment of American Indian children: A viable alternative. American Indian and Alaskan Native. *Mental Health Research, 10*, 21–33.

Pontón, M.O., and León-Carreón, J. (Eds.) (2001). *Neuropsychology and the Hispanic patient*. Mahwah, NJ: Lawrence Erlbaum and Associates.

Pontón, M.O. (2001a). Hispanic culture in the United States. In: Pontón, M.O., and León-Carrión, J. (eds.) *Neuropsychology and the Hispanic patient* (pp. 15–38). Mahwah, NJ: Lawrence Erlbaum and Associates.

Pontón, M.O. (2001b). Research and assessment issues. In: Pontón, M.O., and León-Carrión, J. (eds.) *Neuropsychology and the Hispanic patient* (pp. 39–58). Mahwah, NJ: Lawrence Erlbaum and Associates.

Pontón, M.O., Gonzalez, J., and Mares, M. (1997). Rehabilitating brain damage in Hispanics. In J. León-Carrión (ed.), *Neuropsychological rehabilitation: Fundamentals, innovations, and directions* (pp.513–529). Delray Beach, FL: GR/St. Lucie Press.

Pontón, M.O., Satz, P., Herrera, L., Ortiz, F., Urrutia, C.P., Young, R., D'Elia, L.F., and Namerow, N. (1996). Normative data stratified by age and education for the neuropsychological Screening Battery for Hispanics (NeSBHIS): Initial report. *Journal of the International Neuropsychological Society, 2*, 96–104.

Portes, A., and Bach, R.L. (1985). *Latin Journey: Cuban and Mexican Immigrants in the United States*. Berkley: University of California Press.

Portes, A., and Borocsz, J. (1989). Contemporary immigration: Theoretical perspectives on determinants and modes of incorporation. *International Migration Review, 23*, 606–630.

Portes, A., and Rumbaut, R.G. (1990). *Immigrant America: A portrait*. Los Angeles: University of California Press.

Poser, U., Kohler, J.A., and Schönle, P.W. (1996). A historical review of neuropsychological rehabilitation in Germany. *Neuropsychological Rehabilitation, 6*, 257–278.

Potocky, M. (1996). Refugee children: How are they faring economically as adults? *Social Work, 41*, 364–373.

Prifitera, A., Saklofske, D.H., and Weiss, L.G. (2005). *WISC-IV clinical use and interpretation*. San Diego: Elsevier Academic.

Prifitera, A., Weiss, L.G., and Saklofske, D.H. (1998). The WISC-III in context. In A. Prifitera, and D.H. Saklofske (eds.), *WISC-III Clinical use and interpretation: Scientist-practitioner perspectives* (pp. 1–38.) San Diego CA: Academic Press.

Prigratano, G.P., Ogano, M., and Amakusa, B. (1997). A cross-cultural study on impaired self-awareness in Japanese patients with brain dysfunction. *Neuropsychiatry, Neuropsychology, and Behavioral Neurology, 10*, 135–143.

Pryor, C.B. (2001). New immigrants and refugees in American schools: Multiple voices. *Childhood Education, 77*(5), 275–283.

Puente, A.E., and Ardila, A. (2000). Neuropsychological assessment of Hispanics. In E. Fletcher-Jonzen, T. Stricklond and C.R. Reynolds (Eds.)., *Handbook of Cross-Cultural Neuropsychology* (pp. 87–104). New York: Kluwer Academic/Plenum Publishers.

Punamaki, R.L. (1996). Can ideological commitment protect children's psychological well-being in situations of political violence? *Child Development, 67,* 55–69.

Punamaki, R.L. (2001). From childhood trauma to adult well-being through psychosocial assistance of Chilean families. *Journal of Community Psychology,* 29(3), 281–303.

Pynoos, R., Steinberg, A., and Wraith, R. (1995). A developmental model of childhood traumatic stress. In D. Cicchetti and D. Cohen (eds.), *Developmental psychopathology, vol 2: Risk, disorder and adaptation* (pp. 72–95). New York: John Wiley and Sons.

Quinn, C. (2001). The developmental acquisition of English grammar as an additional language. *International Journal of Language and Communication Disorders, 36,* 309–314.

Ramírez, J., Yuen, S., Ramey, D., and Billings, D. (1991). *Final report: longitudinal study of structured English immersion strategy, early-exit and late-exit bilingual education programs for language-minority children.* (Vols. I, II) (No. 300-87-0156). San Mateo, CA: Aguirre International.

Ramón y Cajal, S. (1889). Sobre las fibras nerviosas de la capa granulos'e del cerebelo. *Internationale Monatschrift fur Antomie und Physiologie, 6,* 158–174.

Reed, L. and Day, J.A. (1995). Efficacy of a language enrichment program with high school students. In C.W. McIntyre and J.S. Pickering (eds.), *Clinical Studies of Multisensory Structured Language Education for Students with Dyslexia and Related Disorders* (pp. 36–43). Salem, OR: IMSLEC.

Reeve, M.E., Groce, N.E., Persing, J.A., and Magge, S.N. (2004). An international surgical exchange program for children with cleft lip/cleft palate in Manaus, Brazil: Patient and family expectations of outcome. *Journal of Craniofacial Surgery, 15,* 170–4.

Reitan, R.M., and Davison, L.A. (1974). *Clinical neuropsychology: Current status and applications.* Washington, DC: Winston.

Rey, G.J., Feldman, E., Rivas-Vasquez, R., Levin, B.E., and Benton, A. (1999). Neuropsychological test development for Hispanics. *Archives of Clinical Neuropsychology, 14,* 593–601.

Reynolds, C.R., and Kamphaus, R.W. (2004). *BASC-2 Behavior assessment system for children second edition manual.* Cricle Pines, MN: American Guidance Service, Inc.

Reynolds, C.R., and Mayfield, J. (1999) Introduction. In S. Goldstein and C.R. Reynolds (eds.), *Handbook of neurodevelopmental and genetic disorders in children.* New York: Guilford Press.

Reynolds, C.R., Kaufman, A.S., and McLean, J.E. (1987). Demographic characteristics and IQ among adults: Analysis of the WAIS-R standardization sample as a function of stratification variables. *Journal of School Psychology, 25,* 323–342.

Reynolds, C.R., Wilson, V.L, and Ramsey, M. (1999). Intellectual differences among Mexican Americans, Papagos, and Whites, independent of g. *Personality and Individual Differences, 27,* 1881–1887.

Reynolds, C.R. (2000). Methods for detecting and evaluating cultural bias in neuropsychological tests. In E. Fletcher-Janzen, T.L. Strickland, and C.R. Reynolds (eds.), *Handbook of cross-cultural neuropsychology.* (pp. 249–286) New York: Kluwer Academic/Plenum Publishers.

Rhodes, R.L., Kayser, H., and Hess, R.S. (2000). Neuropsychological differential diagnosis of Spanish-speaking preschool children. In E. Fletcher-Janzen, T.L. Strickland, and C.R. Reynolds (eds.), *Handbook of cross-cultural neuropsychology* (pp. 317–333). New York: Kluwer Academic/Plenum Publishers.

Richman, N. (1993). Children in situations of political violence. *Journal of Child Psychology, Psychiatry and Allied-Disciplines, 34,* 1286–1302.

Ries, J.. Potter, B., & Llorente, A. (2007). Multicultural aspects of pediatric neuropsychological intervention and rehabilitation. In S.J. Hunter and J. Donbers (Eds.), *Pediatric Neuropsychological Intervention* (pp. 47–67). New York: Cambridge Univ. Press.

Robertson, L.C., Lamb, M.R., and Knight, R.T. (1988). Effects of lesions of temporal-parietal junction on perceptual and attentional processing in humans. *Journal of Neuroscience, 8*, 3757–3769.

Rogers, R. (1997). *Clinical assessment of malingering and deception* (2nd ed.). New York: Guilford Press.

Rogler, L.H. (1996). Framing research on culture in psychiatric diagnosis: The case of the DSM-IV, *Psychiatry, 59*, 145–155.

Rogler, L.H. (1994). International migrations: A framework for directing research. *American Psychologist, 49*, 701–708.

Roid, G.H. (2003). *Stanford-Binet Intelligence Scale* (5th ed). Itasca, IL: Riverside.

Romaine, S. (1995). *Bilingualism.* (2nd ed.). Oxford, England: Blackwell.

Rorer, L.G., and Dawes, R.M. (1982). A base-rate bootstrap. *Journal of Consulting and Clinical Psychology, 50*, 419–425.

Rosa, E.M., and Leow, R.P. (2004). Awareness, different learning conditions, and second language development. *Applied Psycholinguistics, 25*, 269–292.

Rosselli, M., and Ardila, A. (2001). Normal and abnormal aging. In: Pontón, M.O., and León-Carrión, J. (eds.) *Neuropsychology and the Hispanic patient* (pp. 341–360). Mahwah, NJ: Lawrence Erlbaum and Associates.

Rosselli, M., Ardila, A., and Rosas, P. (1990). Neuropsychological assessment of illiterates: II. Language and praxic abilities. *Brain and Cognition, 12*, 281–296.

Rothman, D.J. (1971). *The discovery of the asylum.* Boston: Little and Brown.

Rourke, B.P., Fisk, J.L., and Strong, J.D. (1986). *Neuropsychological assessment of children: A treatment oriented approach.* New York: Guilford Press.

Rousseau, C., Drapeau, A., and Corin, E. (1996). School performance and emotional problems in refugee children. *American Journal of Orthopsychiatry, 66*, 239–251.

Rousseau, C., Drapeau, A., and Corin, E. (1997). The influence of culture and context on the pre- and post-migration experience of school aged refugees from Central America and Southeast Asia in Canada. *Social Science and Medicine, 44*, 1115–1127.

Rousseau, C. (1993). *The place of the unexpressed: Ethics and methodology for research with refugee children. Canada's Mental Health, 41*, 12–16.

Rousseau, C. (1995). The mental health of refugee children. *Transcultural Psychiatric Research Review, 32*, 299–331.

Rousseau, C., and Drapeau, A. (1998). Parent-child agreement on refugee children's psychiatric symptoms: A transcultural perspective. *Journal of the American Academy of Child and Adolescent* Psychiatry, 37, 629–636.

Rousseau, C., Said, T.M., Gagne, M.J., and Bibeau, G. (1998). Resilience in unaccompanied minors from the north of Somalia. *Psychoanalytic Review*, 85(4), 615–637.

Roysircar, G. (2004). Acculturation and ethnic identity concerns with immigrant and international student clients. In T.B. Smith (ed.), *Practicing multiculturalism: Affirming diversity in counseling and psychology* (pp. 256–275). New York: Allyn and Bacon.

Rudic, N., Rakic., V., Ispanovic-Radojkovic, V., Bojanin, S., and Lazic, D. (1993). Refugee children and young people in collective accommodation. In P. Kalicanin and J. Bukelic (eds.), *The stresses of war* (pp.85–89). Belgrade: Institute for Mental Health.

Rumbaut, R.G. (1991). The agony of exile: A study of the migration and adaptation of Indochinese refugee adults and children. In F.L. Ahearn and J.L. Athey (eds.), Refugee children: theory, research and services. *The Johns Hopkins series in contemporary medicine and public health* (pp. 53–91). Baltimore, MD: The Johns Hopkins University Press.

Russell, W.R., and Witty, C.W.M. (1952). Studies in traumatic epilepsy: Factors influencing incidence of epilepsy after brain wounds. *Journal of Neurology, Neurosurgery, and Psychiatry, 15*, 93–98.

Ryan, J.J., Carruthers, C.A., Miller, L.J., Souheaver, G.T., Gontkousky, S.T., and Zehr, M.D. (2003). Exploratory factor analysis of the Wechsler Abbreviated Scale of Intelligence (WASI) in adult standardization and clinical samples. *Applied Neuropsychology, 10*, 252–256.

Sack, W.H., Angell, R.H., Kinzie, D., and Rath, B. (1986). The psychiatric effects of massive trauma on Cambodian children: II. The family, the home, and the school. Journal of the American Academy of Child and Adolescent Psychiatry, 25, 377–383.

Sack, W.H., Clarke, G., Him, C., Dickason, D., Goff, B., Lanham, K., and Kinzie, J.D. (1993). A 6-year follow up study of Cambodian refuges adolescents traumatized as children. *Journal of the American Academy of Child and Adolescent Psychiatry, 32*, 431–437.

Sack, W.H., Clarke, G.N., and Seeley, J. (1995). Posttraumatic stress disorder across two generations of Cambodian refugees. *Journal of the American Academy of Child and Adolescent Psychiatry, 34*, 1160–1166.

Sack, W.H., Clarke, G.N., and Seeley, J. (1996). Multiple forms of stress in Cambodian adolescent refugees. *Child Development, 67*, 107–116.

Sack, W.H., Him, C., and Dickason, D. (1999). Twelve-year follow-up study of Khmer youths who suffered massive war trauma as children. *Journal of the American Academy of Child and Adolescent Psychiatry, 38*, 1173–1179.

Sack, W.H., McSharry, S., Clarke, G.N., Kinney, R., Seeley, J., and Lewinsohn, P. (1994). The Khmer Adolescent Project: I. Epidemiologic findings in two generations of Cambodian refugees. *Journal of Nervous and Mental Disease, 182*, 387–395.

Sack, W.H., Seeley, J.R., Clarke, G.N. (1997). Does PTSD transcend cultural barriers? A study from the Khmer adolescent refugee project. *Journal of the American Academy of Child and Adolescent Psychiatry*, 36, 49–54.

Saigh, P.A. (1991). The development of posttraumatic stress disorder following four different types of traumatization. *Behaviour Research and Therapy, 29*, 213–216.

Salvia, J.M., and Ysseldyke, J.E. (2001). *Assessment* (8th ed). Boston, MA: Houghton Mifflin Company.

Sanua, V.D. (1970). Immigration, migration, and mental illness: In E.B. Brody (ed.)., *Behavior in New Environments: Adaptation of Migrant Populations* (pp. 291–322). Beverly Hills, CA: Sage Publications.

Sastry, P.S. (1985). Lipids of nervous tissue: Composition and metabolism. *Progress in Lipid Research, 24*, 69–176.

Sattler, J.M. (2001). *Assessment of children*. Revised and updated fourth edition. San Diego, CA: Jeromre M. Sattler, Publisher, Inc.

Sattler, J.M., and Winget, B.M. (1970). Intelligence testing procedures as affected by expectancy and IQ. *Journal of Clinical Psychology, 26*, 446–448.

Sattler, J.M. (1998). *Clinical and forensic interviewing of children and families: Guidelines for the mental health, education, pediatric, and child maltreatment fields*. San Diego. CA: Jerome M. Sattler, Publisher, Inc.

Satz, P. (1993). Brain reserve capacity on symptom onset after brain injury: A formulation and review of the evidence for threshold theory. *Neuropsychology, 7*, 273–295.

Savin, D., Sack, W.H., Clarke, G.N., Meas, N., and Richart, I. (1996). The Khmer adolescent project: III. A study of trauma from Thailand's Site II refugee camp. *Journal of the American Academy of Child and Adolescent Psychiatry, 35*, 384–391.

Scar, S., and Weinberg, R.A. (1978). The influence of family background on intellectual attainment. *American Sociological Review, 43*, 674–692.

Schwarz, E.D., and Kowalski, J.M. (1991). Malignant memories: PTSD in children and adults after a school shooting. *Journal of the American Academy of Child and Adolescent Psychiatry, 30*, 936–944.

Sellers, A.H., Burns, W.J., and Guyrke, J. (2002). Differences in young children's IQ's on the Wechsler Preschool and Primary Scale of Intelligence – Revised as a function of stratification variables. *Applied Neuropsychology, 9*, 65–73.

Semel, E., Wiig, E.H., and Secord, W.A. (2003). *Clinical Evaluation of Language Fundamentals* (4th ed.). San Antonio, TX: PsychCorp.

Servan-Schreiber, D., Le Lin, B., and Birmaher, B. (1998). Prevalence of posttraumatic stress disorder and major depressive disorder in Tibetan refugee children. *Journal of the American Academy of Child and Adolescent Psychiatry, 37*, 874–879.

Seymour, H.N., and Roeper, T. (1999). Grammatical acquisition of African American English. In O.L. Taylor and L.B. Leonard (eds.), *Language acquisition across North America: Cross cultural and cross-linguistic perspectives* (pp. 109–152). San Diego, CA: Singular Publishing Group, Inc.

Shepherd, M.J. (2001). History lessons. In A.S. Kaufman and N.L. Kaufman (eds.), *Specific learning disabilities and difficulties in children and adolescents*. New York: Cambridge University Press.

Shepherd, I., and Leathem, J. (1999). Factors affecting performance in cross-cultural neuropsychology: From a New Zealand biocultural perspective. *Journal of the International Neuropsychological Society, 5*, 83–84.

Sheridan, S.M., and Gutkin, T.B. (2000). The ecology of school psychology: Examining and changing our paradigm for the 21st century. *School Psychology Review, 29*, 485–501.

Shonkoff, J.P., and Phillips, D.A. (eds.). (2000). Communicating and learning. In *From neurons to neighborhoods: The science of early childhood development* (pp. 124–162). Washington, DC: National Academy Press.

Shorris, E. (1992). *Latinos*. New York: Norton.

Silove, D., Sinnerbrink, I., Field., Manicavasagar, V., and Steel, Z. (1997). Anxiety, depression and PTSD in asylum seekers: Associations with pre-migration trauma and post-migration stressors. *British Journal of Psychiatry, 170*, 351–357.

Simpson, G., Mohr, R., and Redman, A. (2000). Cultural variations in the understanding of traumatic brain injury and brain injury rehabilitation. *Brain Injury, 14*, 125–40.

Sinnerbrink, I., Silvone, D., Field, A., Steel, Z., and Manicavasagar, V. (1997). Compounding of pre-migration trauma and post-migration stress in asylum seekers. *The Journal of Psychology, 131*, 463–470.

Slomine, B.S., McCarthy, M.L., Ding, R. et al. (2006). Health care utilization and needs after pediatric traumatic brain injury. *Pediatrics, 117*, 663–674.

Smedley, A. (1993). *Race in North America: Origin and evolution of a world view*. Boulder, CO: Westview.

Sohlberg, M.M., and Mateer, C.A. (2001). Variables contributing to neurological and neurobehavioral recovery. In M.M. Sohlberg and C.A. Mateer (eds.). *Cognitive rehabilitation: An integrative neuropsychological approach* (pp. 59–88). New York: Guilford Press.

Sourander, A. (1998). Behavior problems and traumatic events of unaccompanied refugee minors. *Child Abuse and Neglect, 22*, 719–727.

Sparrow, S.S., Balla, D.A., and Cicchetti, D.V. (1984). *Vineland Adaptive Behavior Scales Interview Edition*. Circle Pines, MN: American Guidance Service.

Speorman, C.E. (1927). *The abilities of man*. New York: McMillan.

Spreen, O., and Strauss, E. (1998). *A compendium of neuropsychological tests: Administration, norms, and commentary* (2nd ed.). New York: Oxford University Press.

Srole, L., Langner, T.S., and Mitchell, S.T. (1962). *Mental health in the metropolis: The Midtown Manhattan Study*. New York: New York University Press.

Stansbury, J.P., Reid, K.J., Reker, D.M., Duncan, P.W., Marshall, C.R., and Rittman, M. (2004). Why ethnic designation matters for stroke rehabilitation: Comparing VA administrative data and clinical records. *Journal of Rehabilitation Research and Development, 41*, 269–278.

Stein, B., Comer, D., Gardner, W., and Kelleher, K. (1999). Prospective study of displaced children's symptoms in wartime Bosnia. *Social Psychiatric Epidemiology, 34*, 464–469.

Sternberg, R.J. (1984). Toward a triarchic theory of human intelligence. *The Behavioral and Brain Sciences, 7*, 269–315.

Sternberg, R.J. (1997). A Triarchic view of giftedness: Theory and practice. In N. Coleongelo and G.A. Danis (Eds.), *Handbook of gifted education* (pp. 43–53). Boston: Allyn and Bacon.

Stuart, S. (2002). Communication: Speech and language. In M.L. Batshaw (ed.), *Children with disabilities* (5th ed.; pp. 229–241). Baltimore, MD: Paul H. Books Publishing Co.

Sue, S., and Zane, N. (1987). The role of culture and cultural techniques in psychotherapy: A critique and reformulation. *American Psychologist, 42*, 37–45.

Suinn, R.M., Richard-Figueroa, K., Len, S., and Vigil, P. (1987). The Suinn-Law Asian Self-Identity Acculturation Scale: An initial report. *Educational and Psychological Measurement, 6*, 103–112.

Summerfield, D. (2000). Childhood, war, refugeedom and trauma: Three core questions for mental health professionals. *Transcultural Psychiatry, 37*, 417–433.

Suzuki, L.A., and Kugler, J.F., (1995). Intelligence and personality assessment: Multicultural perspectives. In J.G. Ponterotto, J.M. Casas, L.A. Suzuki, and C.M. Alexander (eds.), *Handbook of multicultural counseling* (pp. 493–515). Thousand Oaks, CA; Sage Publications.

Tager-Flusberg, H., and Sullivan, K. (1998). Early language development in children with mental retardation. In J.A. Burack, R.M. Hodapp, and E. Zigler (eds.), *Handbook of mental retardation and development* (pp. 208–239). New York: Cambridge University Press.

Tannen, D. (1980). Spoken/written language and the oral/literate continuum. In *Proceedings of the 6th annual meeting, Berkely Linguistic Society* (pp. 207–218).

Taylor, O.L. (1999). Cultural issues and language acquisition. In O.L. Taylor and L.B. Leonard (eds.), *Language acquisition across North America: Cross-cultural and cross-linguistic perspectives* (pp. 21–37). San Diego, CA: Singular Publishing Group, Inc.

Teeter, P.A., and Semrud-Clikeman, M. (1997). *Child Neuropsychology. Assessment and interventions for neurodevelopmental disorders*. Boston: Allyn and Bacon.

Thabet, A.A., Abed, Y., and Vostanis, P. (2004). Comorbidity of PTSD and depression among refugee children during war conflict. *Journal of Child Psychology and Psychiatry, 45*, 533–542.

Thabet, A.A., and Vostanis, P. (2000). Post traumatic stress disorder reactions in children of war: A longitudinal study. *Child Abuse and Neglect, 24*, 291–298.

Thurstone, L.L. (1938). *Primary mental abilities*. Chicago: University of Chicago Press.

Tomás Rivera Policy Institute. (2003). *El sueño de su casa: The home ownership potential of Mexican-Heritage Families*. Los Angeles: Author.

Tousignant, M., Habimana, E., Biron, C., Malo, C., Sidoli-LeBlanc, E., and Bendris, N. (1999). The Quebec adolescent refugee project: psychopathology and family variables in a sample from 35 nations. *Journal of the American Academy of Child and Adolescent* Psychiatry, *38*, 1426–1432.

Tulsky, D.S., Saklofske, D.H., Wilkins, C., and Weiss, L.G. (2001). Development of a general ability index for the Wechsler Intelligence Scale-Third Edition. *Psychological Assessment, 13*, 566–571.

Unger, J.B., Gallaher, P., Shakib, S., Ritt-Olson, A., Palmer, P.H., and Johnson, A.C. (2002). The AHIMSA Acculturation Scale: A new measure of acculturation for adolescents in multicultural society. *Journal of Early Adolescence, 22*, 225–251.

United Nations High Commissioner for Refugees. (1992). *Handbook on procedures and criteria for determining refugee status under the 1951 convention and the 1967 protocol relating to the status of refugees*. Geneva: United Nations High Commissioner for Refugees.

United Nations High Commissioner for Refugees. (2001). *Refugees by numbers*. New York: United Nations High Commissioner for Refugees.

U. S. Census Bureau. (1998). *Statistical Abstract of the United States: 1998*. http://www.Census.gov.

U.S. Census Bureau. (March, 2004). U.S. Interim Projections by Age, Sex, Race and Hispanic Origin. http://www.census.gov/ipc/www/usinterimproj/ Washington DC: Author.

United States Census Bureau (2003). Poverty status of the population in 1999 by sex, age, Hispanic origin. and race. March 2000. See http:www.census.gov/populations/socdemo/hispanic/pp1–171/Tab14–1.pdf.

U.S. Census Bureau. (2001). *Census 2000 Brief*. Washington, DC: U.S. Bureau of the Census.

U.S. Department of Health and Human Services. (2004). Health disparities experienced by Hispanics. Washington, DC: Author.

U.S. Immigration and Naturalization Service. (1975). *1974 statistical yearbook of the Immigration and Naturalization Service.* Washington, DC: U.S. Government Printing Office.

U.S. Immigration and Naturalization Service. (1981). *1980 statistical yearbook of the Immigration and Naturalization Service.* Washington, DC: U.S. Government Printing Office.

U.S. Immigration and Naturalization Service. (1991). *1990 statistical yearbook of the Immigration and Naturalization Service.* Washington, DC: U.S. Government Printing Office.

Uomoto, J.M., and Wong, T.M. (2000). Multicultural perspectives on the neuropsychology of brain injury assessment and rehabilitation. In E. Fletcher-Janzen, T. Strickland, and C.R. Reynolds (eds.), *Handbook of cross-cultural neuropsychology* (pp. 169–184). New York: Kluwer Academic/Plenum.

Valencia, R.R., Suzuki, L.A., and Salinas, M.F. (2001). Test bias. In: R.R. Valencia and L.A. Suzuki (eds.), *Intelligence testing and minority students: Foundations, performance factors, and assessment issues.* Thousand Oaks, CA: Sage.

van Gorp, W.G., Myers, H.F., and Drake, E.B. (2000). Neuropsychology training: Ethnocultural considerations in the context of general competency training. In E. Fletcher-Jaugen, T.L. Strickland, and C.R. Reynolds (Eds), *Handbook of Cross-cultural Neuropsychology* (pp. 19–27). New York: Kluwer/Plenum Publishers.

Vázquez, J.Z. (1994). *Una historia de Mexico [A history of Mexico].* Mexico City: Editorial Patria.

Verney, S.P., Granholm, E., Marshall, S.P., Malcarne, V.L., and Saccuzzo, D.P. (2005). Culture-fair cognitive assessment. Information processing and psychophysiological approaches. *Assessment, 12,* 303–319.

Vygotsky, L., and Luria, A. (1930/1993). *Studies on the history of behavior: Ape, primitive, and child.* Ed. and trans. Victor I. Golod and Jane E. Knox. Hillsdale, NJ: Lawrence Erlbaum and Associates.

Wagner, R.K., Torgesen, J.K., and Rashotte, C.A. (1999). *The Comprehensive Test of Phonological Processing* (CTOPP). Austin, TX: Pro-Ed.

Waniganayake, M. (2001). From playing with guns to playing with rice: The challenges of working with refugee children. An Australian perspective. *Childhood Education, 77,* 289–294.

Warner, C., and Nelson, N.W. (2000). Assessment of communication, language, and speech: Questions of "What to do next?" In B.A. Bracken (ed.), *The psychoeducational assessment of preschool children* (pp. 145–185). Boston: Allyn and Bacon.

Wartofsky, M. (1983). The child's construction of the world and the world construction of the child: From historical epistemology to historical psychology. In F.S. Kessel and A.W. Sigel (eds.), *The child and other cultural inventions* (pp. 188–215). New York: Praeger.

Watanabe, Y., Shiel, A., McLellan, D.L., Kurihara, M., and Hayashi, K. (2001). The impact of traumatic brain injury on family members living with patients: A preliminary study in Japan and the U. K. *Disability and Rehabilitation, 23,* 370–378.

Wechsler, D. (1949). *Manual for the Wechsler Intelligence Scale for Children.* New York: The Psychological Corporation.

Wechsler, D. (1950). Cognitive, Conative, and non-intellective intelligence. *American Psychologist, 5,* 78–83.

Wechsler, D. (1974). *Manual for the Wechsler Intelligence Scale for Children-Revised.* San Antonio, TX: The Psychological Corporation.

Wechsler, D. (1991). *Manual for the Wechsler Intelligence Scale for Children-Third Edition.* San Antonio, TX: The Psychological Corporation.

Wechsler, D. (1968) *Escala de Inteligencia Wechsler para Adultos.* New York: Psychological Corporation.

Wechsler, D. (1997). *Wechsler Adult Intelligence Scale-Third Edition Administration and Scoring Manual.* San Antonio: The Psychological Corporation.

Wechsler, D. (1999). *Manual for the Wechsler Abbreviated Scale of Intelligence*. San Antonio, TX: Harcourt Assessment.

Wechsler, D. (2003). *Manual for the Wechsler Intelligence Scale for Children-Fourth Edition*. San Antonio, TX: The Psychological Corporation.

Wechsler, D. (2004). Manual for the WISC-IV Spanish: Wechsler Intelligence Scale for Children - Fourth Edition - Spanish (2004). San Antonio, Texas: Harcourt Assessment.

Wechsler, D., Kaplan, E., Fein, D., Kramer, J., Morris, R., Delis, D., et al. (2004). *WISC-IV Integrated Wechsler Intelligence Scale for Children Fourth Edition - Integrated Technical and Interpretative Manual*. San Antonio Texas: Harcourth Assessment, Inc.

Weine, S. M., Becker, D.F., McGlashan, T.H., and Laub, D. (1995). Psychiatric consequences of "ethnic cleansing": Clinical assessments and trauma testimonies of newly resettled Bosnian refugees. *American Journal of Psychiatry,* 152(4), 536–542.

Weine, S., Becker, D.F., McGlashan, T.H., and Vojvoda, D. (1995). Adolescent survivors of "ethnic cleansing": Observations on the first year in America. *Journal of the American Academy of Child and Adolescent Psychiatry*, 34, 1153–1159.

Weinick, R.M., Zuvekas, S.H., Cohen, J.W. (2000). Racial and ethnic differences in access to and use of health care services, 1977 to 1996. *Medical Care Research and Review, 57*, 36–54.

Wernicke, C. (1874). *Der Aphasische Symptomencomplex*. Breslau: Cohn and Weigert.

Westermeyer, J. (1991). Psychiatric services for refugee children: An overview. In F.L. Ahearn and J.L. Athey (eds.), Refugee children: theory, research and services. *The Johns Hopkins series in contemporary medicine and public health* (pp. 127–162). Baltimore, MD: The Johns Hopkins University Press.

Whelan, T.B. (1999). Integrative developmental neuropsychology: A general systems and social-ecological approach to the neuropsychology of children with neurogenetic disorders. In S. Goldstein and C.R. Reynolds (eds.), *Handbook of neurodevelopmental and genetic disorders in children* (pp. 84–98). New York: Guilford Press.

Wiig, E.H., Secord, W.A., and Semel, E. (2004). *Clinical Evaluation of Language Fundamentals Preschool* (2nd ed.). San Antonio, TX: PsychCorp.

Winick, M., and Noble, A. Cellular response in rats during malnutrition at various age. *Journal of nutrition, 89*, 300–3006.

Winick, M., and Rosso, P. (1969). Head circumference and cellular growth of the brain in normal and marasmic children, *Journal of Pediatrics, 74*, 774–778.

Wolff, P.H., Bereket, T., Egasso, H., and Tesfay, A. (1995). *The orphans of Eritrea: A comparison study. Journal of Child Psychology, Psychiatry and Allied Disciplines, 36*, 633–644.

Wong, T.M., Strickland, T., Fletcher-Janzen, E., Ardila, A., and Reynolds, C.R. (2000). Theoretical and practical issues in neuropsychological assessment and treatment of culturally dissimilar patients. In E. Fletcher-Janzen, T. Strickland, and C.R. Reynolds (eds.), *Handbook of cross-cultural neuropsychology* (pp. 3–18). New York: Kluwer Academic/Plenum Publishers.

Woodcock, R.W. (1981). *Bateria Woodcock de Proficiencia en el Idioma*. Allen, Texas: DLM Teaching Resources.

Woodcock, R.W., and Muñoz-Sandoval, A.F. (2001). *Woodcock-Muñoz Language Survey Normative Update*. Itasca, IL: Riverside Publishing.

Woodcock, R., McGrew, K., and Mather, N. (2001). *Woodcock-Johnson III*. Itasca, IL: Riverside Publishing.

Woodcock, R.W. (1991). *Woodcock Language Proficiency Battery – Revised English and Spanish Form*. Itasca, IL: Riverside Publishing.

Woodcock, R.W., and Johnson, M.B. (1989). *Woodcock-Johnson Tests of Cognitive Ability –* Itasca, IL: Riverside Publishing.

Woodcock, R.W., and Muñoz-Sandoval, A.F. (1993a). *Woodcock-Muñoz Language Survey, English Form*. Itasca, IL: Riverside Publishing.

Woodcock, R.W., and Muñoz-Sandoval, A.F. (1993b). *Woodcock-Muñoz Language Survey, Spanish Form*. Itasca, IL: Riverside Publishing.

Woodcock, R.W., and Muñoz-Sandoval, A.F. (1995). *Woodcock Language Proficiency Battery –* Revised–Spanish. Itasca, IL: Riverside Publishing.

Woodcock, R.W., Muñoz-Sandoval, A.F., McGrew, K., Mather, N., and Schrank, F. (2004a). *Batería Woodcock-Muñoz Pruebas de habilidad cognitiva* (3rd ed.). Itasca, IL: Riverside Publishing.

Woodcock, R.W., Muñoz-Sandoval, A.F., McGrew, K., Mather, N., and Schrank, F. (2004b). *Batería Woodcock-Muñoz Pruebas de aprovechamiento* (3rd ed.). Itasca, IL: Riverside Publishing.

World Health Organization. (1998). *The World Health Report. Geneva: Author.*

Wu, T. (2004). A culturally sensitive health care practice model – Theory construction and its testing. *The American Journal of Chinese Medicine, 32* (3), 467–485.

Yamane, T. (1967). *Elementary sampling theory.* Englewood Cliffs, NJ: Prentice-Hall.

Yeates, K.O., Taylor, H.G., Woodrome, S.E., Wade, S.L., Stancin, T., and Drotar, D. (2002). Race as a moderator of parent and family outcomes following pediatric traumatic brain injury. *Journal of Pediatric Psychology, 27,* 393–403.

Zhimin, L. (2003). Self-care in Chinese school-age children with nephrotic syndrome. *American Journal of Maternal and Child Nursing, 28,* 81–85.

Zimmerman, I.L., Steiner, V.G., and Pond, R.E. (2002). *Preschool Language Scales* (4th ed.). San Antonio, TX: Psychological Corporation.

Zindi, F. (1994). Differences in psychometric performance. *The Psychologist: Bulletin of the British Psychological Society, 7,* 549–552.

Appendix
Sample Report

Identifying Information and Reason for Referral

E.P. is a 27-year-old, right-handed, Hispanic (foreign national born in a province in Southern Mexico[1] from a Nahuatl indigenous background), single male. He attended school in the U.S. (e.g., Good High School in Odessa, Texas), but he did not complete high school (or achieve a GED) after he immigrated (by himself without any reported assistance) to be reunited with his family approximately 10 years ago. He appeared to have attended school for approximately 10–11 years in rural school districts, where the quality of education was below national standards in the U.S. and Mexico. He was employed as an unskilled laborer (e.g., construction aid, cook) in the U.S. a portion of his life prior to his incarceration.

Mr. P was referred by a Texas State Court (subsequent to a request from the Office of the Public Defender for No Where County, Texas) for neuropsychological evaluation in an attempt to assess his present level of cognitive functioning and determine whether he suffers from encephalopathy and mental retardation. Mr. P has been charged with multiple counts of murder in the first degree, and the State of Texas is seeking the death penalty. He is reportedly receiving psychotropic medication at this time (verified through medical records from his detention center), including Ritalin (15 mg/day) and Lexapro (10 mg/day).

Relevant History/Background Information and Review of Records

Mr. P was charged with multiple counts of first-degree murder as a result of homicides committed during multiple shootings and armed robberies during a period of 48 hours while under the influence of controlled substances, including methamphetamine (corroborated from independent laboratory records). During the course of such shootings he was able to elude capture through the use of facial

---

[1] All demographic and other identifying information have been modified to protect his identity.

camouflaging. During the clinical interview, he admitted that such events occurred, but he reportedly was not able to recall details about the incidents. A review of police reports and records, interviews with news media sources involved in the case and review of videotapes provided, verbal reports obtained from eyewitnesses, and verbal reports from defense counsel supported the occurrence of the alleged events. Furthermore, Mr. P reportedly confessed and was subsequently charged with the aforementioned capital offenses. He admitted to a history of previous involvement with the law, particularly in 1999, when he was arrested and charged with the assault of a Texas State Trooper and an Oklahoma Police Officer (verified through court records). He subsequently served approximately 12 months in jail for those offenses. Review of records failed to reveal the presence of other criminal behavior, except petty theft. When asked, he indicated behaving appropriately while incarcerated at the present center, information consistent with data provided by the detention center's warden and review of records.

Mr. P was able to correctly recall portions of his history, but some information had to be obtained from records provided by a detective working for defense counsel and data obtained from affidavits ascertained during a trip to his native country by this clinician from individuals familiar with Mr. P's past. Family members were interviewed but not his biological mother, as she perished in an automobile accident 12 years ago. These individuals did not note developmental delays in early motor functions but did note difficulties in speech development, although the reports were sketchy. For example, one of his sisters noted that he exhibited appropriate vocabulary and speech and language development, but that his articulation was not within normal limits, thus making him difficult to understand by individuals outside his home (dysarthria). No other information was remarkable or available in this regard. In addition, it appears as if Mr. P exhibited mild adaptive delays in self-help skills as he was growing up, and his sisters reportedly helped Mr. P to dress and bathe past the age of expectation (reportedly until about the age of 8 years, delayed even within a cultural context). With regard to past family medical history, several members of his family noted the presence of "alcoholism and psychiatric disorders," the latter predominantly associated with severe mood disturbances, including anxiety, recurrent unipolar depression and possible bipolar disorder, and postpartum depression, all requiring treatment, and in some instances inpatient hospitalization. The interview with these family members also revealed that Mr. P had an impoverished background that included physical and sexual abuse, malnutrition, and neglect. He also experienced poor living conditions in his native country, and quality of housing was poor and without basic necessities such as running water and other services as he was growing up in rural southern or suburban northern Mexico. With regard to the reported past abuse, according to his sisters, Mr. P was reportedly physically abused as a child (statutory rape) "by a woman" who had sexual contact with him at the age of 12 years for an extended period of time ("a neighbor" of his family that resided close to them). His siblings additionally reported that he had been exposed to a significant amount of violence as he grew up in his home, the result of marital violence between his parents ("his mother was regularly beaten and raped by his father while he was intoxicated," and Mr. P was exposed to these events), and physical violence perpetuated upon him by his father, including severe and "odd" punishments (hit with tree branches and power extension cords, made to kneel on the blades of a saw or corn kernels until his knees bled, etc.).

During the clinical interview, Mr. P reported selected aspects of his medical history, most important and relevant to this case, his history of multiple brain injuries as he fell from a moving vehicle and a severe TBI that occurred in a motorcycle-automobile collision in which he lost consciousness for an extended period of time (GCS=3 upon arrival at the hospital; 12 unconscious days; extended PTA; all corroborated by existing hospital records). Mr. P's family also reported several incidents during his childhood that might have resulted in neurological involvement, including an incident resulting in a concussion in which he was hit in the head as a small child by a beast of burden. However, except for the motorcycle accident, the family did not seek medical care for those incidents due to economic factors and the nonavailability of "formal medical care in Mexico"; only a verbal report from a local healer ("curandera") was available. However, a record documenting the car accident was recently located by defense counsel, an event in which one individual may have perished, supporting the report provided by the client and his family related to the severity of the incident. He also reported occasional headaches, events treated with over-the-counter analgesics. Imaging was conducted in the past, but reports from those procedures were not available. However, hospital records (daily medical notes) from his extended hospitalization noted above indicated the presence of a remarkable CT scan indicative of "frontal bilateral diffuse involvement." A repeat scan was not conducted.

With regard to past psychiatric history, Mr. P reported the presence of auditory hallucinations while incarcerated and prior to incarceration, and it is possible that he may have received psychiatric and/or psychological care prior to his incarceration, but records of such treatment(s) are not available. These hallucinations predated his current psychopharmacological treatment. However, it appears as if he has experienced bouts of depression which may have gone untreated in the past bouts of depression with psychotic features, probably exacerbated by his past drug use. Such events were differentially diagnosed from cultural issues that may explain such events such as his participation in "brujería," which he admitted during the clinical interview. He has received psychiatric care while incarcerated and is currently receiving medication as noted above but has never received protracted psychotherapy throughout his life.

Review of academic records obtained during a visit by this clinician and his mitigation specialist to his past school districts in Mexico revealed the presence of significant variability in school performance. Records provided suggest that Mr. P attended first through sixth grades at a primary rural school in Mexico (grades and similar academic information is not available). He attended secondary school (grades seven through nine) at a secondary suburban school in northern Mexico.

According to his report cards, Mr. P received the following grades in his first year of secondary school, (translating grades from the Mexican educational system to the U.S. educational system, a posture that may have diminished validity): B in Spanish, B in math, C in additional Spanish instruction, B in biology, B in philosophy, B in chemistry, B in history, B in geography, A in civics, B in PE, A in Art, and a B in a metal works course. His grades from his second year of secondary school indicate that he received the following grades: C in Spanish, C in math, B in additional Spanish instruction, C in biology, C in physics, C in chemistry, C in history, B in geography, C in civics, B in PE, B in art, and a C in a technology course. The next year's grades from secondary school indicate that he received the following grades: C in Spanish, C in math, C in additional Spanish instruction, C in biology, B in physics, C in chemistry, C in history, C in geography, C in civics, B in PE, A in art, and a B in a technology course. School records appear to indicate that Mr. P's GPA from secondary school was B-C (7.6/10). His record from the equivalent of high school in the U.S. (grades 10 through 12) while living in Mexico, indicate that he received the following grades while in the 10th grade: C in reading and editing, C in languages, C in philosophy, C in sociology, and A in Art History. However, there are reports that either his family or colleagues may have assisted him throughout his academic career while in Mexico. Subsequent to arrival in the U.S., Mr. P attended high school as an ESL. student. He was not placed in special education; however, according to school officials, there was no "Special Education available for Spanish-speaking students at that time in TX," and "psychoeducational testing was only conducted upon parental request," a request never entertained by his family. Therefore, no psychoeducational assessments are available. At that time he received the following grades for the first semester of 11th grade: C in Reading II, B in ESL, F in American History, B in Algebra I, and an A (PE). Mr. P received an "N" for his classes for second semester 11th grade. The "N" may indicate that no grade was issued due to his increased absences (as high as 23 absences in two of his classes). The same records indicate that he was not in school the next year (12th grade) and that he dropped out at that time. No efforts were made by his school district or his family to have him enroll in school again.

The interview with Mr. P failed to reveal any type of military service in the U.S., information later confirmed by this clinician's personnel through a contact with the U.S. Military Clearing House. The interview with Mr. P revealed a history of employment in unskilled positions. He reportedly was employed in the U.S. in the construction industry building "streets and houses." He essentially was a carpenter, as described by one of his former supervisors who was willing to assist in the case. He was also employed as a "cook" in restaurants. However, he did well in these positions and rose to "cook manager" in one position, and his performance in all of the above was reportedly very good according to his former supervisors, all of whom missed "his performance" after he left them. He was unable to remember any other specific employment experiences, yet noted having worked in other places. Records were not available.

With regard to interpersonal relationships, Mr. P indicated that he was single. When asked, he indicated that he had two children ages one and seven years. His "girlfriend" reportedly left him and is now with "another man." He has no contact with his children or his former partner. He also indicated leaving his first girlfriend because "she fought and drank too much." No other romantic relationships were reported. Social problems were not reported while in school in the U.S., where his "drug use" began as he interacted with his friends, the "wrong crowd." He reported having used several controlled substances (PCP, marijuana, and meta amphetamine) for a protracted period of time and substantial amounts of alcohol but did not recall frequency or specific magnitude of use. He was able to recall the approximate onset (age 9 years for alcohol, and age 17 years for all other drugs).

Review of psychological records from evaluations while incarcerated indicated that Mr. P had undergone a previous psychological evaluation[2] in April of 2002 under the care of Dr. Nogood. At that time, Mr. P was administered the WAIS-III (translated from English into Spanish) in which he obtained a Full Scale IQ score of 70. At that time, he also obtained respective Verbal and Performance Scale Indices scores of 73 and 73. Acculturation or language proficiency measures were not administered at that time.

On June 2004, Dr. Worst, a forensic state psychologist, evaluated Mr. P's competency. This evaluation reportedly lasted approximately 15 minutes. Dr. Worst stated that she was unable to determine if Mr. P met the statutory requirements for competence, in part due to the client's primitive English communication skills. Dr. Worst reportedly conducted a second evaluation in July 2002. This evaluation was conducted through an interpreter (despite the fact that such a course of action should not be taken in forensic evaluations, not to mention one where capital punishment is being sought). The evaluation lasted approximately one hour and 30 minutes and was conducted prior to Mr. P's being medicated. As a result of this evaluation, Dr. Worst reported that Mr. P's intellectual functioning (assessed in English through a translator) was grossly estimated to be in the low range of functioning, but provided no scores or an explanation how she arrived at such a diagnostic conclusion. When asked for her opinion, as noted in Mr. P's report, the interpreter stated that Mr. P used "basic Spanish," "poor grammar," and "incomplete sentences." According to records provided, the "interpreter (not a health care worker) estimated Mr. P's functioning to be 'low' due to 'drugs.'" Raw data had been reportedly lost and were not available.[3]

---

[2] It should also be noted that none of the aforementioned evaluations, despite their forensic nature, ever addressed the issue of response bias, a posture inconsistent with current minimum standards of practice.

[3] Just as egregious and unethical, an interpreter was employed and/or the use of English was employed as a way of communicating with an individual who is predominantly fluent in Spanish, and this information used as the basis for many of the "expert" opinions expressed, despite significant literature indicating that such a course of action should not be taken, particularly in this case in which capital punishment was under consideration.

Behavioral Observations

Mr. P was evaluated in an attorney-client contact room within the confines of a state prison. He was evaluated without upper extremity restraints. The entire examination was conducted in Spanish, as he is predominantly fluent using Spanish (see below). Although the court had explained the purpose of this examination, similar to the introduction provided prior to the start of his evaluation by defense counsel, ethical (consent) and legal (limits of confidentiality) and other information was initially addressed with the client by this clinicion. During the initial interview and the evaluation, his speech was slow but coherent. The content of his speech was impoverished for someone his age (e.g., rudimentary vocabulary), and he exhibited moderate dysarthria. He was well oriented to person, time, and place.

Although Mr. P initially appeared to be somewhat apprehensive initially, he slowly acclimated to the assessment situation and appeared to put forth appropriate effort on all tasks. He initiated conversations about his present condition (incarceration, where he is reportedly being treated well).

In response to confrontational questions surrounding his present condition, he exhibited significant remorse but he indicated that he was unable to remember specifics related to the events that took place. He noted having seen the videos, and agreed that it was him, but reported not being able to "remember being there." A discussion of his childhood did not elicit blunt affect. Overall, affect appeared to be within normal limits. Mood appeared to be within normal limits (he is being medicated). The assessment environment was quiet throughout most of the examination, thus reducing threats to the validity of this evaluation. Mr. P was asked to show the examiner scars found in his knees from the reported abuse, and he reluctantly agreed, displaying significant scarring from such incidents. He refused to talk about his parents' marital difficulties and his own sexual abuse as he was growing up but did not deny them.

Mr. P's demeanor was observed outside of the one-on-one testing situation when he took small breaks during the course of the two-day evaluation to use the restroom (he had lunch in the test room). During these observational periods, he was at all times appropriate from a behavioral standpoint consistent with his imprisonment records of unremarkable behavior. Although Mr. P did not wear upper extremity cuffs, at no time did this examiner feel unsafe in the exam room while assessing this individual.

Procedures and Tests Administered

Batería Woodcock-Muñoz-Pruebas de Aprovechamiento-Revisada (Letter-Word
    Identification and Reading Understanding only) (WMPA-R)
Batería Woodcock-Muñoz-Pruebas de Habilidad Cognitiva-Revisada (WMPHC-R)
Beck Anxiety Inventory (Spanish version)

Beck Depression Inventory (Spanish version)
Clinical Interview with the Patient (Spanish)
Color Trails Test 1 & 2 (CTT) (Spanish Instructions and American Norms)
Draw-A-Person Test (Spanish Instructions)
Grooved Pegboard Test (Spanish Instructions and American Norms)
Judgement of Line Orientation, Form H (Spanish Instructions and North American
    Norms)
Multilingual Aphasia Examination (Spanish Token Test) (Spanish Administration,
    American Norms)
Pontón-Satz Boston Naming Test (Spanish Instructions and Hispanic Norms)
    (BNT)
Reitan-Kløve Sensory Perceptual Examination - Except Tactile Form
    Recognition –Spanish Instructions and North American Norms
Rey 15-Item Memory Test (Spanish Instructions)
Rey 15-Word Memory Test (Modified-Spanish Instructions)
Rey-Osterrieth Complex Figure Test (Copy and 30' Delayed Recall) (Spanish
    Instructions and Hispanic Norms)
Stroop Interference Test (Spanish Version, American Norms)
Symptom Validity Test – (SVT) (Spanish Instructions)
Test of Nonverbal Intelligence-Second Edition (TONI-2) (North American Norms and
    Norms from Studies with Hispanic and Aboriginal Populations)
WHO-UCLA Auditory Verbal Learning Test (WHO-UCLA-AVLT) (Spanish Version)
    (Hispanic Norms)

Assessment Results

Assessment Validity

Due to the legal nature of this case, coupled with the fact that Mr. P may have
been motivated to present himself in a good light (or ill) as a result of his
impending legal proceedings, several procedures believed to be sensitive to the
presence of feigned symptom exaggeration and/or response bias were administered. The results of these procedures revealed that Mr. P was being straightfor-
ward and honest in his responses to test items. He performed within the range
of expectation on the Rey 15-Item Memory Test (Score = 15/15). Similarly, his
scores on the DCT fell within normal limits (50th to 75th percentile). On a
more complex probabilistic procedure (SVT), his performance fell within
expectation, as he obtained a perfect score on all three trials. Other tests indices
obtained throughout the assessment also supported a hypothesis suggesting the
presence of appropriate effort, including better recognition than recall during
memory tasks, lower levels of performance on increasingly more difficult test
items consistent with expectation, as well as expected performance and other

test indices (validity indices). The level of rapport established with this individual also was appropriate.

However, it should be noted that limitations are associated with this component of his examination, as there are no norms for individuals from his ethnic (not racial) background on the SVT and the DCT.

Current Academic Functioning (Reading, Mathematics, Written Language) and Acculturation Level

Informal assessment to examine his level of acculturation revealed little assimilation of American customs and values. He uses "English" only when required by his environment, and never used this language in his home or daily living activities prior to or after his incarceration. While attending school, his friends were not bilingual, and all were monolingual Spanish-speaking pupils. All other informal indices revealed the presence of little acculturation including his social contacts, leisure activities, etc.

A more formal approach was taken to address his level of acculturation. This posture was necessary because despite the fact that Mr. P was "Hispanic," and he only spoke "Spanish," his family came from a Nahuatl[4] aboriginal background from Mexico. However, as he noted, his "parents never learned that language" and were only exposed to Spanish. He never had contact with his grandparents because his family moved to a larger city in northern Mexico, and therefore had no exposure to the indigenous language, except in passing as a child during contacts with other members of his family. Hence, all his immediate family spoke Spanish in the home and for all other activities. A formal scale of acculturation (Marin Acculturation Scale) supported this finding (score = 13).

Because of his academic record, Mr. P was administered subtests from the WMPA-R (Letter-Word Identification [Identificación de Letras y Palabras] and Passage Comprehension [Comprensión de Textos]) in an attempt to assess his reading skills, skills necessary in portions of this evaluation. On this measure, his performance fell at an 11.1 grade-equivalent score in reading decoding and an 9.1 grade-equivalent level in reading comprehension. On a math computation test [Cálculo], he obtained a grade-equivalent score of 12.1. His score on a test of written language [Muestras de Redacción] fell in the 8.1 grade equivalent level (although Standard Scores are preferable, grade equivalents are only shown as estimates, and were requested by counsel). Finally, an attempt was made to assess his academic achievement levels in English, but such an assessment was desisted because he was not able perform the initial decoding test, as his level of English fluency and proficiency was very low.

---

[4] Consultation was sought by this clinician with a colleague familiar with the client's cultural background in an attempt to better understand Mr. P's background, including his family's aboriginal background, consistent with APA's Principles of Psychologists.

Altogether, these findings, coupled with his lack of English proficiency, prompted the evaluation to be conducted in Spanish.

Intellectual Functioning (Estimates)

Mr. P was administered the WMPHC-R, an aptitude test (this procedure was selected as a result of its extensive normative sample, including oversampling of individuals from Mexican backgrounds, its standardized Spanish version, and the lack of more appropriate tests available in the U.S. with Hispanic samples from Mexican backgrounds at the time this assessment was conducted). On this intellectual instrument, he obtained an overall score of 78 (71 to 85), placing his overall performance (Broad Cognitive Ability) within the 6th percentile and within the Borderline range of intellectual abilities when compared to his same-age peers. However, when controlling for his educational level, his overall score fell in the Dull Normal range (82; 12th percentile). He obtained the following Standard Scores (SS) (mean = 100; standard deviation = 15):

Subtest	Process assessed	SS	%ile
Memory for Names	aud.-visual association	69	2nd
Memory for Sentences	attention/memory	68	2nd
Visual Matching	processing speed	76	5th
Incomplete Words	auditory processing	88	21st
Visual Closure	visual processing	108	70th
Picture Vocabulary	crystallized intellect	74	4th
Analysis-Synthesis	fluid intellect/reasoning	90	25th

His performances on WMPHC-R subtests merits further attention because they capture the essence of this individual's cognitive profile. Unfortunately, such variability precludes an accurate gauge of his overall ability because it interferes with the test capacity to capture a unitary construct measuring intellectual skills. His score on subtests requiring significant attention and memory skills (Memory for Sentences) and auditory-visual associative skills (Memory for Names) fell within the impaired range. His scores on measures assessing visual processing speed (Visual Matching), crystallized reasoning (Picture Vocabulary), and auditory processing (Incomplete Words) fell within the borderline to low average range. In contrast, his scores on subtests assessing fluid intellect (Analysis-Synthesis) and visual processing (Visual Closure) fell within the average range. The discrepancies between select sets of scores are such that they are statistically and clinically significant as a result of their level of significance and low base rates.

He was also administered the TONI-2 (this test was administered for several reasons, including a lower reliance on language skills and the fact that studies with this measure have been conducted in Mexico and the U.S. with Hispanic populations; the reader is asked to think of other reasons). On this test, a measure of non-verbal intellect, he obtained a score of 88 ± 3 (95% confidence interval; Below Average). It should be noted that his WMPHC-III subtest score on a measure of fluid reasoning (Analysis-Synthesis) is qualitatively and quantitatively consistent with his TONI-2 score.

Attention and Concentration

Mr. P was administered several measures to investigate attention and concentration skills. His performance on a measure assessing his ability to visually concentrate (Color Trails Test 1) fell within the impaired range when compared to 18- to 29-year-olds with 9 to 11 years of education (198 secs; <1st percentile). His score on a more difficult procedure requiring visual concentration and sequencing (Color Trails Test 2) using the same demographics also fell in the impaired range (231 sec; <1st percentile). His interference score on this measure fell within normal limits (0.16; >16th percentile).

His performance fell within the low average range (16th percentile) on a measure of auditory attention (WMPHC-R, Inversión de Números) as he repeated digits backward when compared to his same age peers. On this measure, he was able to consistently repeat three digits backward, and inconsistently repeat four digits backward.

Language/Auditory Processing (Screening)

Although Mr. P spoke fluently, and his speech was coherent and normal in prosody, he exhibited significant dysarthria. His score (22/30) on a task requiring confrontational naming (BNT) fell in the range of expectation (35th percentile, average) when compared to norms for Hispanic individuals with 11 to 15 years of education. Functional and phonemic cues did not aid his performance on this test. He scored in the average range (50th percentile) on the Spanish Token Test, a measure of receptive language.

Visual Spatial Skills and Perceptual Organization

On a complex visuomotor procedure requiring perceptual organization and visual processing (Copy, Rey-Osterreith Complex Figure), Mr. P obtained a score of 28/36, placing his performance within the low end of the average range (26th percentile) when compared to individuals with similar educational and cultural backgrounds. On this task, he exhibited significant organizational difficulties, and he missed or distorted several components of the drawing as he copied it. Mr. P also was administered a motor-free visuoperceptual measure assessing his ability to determine angular distances between lines (JLO). On this measure, his score (20/30) fell within the "moderately defective" range (4th percentile) when compared to 16- to 49-year-olds.

Learning and Memory Functions

Verbal Memory

Mr. P's verbal memory was assessed using a rote verbal memory as he performed a list learning task (WHO-UCLA AVLT-SV). On this measure his score fell within the impaired range (<1st percentile) on the fifth recall of the original list (Trial V), a measure of overall learning. Similarly, his score fell in the impaired range (<1st percentile) on indices assessing short and long free delayed recall. All these indices were corrected for individuals with his same low educational level (11 to 15 years to use the most appropriate approach). While learning the word list, he predominantly used a primacy and recency approach as expected, providing further support for the validity of this assessment. He exhibited no retroactive or proactive interference.

Visual Memory

Mr. P's performance on a visual learning and memory task (Rey-Osterrieth Complex Figure, 30-minute Delayed Recall) fell within the impaired range (5/36; 1st percentile) when compared to peers with similar educational and cultural backgrounds.

Motor/Sensory Skills

Informal lateral preference assessment (use of hand to write, throw a ball [pantomimed], etc.) suggests that Mr. P is right-hand dominant. Using this information, his motor/sensory functioning was assessed. On the Grooved Pegboard Test, a test requiring fine motor coordination and dexterity, his scores fell within the impaired range with his right (dominant) and left (nondominant) hands (preferred hand 43rd percentile; nondominant hand = 56th percentile) when compared to 20- to 39-year-old males with less than a high school education. There was a nonsignificant raw score lateralizing discrepancy of 10% favoring his preferred hand. His performance on the Sensory Perceptual Exam revealed no errors.

Executive Skills Functioning

On Color Trails Test 2, a test requiring inhibition and shifting of set, his score using appropriate demographics (compared to 18- to 29-year-olds with 9 to 11 years of education) fell in the impaired range (231 sec; <1st percentile). His interference score on this measure fell within normal limits (1.24 >16th percentile), suggesting that many of his difficulties may be due to complex attentional difficulties. In addition, he exhibited significant difficulty in organization and planning while performing the copy portion of the Rey-Osterrieth Complex Figure. He scored in the impaired range when compared to same age peers on the three components (color naming [1st percentile], word reading [2nd percentile], and color-word reading [<1st percentile]) of another procedure assessing the ability to inhibit a common response for a more complex response (Stroop Interference Test). His impaired score on this measure fell in the impaired range despite the fact that he exhibited reading-decoding at an 11th-grade level.

Behavioral/Emotional/Personality Functioning

During this assessment, Mr. P was asked to complete the Draw-A-Person Test a measure administered to investigate his cognitive level. His drawing of a person was unremarkable from a developmental standpoint. Using the Goodehough-Harris system, his performance is similar to that produced by other adults. He also completed the Beck Anxiety and Depression Inventories. On these measures, he obtained scores of 5 and 6, respectively. Although not diagnostic, these scores suggest that he is not experiencing anxious or depressive symptoms while medicated.

Summary and Clinical Impressions

E.P. is a 27-year-old, right-handed, Hispanic male. He attended school, but he did not complete high school in Mexico or the U.S., and he appears to have attended school for approximately 11 years between Mexico and the U.S. He immigrated by himself to the U.S. to be reunited with his family approximately a decade ago but has exhibited little acculturation and assimilation. He was employed as an unskilled laborer a portion of his life prior to his incarceration, including employment in the construction and food service industries. Mr. P experienced significant psychosocial stressors early in life, including possible abuse. Most important, he sustained several severe head injuries in which he lost consciousness for an extended period of time. He was referred for a neuropsychological evaluation in an attempt to assess his present level of cognitive functioning, and rule-out encephalopathy and mental retardation. Mr. P has been charged with murder in the first degree, and the State is seeking the death penalty. He is presently in a detention center. He is receiving psychotropic medication.

The present results revealed overall intellect within Borderline range of intellectual abilities. Within this overall level of functioning, his profile exhibited significant variability. A number of subtests scores fell in the impaired to borderline range, whereas others fell in the low average to average range. On another measure of nonverbal intellectual skills his score fell in the average range consistent with a subtest assessing fluid reasoning skills on the comprehensive measure of intellectual skills. It is important to note that studies conducted in Mexico[5] and Chile[6] with Spanish-speaking populations, as well other populations with limited English proficiency, have revealed scores within the average range in healthy populations. Therefore, his overall score on the comprehensive intellectual measure suggests the presence of dampened intellect, even for an individual with his educational background. It is also important to note, as it provides consistent information, that his present scores are similar to those obtained on a translated version of another comprehensive intellectual skills test conducted while imprisoned. However, his score on that evaluation was probably not as valid as a result of the use of a translator and use of an unstandardized translation of a test, and his current assessment most likely reflects a more accurate score related to his overall aptitude. It is also important to note that his current pharmacological treatment is unable to account for his below-average intellectual skills, as his medication is having a positive therapeutic effect.

The patient's neuropsychological performance fell within the range of expectation on selected domains when compared to individuals with similar chronological age, and where possible, when compared to individuals with similar levels of educational attainment (these types of comparisons are important to rule-out artificial dampening effects on performance as a result of educational level), and in some instances using Hispanic norms with large representation of individuals living in the U.S. from Mexico. The present results revealed performance within the range of expectation on selected measures of auditory attention, language (expressive and receptive), sensory-perceptual abilities and fine motor skills. In contrast, the results of this examination revealed relative weaknesses or blatant deficits on measures of complex visual attention and working memory, select aspects of complex visual processing, verbal and visual memory abilities (severely impaired) and executive skills (impaired). His impaired scores on measures assessing memory and executive skills are such that they fell in the first percentile, even when corrected for age and education, not to mention cultural factors in some instances. In addition, some of his scores (e.g., Stroop Interference) fell in the impaired range despite the fact that underlying skills (reading) were at a level inconsistent with his poor performance. These findings have significant diagnostic implications (see below).

---

[5] See Garcia, A. (1988). Investigación del test no verbal inteligencia (TONI) en la ciudad de Chihuahua. *Unpublished thesis,* UAC, Chihuahua, Mexico.

[6] See Siriany, A. (1989). Developing a slide projection group administration procedure for the TONI. *Unpublished manuscript,* Universidad Austral de Chile, Valdivia, Chile.

Behavioral and emotional indicators obtained during this examination revealed that Mr. P is probably not experiencing significant psychological distress at this time. Measures assessing anxious and depressive symptomatology fell within the normal range. However, he is currently being medicated, and his treatment appears to be having positive impact on his overall level of functioning. Nevertheless, it is my clinical opinion that his mood difficulties preceded his incarceration if his history is taken into consideration., particularly his past family history.

With regard to diagnostic impressions and rule-outs, these issues are difficult to address. In particular mental retardation[7] (MR) is a difficult issue to address in this individual for several reasons. On the one hand, he exhibited impaired performance on an intellectual measure while undergoing evaluation by the State's forensic psychologist. Similarly, some aspects of his adaptive history also would argue in favor of MR as specified by the AAMR, including his inability to safely care for himself and his poor adaptation, not to mention delayed self-care as he was growing up as described by his sisters, even for an individual from his ethnic background. Unfortunately, no previous assessments were ever located for this individual, precluding a determination of the onset of his cognitive difficulties (there is no question that selected adaptive delays had an onset in childhood), noting an onset before the age of 18 years as delineated by the AAMR. Similarly, although the measure administered by the forensic psychologist revealed impaired intellect, the scores obtained from that evaluation are in all likelihood invalid as a result of the inappropriate assessment posture taken during the course of that examination.[8] His current level of intellectual functioning would argue against the presence of MR, despite the fact that his overall score is below average (it is not impaired even when several factors are taken into consideration including the Flynn Effect and AAMR Criteria allowing scores as high as 75 to meet criteria as a result of measurement error). In addition, it is difficult to gauge his current level of adaptation because it is provided by the State Correctional System, and quite frankly, his current environment is one of the best he has ever enjoyed when his history is taken into consideration. Because there are no measures to retrospectively assess adaptation, and adaptive skills are difficult to assess retrospectively (verbal report may be inaccurate and there are no valid and reliable formal measures to do so for this individual), coupled with the inability to assess these abilities while an individual is incarcerated, a question remains whether a hypothesis of adaptive deficits is supported by his history. With this in mind, many unbiased and independent sources of information coincide to support a postulate suggesting a lack of adaptive delays in most areas since childhood with the exception of self-care and possibly safety. Although

---

[7] According to the AAMR and its definition, used herein, mental retardation is considered when significant and "concurrent limitations, both in intellectual functioning and in adaptive skills originates before the age of 18." By impairments, scores two standard deviations or below are considered deficient.

[8] Aside from cross-cultural issues already mentioned (e.g., translation of a test), it should also be noted that no mention was made of the possibility that he may have been suffering from a profound depressive episode, or other condition(s), including dementia, PTSD, etc.

self-report and reports from family members could be considered biased, review of records indicated the presence of a lack of delays in adaptation in most areas. His records revealed an appropriate academic history, and his level of academic attainment is inconsistent with that usually attained by individuals with MR, including Mild MR. Similarly, although his vocational history is marked by employment in unskilled jobs, his performance in those jobs was appropriate and such a finding also supports a postulate indicative of a lack of vocational adaptive delays. In this regard, he was employed throughout his life prior to being incarcerated with significant occupational stability, and he did quite well in some those positions. Similar conclusions can be reached regarding his history of interpersonal relationships (e.g., friends in school, etc.). Thereforc, altogether, although he currently suffers from below-average intellect, and there is a significant history of adaptive delays in two reported domains, he does not appear to have suffered from impaired intellect as a child, clearly before the age of 18 years. Hence, with a reasonable degree of certainty, Mr. P's profile does not meet the diagnostic criteria for mental retardation as set forth by the AAMR because of my inability to concretely note that his intellectual impediments began before the age of 18 years (the third AAMR prong) and because his intellectual impediments do not rise to an impaired level even during the course of his current intellectual assessment, coupled with the fact that he may only have exhibited adaptive delays in limited areas. Finally, there are other phenomenological issues to consider that support such a diagnostic posture, including the fact that Mr. P was able to elude police for a period of approximately 48 hours as a result of camouflaging he used during the two days in which the reported shootings and robberies took place, as well as the fact that he was able to immigrate to the U.S. by himself without any assistance.

With regard to the "organicity" rule-out, the pattern of neuropsychological performance observed during the course of this evaluation suggests that Mr. P suffers from organic brain damage (encephalopathy). Such a hypothesis is supported by the preponderance of his scores on several domains and his history, particularly the protracted and severe use of use of controlled substances and his head injuries. Therefore, it is impossible to rule-out the presence of static encephalopathy (brain damage) at this time.[9]

Although he is said to have participated in an event that led to the tragic deaths of several individuals, he apparently committed these acts without previous planning under the influence of controlled substances in the course of two days. Specific information obtained during the course of this evaluation indicates that these individuals came in contact with Mr. P at random and that he did not choose

---

[9] Although not requested by the referral source or required and therefore not provided, using DSM-IV, a dementia could have been considered as a diagnostic alternative to MR, or as a stand-alone diagnosis. For example, a dementia due to multiple etiologies (e.g., head injuries, drug use) could have been considered, particularly within the context of his deficits in executive skills and impaired visual and auditory memory. Diagnostic consideration should also be given to PTSD and other diagnoses.

these victims as a result of any previous acrimonious contact with them. In my opinion, he does not posses the mental capacity to have planned such incidents. His executive scores merit additional attention because they have direct bearing on the present situation. Aside from supporting a hypothesis suggesting the presence of dampened cognition, his deficits in executive skills are also partially responsible for the present condition, and individuals with these profiles have been known to be at greater risk to use poor judgment and impulsivity, particularly when under the effects of powerful controlled substances such as methamphetamine and a depressive disorder.

In summary, with a reasonable degree of scientific certainty, it is my impression that Mr. P's profile does not meet criteria for MR. Although his profile does not meet criteria for mental retardation, it is not possible to rule out the presence of encephalopathy at this time (organic brain disorder).

Thank you for referring this individual for evaluation. If I can be of further assistance, I remain available for further consultation.

Index

Printed in the United States of America.